Pharmacokinetics of Cardiovascular, Central Nervous System, and Antimicrobial Drugs

Pharmacokinetics of Cardiovascular, Central Nervous System, and Antimicrobial Drugs

Peter G. Welling
Warner-Lambert/Parke-Davis, Ann Arbor, U.S.A.
Francis L. S. Tse
Sandoz Research Institute, East Hanover, U.S.A.

The Royal Society of Chemistry
Burlington House, London W1V 0BN

British Library Cataloguing in Publication Data

Welling, Peter G.
 Pharmacokinetics of cardiovascular, central
nervous system, and antimicrobial drugs.
 1. Pharmacokinetics
 I. Title   II. Tse, Francis L.S.
 615'.7   RM301.5

ISBN 0-85186-937-8

Printed in Great Britain by
Whitstable Litho Ltd., Whitstable, Kent

Contents

Peter G. Welling, Ph.D., D.Sc.

Warner-Lambert/Parke-Davis

Pharmaceutical Research

2800 Plymouth Road

Ann Arbor, Michigan 48105

Francis L. S. Tse, Ph.D.

Sandoz Research Institute

Sandoz Inc.

Route 10

East Hanover, New Jersey 07936

Introduction

During the last 20 years the drug industry and the practice of medicine have expanded at an incredible rate. This has been due to the combined influences of a number of factors, including rapid advances in pharmacology and pathology, and accompanying advances in such diverse areas as pharmacodynamics, pharmacokinetics, and the development of sophisticated drug delivery systems. The last of these has been the focus of frenzied activity during the last ten years, and is likely to continue for some time. More recent advances in immuno-pharmacology and the use of monoclonal antibodies have provided further impetus to the quest for new drugs in many therapeutic areas.

As the number, selectivity, and potency of therapeutic agents have increased, so has the need to understand more precisely how these agents are handled by the body and what influence this has on their therapeutic efficacy. The recent rapid expansion of the drug indus-try, and the need to understand and hopefully regulate various aspects of drug absorption, distribution, metabolism, and excretion (ADME) have provided the perfect spawning ground for the disciplines of pharmacokinetics and biopharmaceutics.

At all levels of drug use, from industrial or academic develop-ment laboratories, to the daily practice of medicine, and to regula-tory practices world-wide, it is recognized that in order to develop, understand, and use a drug with optimum benefit to the patient the multifactorial, qualitative and quantitative aspects of its ADME characteristics must be clearly understood.

During the ten years from 1970 to 1979 one of us (PGW) had the opportunity to prepare a series of review articles for the Chemical

Society, later the Royal Society of Chemistry, on the subject of drug kinetics.[1-5]   Each of these review articles covered a two year period and provided a broad, but necessarily not exhaustive, coverage of pharmacokinetic and biopharmaceutic literature for many therapeutic drug classes.

This exercise was rewarding for the writer, and hopefully also for the reader, in providing a continuous update in this rapidly developing and changing area of research.   On completion of the reviews it appeared logical to compile them into one text so as to provide a comprehensive review of the subject during one decade.

Space does not permit this to be done for all drug classes. Therefore, in order to provide maximum coverage and also to limit this book to a reasonable size, three major drug classes were selected, cardiovascular agents, drugs acting on the central nervous system (c.n.s.), and antimicrobial agents. These three classes are clearly unrelated to each other, but nonetheless represent three major therapeutic areas that have undergone dramatic changes during recent years.

Owing to the time that has elapsed since completion of the last review, covering the period 1978-79, coverage in this book has been exanded by three additional years to include a total period of 13 years, from 1970 through 1982.

The book is thus divided into three major sections, each being devoted to a single drug class. Specific drug groups within each class are indicated by separate subheadings. As in the original reviews, each drug, or group of drugs when they are considered together, will be discussed in the order of absorption, distribution, metabolism, and excretion, provided information is available. Within each of these sections information is presented in the approximate order in which it appeared in the literature.

Because of the huge volume of literature that has been generated on the pharmacokinetics of cardiovascular, central nervous system, and antimicrobial agents, no attempt has been made to provide an exhaustive coverage of the literature. Such information can be obtained from computerized searches. Rather, we have attempted, by selective reviewing, to describe the trends that have occurred in pharmacokinetic and biopharmaceutic studies for three major drug classes during a large segment of the relatively short history of this important and ever-changing subject.

References

1. P.G. Welling, 'Foreign Compound Metabolism in Mammals', ed. D.E. Hathway, The Chemical Society, London, 1972, Vol. 2, p. 412.

2. P.G. Welling, 'Foreign Compound Metabolism in Mammals', ed. D.E. Hathway, The Chemical Society, London, 1975, Vol. 3, p. 107.

3. P.G. Welling, 'Foreign Compound Metabolism in Mammals', ed. D.E. Hathway, The Chemical Society, London, 1977, Vol. 4, p. 1.

4. P.G. Welling, 'Foreign Compound Metabolism in Mammals', ed. D.E. Hathway, The Chemical Society, London, 1979, Vol. 5, p. 1.

5. P.G. Welling, 'Foreign Compound Metabolism in Mammals', ed. D.E. Hathway, The Chemical Society, London, 1980, Vol. 6, p. 1.

1 Cardiovascular Drugs

Cardiac Glycosides and Other Cardiotonic Agents

Digoxin

The perennial problem of digoxin toxicity associated with its narrow therapeutic index and variable p.o. bioavailability, and also the advent of the radioimmunoassay, have given rise to a large number of studies concerning digoxin absorption,[1-7] relationships between bioavailability and _in vitro_ dissolution profiles,[8-14] tablet disintegration,[15] and the influence of particle size on digoxin bioavailability.[16,17]

Some studies have indicated only small differences,[18-20] while others have indicated larger differences[21-23] in digoxin availability from oral dosage forms. Digoxin absorption is generally[24-27] but not always[28] superior from a solution or elixir compared to tablets, and absorption from both solid and solution dosage forms is not markedly affected by accompanying food.[29]

Differences in digoxin availability from solid dosage forms can be quite large. A study on four commercial products available in the United States yielded a seven-fold difference in serum digoxin levels between two of the products with other brands giving intermediate values.[30] The product yielding lowest serum levels did not comply with United States Pharmacopeia specifications for potency.[31,32] It has been suggested that blood levels alone may give erroneous bioavailability data for digoxin and should be supplemented by cumulative urinary excretion studies.[33]

Several studies have reported superior absorption of digoxin from solutions contained in capsules compared with tablet formulations or conventional solutions.[34-36] In one of these studies the intriguing observation was made that urinary excretion of digoxin following a 3 h i.v. infusion was 21% greater than that following a 1 h infusion of the same quantity of drug.[35] This inexplicable phenomenon has implications for the use of digoxin injections as primary standards in bioavailability testing.

The superior availability of digoxin from an encapsulated solution compared with tablets and solutions has been demonstrated also when doses are given following a substantially high-fat meal.[37] Mean serum digoxin levels obtained in 12 individuals are shown in Figure 1.1. Following a single 0.4 mg dose, capsules produced peak serum digoxin levels of 2.7 ng ml^{-1} at 50 min compared with 1.6 ng ml^{-1} at 68 min from tablets, and 1.6 ng ml^{-1} at 73 min from a solution. Faster absorption of digoxin was obtained from a digoxin-hydroquinone complex, compared with conventional tablets in man,[38] whereas digoxin absorption was inhibited in subjects who were receiving sulphasalazine,[39] and also in patients with progressive systemic sclerosis.[40]

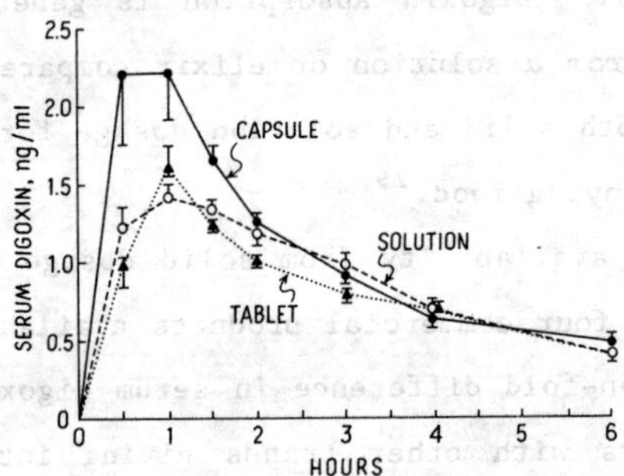

Figure 1.1 Mean serum digoxin concentrations in twelve normal subjects 0 to 6 h after administration of 0.4 mg of each of three digoxin formulations (capsule, solution, or tablet) following a high-fat meal. Bars indicate 1 SEM. (Reproduced by permission from <u>Clin.</u> <u>Pharmacol. Ther.</u>, 1977, <u>21</u>, 278)

Apart from product[41,42] variations, the absorption of orally administered digoxin may be influenced also by other drugs,[43] antacids or antidiarrheal agents,[44-46] and by drugs affecting biliary excretion of gastric motility,[47-49] although the latter effect may occur only with slowly dissolving formulations.[50]

Other studies using solubilized ^{3}H-digoxin show that digoxin absorption is not greatly affected by gastric ulcers.[51] When the drug is dosed as a solution, 40-60% is absorbed from the stomach and the proximal small intestine.

In examining the influence of a kaolin-pectin suspension on digoxin absorption, Albert et al.[52] calculated digoxin relative bioavailability assuming constant nonrenal drug clearance as in equation 1.1:

$$\frac{F^t}{F^s} = \frac{AUC^{\infty,t}}{AUC^{\infty,s}} - \frac{AUC^{\infty,t}}{D^t} (Cl^s_R - Cl^t_R) \tag{1.1}$$

nonrenal clearance varying in proportion to renal clearance, as in equation 1.2:

$$\frac{F^t}{F^s} = \frac{AUC^{\infty,t}}{AUC^{\infty,s}} \left(\frac{Cl^t_R}{Cl^s_R}\right) \tag{1.2}$$

and constant plasma clearance, as in equation 1.3:

$$\frac{F^t}{F^s} = \frac{AUC^{\infty,t}}{AUC^{\infty,s}} \tag{1.3}$$

In the equations, F^t/F^s is the bioavailability ratio of the test (kaolin-pectin) and standard treatments, AUC^{∞} is the area under the plasma concentration-time curve through infinity, and Cl_R is the renal clearance. Application of equations 1.1, 1.2, and 1.3 yielded respectively bioavailability ratios of 0.82, 0.86, and 0.84 when kaolin-pectin was administered 2 h before digoxin, and 0.95, 1.0, and 0.90 when kaolin-pectin was given 2 h after digoxin, indicating only slight drug interactions. However, when the kaolin-pectin and digoxin were given together, the mean digoxin bioavailability was reduced to 0.4. Although a slower absorption rate of digoxin may have a marked effect on plasma levels of drug shortly after a single dose, this effect is attenuated with repeated dosing due to the long biological $t_{0.5}$ of digoxin.

Large intersubject variations in serum digoxin concentration profiles, due to erratic absorption or distribution, have been observed in patients suffering from congestive heart failure.[53,54] The erratic bioavailability could also be due to a varying degree of digoxin degradation in the stomach as a function of gastric pH. Gault et al.[55] reported that 90 min after administration of ^{3}H-digoxin with maximum acid secretion stimulated by pentagastrin, nearly all of the radioactivity remaining in the stomach was present as hydrolysis products, mainly digoxigenin. Gastric acid stimulation also resulted in a marked increase in urinary metabolites in the same subjects.[56] However, a recent study in which ten healthy volunteers received 0.75 mg digoxin tablets confirmed that food ingestion had no effect on the absorption of the unchanged glycoside.[57]

Double peaks that have been reported in digoxin plasma levels after p.o. doses[58] may be due to absorption of dihydrodigoxin formed by bacteria in the lower intestine.[59] Similar observations of double peaks in circulating lanatoside C after p.o. doses have been attributed to bacterial metabolism of the relatively poorly absorbed lanatoside C to the more readily absorbed digoxin.[60-61] This acid-catalysed conversion is reduced in the presence of antacids.[62] Low recovery of ^{3}H-digoxin and its metabolites in the lymph of patients undergoing thoracic duct drainage indicates the lymphatic channels provide a minor pathway for digoxin absorption.[63]

The distribution space of digoxin in man, from the relationship $V\beta = Dose/\beta \cdot \int_0^\infty C$ appropriate to the two-compartment model, is <u>ca.</u> 5.3 1 kg^{-1} whereas for lanatoside C is 4.4 1 kg^{-1}.[64] The distribution space for digoxin decreases in patients with renal failure, and this may be attributed either to a decrease in the volume of extracellular fluid or to a decrease in the extent of drug-tissue binding.[65]

Accumulation of digoxin and ouabain in the mouse liver is reduced by probenecid, leading to considerable redistribution of drug in the body.[66] The mechanistic basis of this probenecid-digoxin interaction is not known. Approximately 30% of circulating digoxin is bound to human serum albumin over the concentration range 0.02 - 14.8 ng ml^{-1}.[67] The number of binding sites is almost infinite, but the binding constant is extremely small with a value of 6.8 x 10^{-4} mol^{-1}. Extensions of earlier studies have shown that a good correlation exists between the positive inotropic effect of digoxin and the amount of drug bound loosely to cardiac microsomal cell fractions. Tightly bound drug did not correlate well with positive inotrophy.[68]

Several studies have correlated blood digitalis levels with therapeutic[69-71] and toxic[72,73] effects. However, toxic reactions from low serum digitalis levels, nontoxic reactions from high serum levels[74] and myocardial resistance to high serum levels have been reported.[75]

Schoenwald[76] has described a relationship between ventricular heart-rate slowing and circulating digoxin levels, and has used this relationship to demonstrate prolonged digoxin absorption over 120 h after p.o. doses. This prolonged and fluctuating absorption suggests that enterohepatic cycling of digoxin in man may be extensive. Circulating levels of digoxin after rapid i.v. injection into human volunteers have been described using a three-compartment model.[77] However, comparison of three- and two-compartment model analyses shows that the disposition rate constants for the second compartment are similar for both models and that the equivalent rate constants for the third compartment of the three-compartment model are extremely high relative to other rate constants. Thus, the third compartment is relatively "shallow" and would not be detected after any other form of digoxin dosage. The "gamma" phase elimination $t_{0.5}$ reported in this study is numerically similar to "beta" phase $t_{0.5}$ generally obtained from two-compartment analysis.[78-80]

A physiological pharmacokinetic model, designed to describe the time curves of plasma and tissue concentrations of digoxin in the dog, was adapted with partial success for use in humans by considering species differences in organ volume and flow rates.[81] The model adequately predicted digoxin levels in patients with moderate uraemia but provided a relatively poor fit in anuric individuals. Preferential uptake of digoxin by particular tissues is demonstrated by reports of a mean myocardial tissue:serum digoxin level ratio of 67 in patients undergoing heart surgery[82] and mean c.s.f:serum digoxin level ratio of 0.3 in infants and in adults receiving digoxin therapy.[83]

Aronson et al.[84,85] investigated the use of digoxin inhibition of ^{86}Rb uptake by human erythrocytes to monitor pharmacodynamic effects of this drug. Good correlations were obtained between distribution characteristics of digoxin and the therapeutic response of patients with atrial fibrillation to changes in erythrocyte ^{86}Rb uptake. The tendency for oral digoxin to induce cardiac dysrhythmia has been shown in dogs to be unrelated to the occurrence of transient peak circulating levels of drug.[86]

Circulating levels of digoxin in man are increased by the presence of quinidine,[87] but are decreased by penicillamine.[88] Increased glycoside levels in the presence of quinidine appear to be associated with displacement of digoxin from tissue binding sites. The decreased glycoside levels due to penicillamine appear also to be due to a redistribution phenomenon as neither the digoxin absorption nor the elimination rate are affected by penicillamine.

Penetration of digoxin into the c.n.s. is poor, and the ratio of c.s.f.:serum levels in patients is 0.14.[89] Even within the brain the distribution of digoxin is variable, as levels in the choroid plexus far exceed those in cerebral grey and white matter. The choroid plexus binds digoxin to an extent similar to the myocardium.[90]

The inotropic effect of digoxin, as measured by changes in the QS_2 index (ΔQS_2I) is closely related to calculated digoxin levels in the slowly distributing (deep) tissue compartment of the kinetic three-compartment model, although it is uncertain whether this is a linear or nonlinear relationship.[91]

The distribution of digoxin into the skeletal muscle, which is affected by cardiac glycosides similarly to the heart,[92] has been examined.[93,94] In healthy subjects receiving 0.13–0.5 mg d^{-1} digoxin, a significant correlation existed between the digoxin concentrations in serum and skeletal muscle (Figure 1.2) as well as between skeletal muscle digoxin concentration and cardiac effect, measured by changes in QS_2I.[93] The estimated half-life of digoxin in skeletal muscle, ca. 2 d, was comparable to that reported for serum digoxin. A similar study conducted in patients during digitalization or during withdrawal of digoxin treatment showed similar, albeit statistically insignificant, correlations between changes in systolic time intervals and steady-state serum or skeletal muscle digoxin concentrations.[94] Bonelli et al.[95] investigated the distribution of digoxin into cerebrospinal fluid (c.s.f.) after 9 d of treatment with β-methyldigoxin or β-acetyldigoxin. Equipotent doses of the two compounds gave rise to similar plasma:c.s.f. digoxin concentration ratios of approximately 3.5:1.

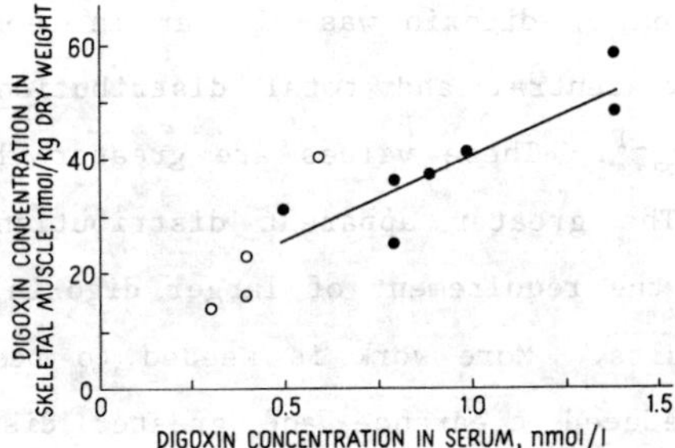

Figure 1.2 Correlation between digoxin concentration in serum and skeletal muscle at the higher dose level (r = 0.87; p < 0.05; n = 7). For comparison data from four subjects at the lower dose level are shown (o). Reproduced by permission from *Eur. J. Clin. Pharmacol.*, 1981, **19**, 89.

Critical analysis of previous work regarding the distribution of digoxin in hyperthyroid patients showed that, contrary to original suggestions, digoxin distribution was similar in normal subjects and hyperthyroid patients, while both renal and nonrenal clearance increased substantially in hyperthyroidism.[96]

It is well established that therapeutic doses of digoxin are higher in infants than in adults. Although the underlying reason for higher dose requirement in infants is uncertain, it appears to have a pharmacological rather than a pharmacokinetic basis. Different studies have shown that therapeutic serum digoxin levels are also higher in infants than in adults,[97] while absorption,[98] protein binding,[99] and elimination characteristics[100] are similar in the two populations. However, in neonates at full-term high circulating digoxin levels may be associated with low renal elimination of glycoside.[101] Therapeutic doses, and also serum levels of digitoxin, are similarly higher in infants than in adults.[102]

Changes in dose-response relationships for digoxin after corrective heart surgery may be related to changing haemodynamic status in neonates, infants, and children.[103] Renal clearances of digoxin were lower and elimination $t_{0.5}$ values were longer in neonates compared with infants, and renal clearance in both neonates and infants was approximately two-fold greater than creatinine clearances.[104] Distribution of digoxin was similar in neonates and infants, with steady-state central and total distribution volumes averaging 1.3 and 9.9 1 kg^{-1}. These values are greater than those reported in adults.[105] The greater apparent distribution volumes reported here may explain the requirement of larger digoxin doses by children compared with adults. More work is needed to resolve the opposing influences of reduced clearance and greater distribution volumes of digoxin on circulating digoxin levels and the greater tolerance to digoxin by infants compared with adults.

Digoxin clearance increases rapidly during the first three months of life, apparently due to development of both renal filtration and tubular secretion processes.[106] Although neonates and very young infants have a high digoxin tolerance, impaired clearance of drug in these populations suggests that some recommended doses, particulary in neonates, may be too high.[107]

In seven premature neonates at a postnatal age of 1 to 9 d, the corrected renal digoxin clearance correlated well with creatinine clearance, with respective mean values of 10.4 and 12.2 ml min^{-1} 1.73 m^{-2}.[108] These values were lower than those of full-term neonates. On the other hand, the $t_{0.5}$, renal clearance, and tissue distribution of digoxin were similar in newborn and adult sheep.[109] While total drug clearance and steady-state distribution volume were higher in newborns than in adults, intersubject variation was substantial.

Although animal models are used frequently to investigate digoxin kinetics, Weidler et al.[110] have shown that considerable species differences can occur. The overall distribution volume of digoxin is larger in cats than in man and dogs, whereas, the elimination rate constant β is significantly larger in dogs than in man and cats.

Evidence has been presented that renal excretion of digoxin is significantly decreased during furosemide induced diuresis.[111] The average digoxin serum $t_{0.5}$ in six healthy individuals increased from 37 h to 86 h, and urinary excretion of digoxin was transiently decreased over 10 h. The mechanism of this interaction is not known, but it may be associated with inhibition of digoxin tubular secretion or reduced renal filtration due to volume depletion. However, some other studies have reported unchanged[112,113] and increased[114] renal clearance of digoxin in the presence of furosemide.

Renal elimination of digoxin increases, and plasma levels of drug decrease, in hyperthyroidism[115] while elimination of digoxin is decreased with increasing age.[116] In seven elderly individuals (mean 81 yr), the plasma $t_{0.5}$ of digoxin was 69 h compared with 37 h in normal controls. The apparent drug distribution volume was similar in the two groups when corrected for body weight.

Both renal and nonrenal digoxin clearances were impaired by quinidine, which significantly reduced total plasma or serum clearance of digoxin in healthy subjects, by ca. 50%.[117-119] The findings were confirmed in studies of patients receiving chronic digoxin therapy.[117,118,120] Serum digoxin levels rose significantly to a new steady-state after administration of quinidine. Furthermore, the positive inotropic effect of digoxin, measured by decreases in the preejection period index (PEPI), was abolished during concomitant treatment with quinidine.[119] Figure 1.3 illustrates such changes in the pharmacodynamics of intravenously administered digoxin in six healthy subjects. Similar suppression of digoxin induced inotropism by amiloride has been reported.[121] Quinine, the 1-isomer of quinidine, also significantly reduced digoxin total body clearance, primarily through a decrease in nonrenal clearance, by an average of 55%.[122] Decreased renal and extrarenal clearances contributed equally to the reduction of digoxin total body clearance during concurrent verapamil administration,[123] while in contrast the related calcium channel antagonist nifedipine showed no overall effect on digoxin elimination in healthy subjects,[124] although it appeared to cause an increase in extrarenal clearance of digoxin and a corresponding decline in the total urinary recovery of the drug. Aspirin also did not

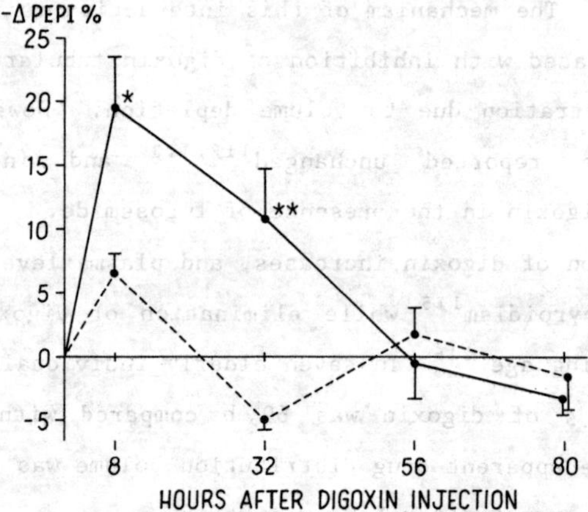

Figure 1.3 The time course of the changes in preejection period index (ΔPEPI) expressed as percentage of control value of PEPI. -ΔPEPI is shown after intravenous digoxin (●——●) and during concomitant quinidine administration (●----●). Mean values and SEM are indicated. *Statistically significant (p < 0.02) difference between ΔPEPI during digoxin administration and ΔPEPI during digoxin and quinidine administration. ** p < 0.01. Reproduced by permission from <u>Clin. Pharmacol. Ther.</u>, 1980, <u>27</u>, 791.

influence the kinetics of a single dose of digoxin with respect to digoxin total body clearance, volume of distribution, elimination $t_{0.5}$, or renal clearance.[125]

A study by Wagner et al.[126] provided evidence of nonlinearity in digoxin pharmacokinetics. In six male volunteers who received 0.5 mg doses of digoxin as a bolus intravenous injection over 2 min, a constant rate intravenous infusion over 1 h, a constant rate intravenous infusion over 3 h, and a solution in 5% dextrose given orally, both the total clearance and the nonrenal clearance of digoxin differed significantly with the method of intravenous administration. With decreasing rate of input of digoxin to the body, total clearance increased from 239 to 366 ml min^{-1} while nonrenal clearance increased from 75 to 151 ml min^{-1}. Ochs et al.[127] studied the kinetics of intravenous digoxin in nine healthy men after a single dose and ten consecutive daily doses. Multiple drug administration resulted in no systematic change in digoxin clearance, but single dose kinetic behavior was poorly predictive of digoxin accumulation and steady-state pharmacokinetics. This phenomenon could not be attributed to variations in digoxin absorption, inasmuch as the drug was given intravenously, but was believed to reflect intrasubject variability of digoxin distribution and clearance.

Although the elimination of digoxin is slowed in renal failure,[128] there is little agreement on the best method of dose adjustment in uraemic patients. Poor correlations were reported between digoxin plasma levels and such physiological parameters as body weight, serum creatinine, creatinine clearance, age, and height in patients with varying renal function.[129] Better correlations have been obtained, however, using urea clearance and blood urea nitrogen values.[130] Jusko et al.[131,132] have shown that digoxin levels can be calculated with some accuracy from the relationship between digoxin and creatinine clearance, assuming Michaelis-Menten type changes in

the apparent drug distribution volume with changing renal function.
Changes in distribution volume were thus described by equation 1.4,
where Cl_{CR} is creatinine clearance, V_A is the minimum volume of

$$V_D = V_A + \frac{V_N Cl_{CR}}{K_D + Cl_{CR}} \qquad\qquad (1.4)$$

distribution expected in renal failure, and V_N and K_D are
Michaelis-Menten constants which provide a maximum value of V_D
approaching $V_A + V_N$ in normal renal function. Further evidence of
reduced digoxin distribution in renal failure was obtained from high
correlations between myocardium:serum digoxin concentration ratios and
creatinine clearance.[133]

Additional evidence has been presented of apparent reduction of
digoxin distribution in the body during renal failure, possibly due to
reduced tissue binding associated with hyperkalaemia, altered tissue
perfusion,[134] or accumulation of uraemic toxins displacing digoxin
from tissue binding sites.[135] The rate of digoxin elimination during
dialysis is controlled not only by the efficiency of the dialyzer but
also by the rate at which drug returns to plasma from body tissues.[136]

Sumner et al.[137] used a three-compartment model to describe
digoxin disposition following i.v. doses to healthy volunteers. The
renal clearance of digoxin was similar to the creatinine clearance,
while extra-renal clearance was approximately one-half of the renal
clearance. A simplified expression was described in the form of
equation 1.5 to calculate digoxin maintenance doses for any degree

$$\text{Maintenance Dose} = \frac{0.0025 \text{ (glomerular filtration rate + 47)}}{\text{fraction of dose absorbed}} \qquad (1.5)$$

of renal function. However, this approach does not allow for changes
in the digoxin distribution volume in uraemia. Methods for predicting
steady-state digoxin levels assuming no changes in distribution
volume, a Michaelis-Menten type relationship between distribution

volume and renal function, and a linear relationship between distribution volume and renal function were examined in 55 patients receiving digoxin.[138] In the first method, steady-state digoxin levels $\overline{C}^{\infty}$ were calculated by equation 1.6 where D is the dose, C_{CR} is

$$\overline{C}^{\infty} = \frac{D \times C_{CR}}{5W} \qquad (1.6)$$

the serum creatinine, and W is ideal body weight. The second and third methods used the relationship in equation 1.7, where F is the fraction of dose absorbed, V is the overall digoxin distribution

$$\overline{C}^{\infty} = \frac{FD}{V \, k_{el} \, \tau} \qquad (1.7)$$

volume, k_{el} is the first order rate constant for digoxin elimination, and τ is the dosage interval. In the second method V is related to creatinine clearance, Cl_{CR}, as in equation 1.4, while in the third method, V is linearly related to Cl_{CR} as in equation 1.8. In equations 1.4 and 1.8, V_A is the minimum digoxin distribution volume

$$V + V_A = b \times Cl_{CR} \qquad (1.8)$$

to be expected in severely uraemic patients, V_N and K_D are Michaelis-Menten type constants, while b is the slope of the line relating volume to Cl_{CR}. Application of the methods yielded the results shown in Figure 1.4. Correlations between calculated and observed digoxin levels were substantially improved by incorporating changes in the distribution volume, while the linear relationship between volume and Cl_{CR} yielded marginally better correlations than the nonlinear relationship. In the same study, the possibility of sex-related differences in digoxin distribution in normal and impaired renal function was considered. Biliary excretion of i.v. digoxin, amounting to 30% of the dose, was confirmed in patients with biliary fistulas.[139] The numerous equations proposed for the prediction of

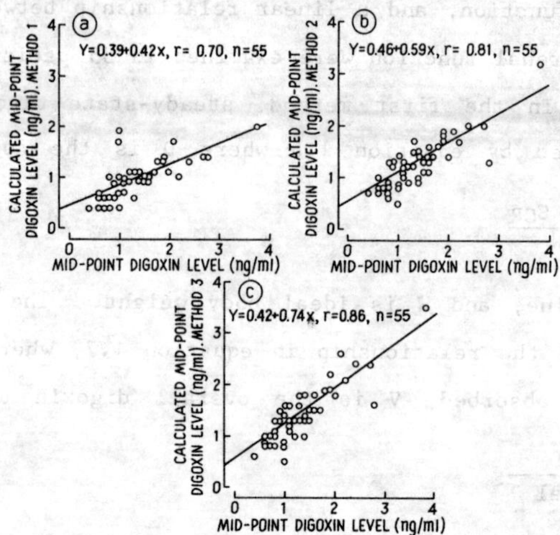

Figure 1.4 Relationship between calculated and observed mid-point digoxin serum levels using method 1 (a), method 2 (b), and method 3 (c). For explanation see text. Reproduced by permission from *J. Clin. Pharmacol.*, 1976, <u>16</u>, 660.

steady-state digoxin levels and the determination of rational dosage regimens were recently evaluated by Tsujimoto et al.[140]

Impaired renal function also influences the clearance of the metabolites of digoxin.[141] In six patients with normal renal function, and six patients with minimal renal function, elimination $t_{0.5}$ values were respectively 40 and 120 h for digoxin, 11.5 and 40 h for the bis-digitoxoside, 8.5 and 12 h for the monodigitoxoside, 2 and 7.5 h for digoxigenin, and 1.2 and 7 h for dihydrodigoxin. There was no major alteration in the drug biotransformation pattern in renal failure. Renal tubular secretion of digoxin is inhibited in hypokalaemia.[142]

Despite changes in digoxin distribution in renal impairment, a linear relationship has been established between the digoxin dose and steady-state plasma levels for any degree of renal function.[143] This is of clinical importance as it permits accurate prediction of drug plasma levels with changing doses in patients with normal or compromised renal function. Both haemodialysis[144] and haemoperfusion[145] may be used to accelerate digoxin clearance in cases of overdose, but their usefulness is limited by the large distribution volume of digoxin in the body, and the small proportion of the body drug load that exists in the circulation. These procedures are most useful during the first 6 to 8 h, when there is a greater percentage of drug in the circulation.

Gibson and Nelson[146] studied the accumulation of digoxin metabolites in renal failure, using nine subjects who required regular dialysis and nine subjects with various degrees of renal function but not requiring dialysis, all of whom had been on digoxin maintenance therapy for at least three months. Trace quantities of one or more of the digoxin metabolites were found in the plasma of all dialysis patients while patients with lesser degrees of renal impairment had either none or only one metabolite in trace amounts, usually digoxigenin-bis-digitoxoside.

Increasing knowledge regarding digoxin kinetics and dose-response relationships has led to attempts by many investigators to put digoxin therapy on a more quantitative basis.[147] Among these are the use of computer programmes[148,149] and also dosage design based on patients' body weight, sex, age, and renal function.[150] High correlations have been obtained between digoxin dosage and plasma concentrations in patients with atrial fibrillation, toxic symptoms appearing at steady-state values of about 1.6 ng digoxin ml^{-1}.[151] There is some disagreement, however, on the validity of correlating circulating digoxin levels with toxic effects.[152-154] Two bizarre instances of poor correlations are provided by patients who had serum levels as high as 20 ng ml^{-1}, and yet who survived with appropriate therapy.[155,156] Digoxin serum levels may not be closely related to toxic or therapeutic effects during the distributive phase of serum level curves, when serum:tissue ratios fluctuate widely, but good dose-effect correlations may be observed during steady-state conditions, when the ratios are relatively stable.[157] Myocardial sensitivity to the toxic effects of digitalis is increased during 24 h following pulmonary by-pass.[158] Comparison of steady-state digoxin levels after i.m. and p.o. doses indicates that digoxin is only 60% absorbed from the p.o. route.[159] This value is lower than those previously reported and may well be a function of formulation.

A monograph for digoxin dose adjustment has been described by Jelliffe and Brooker,[160] while some aspects of digoxin pharmaco-kinetics and metabolism in normal and uraemic subjects have been reviewed by Marcus.[161] Loading and maintenance doses of digoxin have been calculated on the basis of plasma levels, total body digoxin, and the amount of drug in the tissue compartment of the two-compartment model.[162] This approach adds a further degree of sophistication to digoxin dose management but, as pointed out by Chiou,[163] the variety and complexity of proposed solutions to the digoxin problem constitute a credibility problem of perhaps greater magnitude.

Biliary excretion of digoxin and metabolites in the rat is influenced by the rate of bile flow, but is at least partially inde-pendent of bile salt flow as excretion is stimulated by phenobarbital and inhibited by ethacrynic acid treatment,[164] neither of which affects bile salt output. Blood-to-bile transport of digoxin and digitoxin appears to involve an active process as excretion occurs against a bile:plasma concentration gradient ranging from 10 to 300 in the rat, rabbit, and dog.[165] More active biliary excretion of cardiac glycosides by the rat may explain the resistence of this species to their toxic properties,[166] although active biliary excretion does not occur in immature animals.[167]

β-Methyldigoxin

Studies on the absorption of β-methyldigoxin have demonstrated that it is rapidly absorbed from ligated guinea-pig intestinal seg-ments,[168] after intraduodenal administration to rats,[169] and p.o. doses of tablets[170] and solutions[171] to human subjects. Most p.o.

dosed β-methyldigoxin is absorbed from the duodenum and jejunum, and
<u>ca</u>. 75-90% of the dose is absorbed, partially as metabolites.
Clinical response is similar following equivalent p.o. and i.v.
doses.[172] Spironolactone has little effect on β-methyldigoxin absorption but diminishes urinary excretion of the cardiac glycoside in
rats. However, metabolic 0-demethylation is increased and biliary
excretion of drug and metabolites is almost quadrupled, reducing the
$t_{0.5}$ of total radioactivity in blood by a factor of four to nine in
treated animals (Figure 1.5).[173-175] Decreased urinary excretion
and greatly increased biliary excretion due to spironolactone have
also been observed with ^{3}H-digitoxin.[176,177]

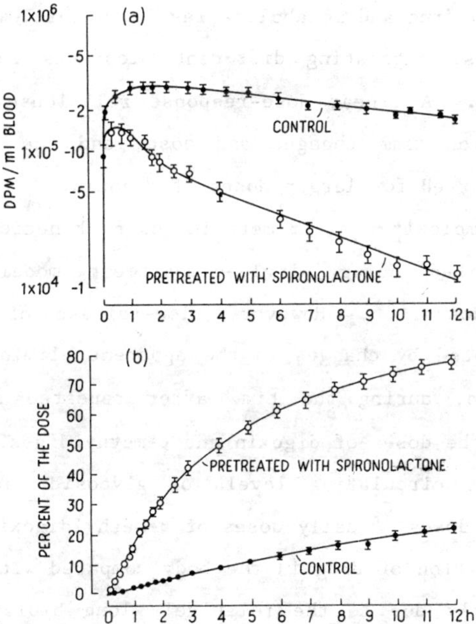

Figure 1.5   (a) Radioactivity in blood after intraduodenal administration of identical doses of [4'''-^{3}H]-
methyldigoxin in spironolactone pretreated o——o and
in control rats ●——●. $\overline{x} \pm S\overline{x}$ (n = 8); (b) cumulative
biliary excretion of radioactivity after intraduodenal
administration of identical doses of [4'''-^{3}H]-methyl-
digoxin in spironolactone pretreated o——o and in
control rats ●——●. Data are expressed as percent of
the dose. $\overline{x} \pm S\overline{x}$ (n = 9). Reproduced by permission
from <u>Arch. Pharmakol</u>., 1973, <u>278</u>, 91.

Plasma levels of ^{3}H-β-methyldigoxin in man were described using a tetraexponential function, with apparent $t_{0.5}$ values of 0.04, 0.33, 3.5, and 41 h.[178] The drug was 10% bound to plasma proteins, but the renal clearance of unchanged drug was 59 ml min^{-1}. Seventy-three percent of orally dosed solutions of ^{3}H-β-methyldigoxin was absorbed as unchanged drug and digoxin, while 60% was absorbed unchanged.[179] First-pass metabolism appeared to be prehepatic and was attributed to gastrointestinal degradation. Drug-related changes in ventricular ejection time correlated with the time course of β-methyldigoxin and also with the active metabolite digoxin in the deepest pharmacokinetic compartment rather than with plasma levels.[180] Changes in heart-rate action correlated with drug and metabolite levels in shallower pharmacokinetic compartments, suggesting different biophases for the two pharmacologic effects. A linear dose-response relationship was obtained between ejection time changes and dose, and the effect was greater than that reported for larger doses of digoxin.

Despite the complexity of β-methyldigoxin kinetics, plasma profiles were described using single-compartment model kinetics following repeated doses.[181] However, slow-release of glycoside from tissue is suggested by changes in the apparent elimination $t_{0.5}$ from 1.7 d to 2.8 d, during the time after repeated dosing had ceased.[182] Although the doses of digoxin and β-methyldigoxin required to produce equivalent circulating levels of glycoside are similar following single i.v. doses[183] daily doses of β-methyldigoxin resulted in a 2.8-fold accumulation of drug in the body compared with 1.8-fold for digoxin, presumably due to the relatively long biological $t_{0.5}$ of β-methyldigoxin.[182]

Digitoxin

A bioavailability monograph has been presented for digitoxin.[184] Binding of digitoxin to plasma proteins was reduced from a normal value of 97.1 to 93.7% (P < 0.0025) in uraemic individuals. Binding was not changed by <u>in vitro</u> addition of procainamide, phenytoin, heparin, or rifampicillin,[185] but was significantly decreased by the presence of heparin <u>in vivo</u> during haemodialysis.[186] It is suggested that <u>in vivo</u> release of fatty acids due to heparin causes displacement of digitoxin, and also digoxin, from albumin-binding sites.

Cumulative renal excretion of digitoxin during 8 d following a single i.v. dose was higher (23% of dose) in nephrotic patients than in controls (16% of dose).[187] Increased renal excretion in nephrotic patients is due to decreased protein binding and also to urinary excretion of bound drug. The elimination kinetics of digitoxin and its metabolites in uraemic patients are reported[188] to be similar to those in healthy individuals, but uraemia-induced changes in both digitoxin metabolism and elimination may decrease the serum $t_{0.5}$ and produce lower serum levels of glycoside.[189]

Although digitoxin is considered to be extensively metabolized in man, studies using ^{3}H-digitoxin have shown that it circulates in the body predominantly in the unchanged form.[190] The prolonged biological $t_{0.5}$ of digitoxin is related to extensive (90-95%) binding to plasma proteins and to the slow rate of hydroxylation to digoxin. Pretreatment with phenobarbital decreased the digitoxin $t_{0.5}$ owing to increased metabolism, decreased protein binding, or a combination of these.[191] Enterohepatic cycling also contributes to the slow decline in digitoxin blood levels. Interruption of enterohepatic cycling of unchanged drug and its metabolites by means of a biliary fistula decreased the drug $t_{0.5}$ in serum from 8.1 to 4.3 d.[192]

Digitoxin $t_{0.5}$ values were also reduced by coadministration of rifampicin in man[193] and spironolactone in rats.[194] In both instances, reduced $t_{0.5}$ values were associated with increased metabolism. In the case of rifampicin, however, a direct influence on renal tubules blocking digitoxin reabsorption was considered as a possible contributing factor.

The effect of age on digitoxin pharmacokinetics was studied in two groups of healthy subjects aged 25-30 yr and 69-79 yr.[195] Plasma digitoxin levels following a single 0.6 mg i.v. dose are shown in Figure 1.6. No statistically significant difference between the groups in digitoxin $t_{0.5}$, apparent volume of distribution, or total clearance was observed.

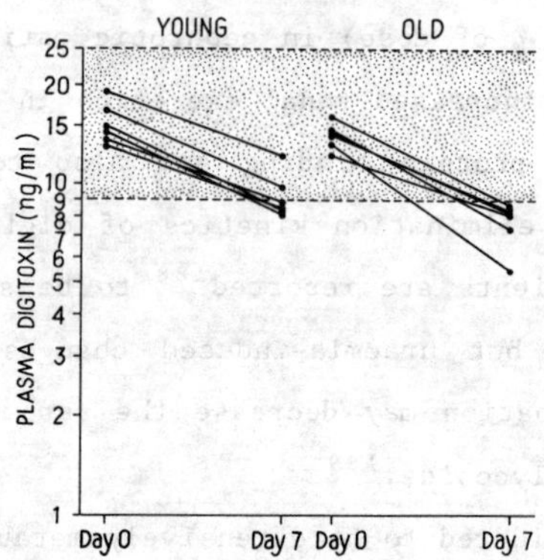

Figure 1.6   Fall in plasma digitoxin levels over 7 d in 6 young and 6 old subjects, calculated from the β elimination phase, following a single intravenous dose of 0.6 mg of digitoxin. The shaded area indicates the therapeutic range.   Reproduced by permission from *Brit. J. Clin. Pharmacol.*, 1981, __11__, 401.

Other Cardiotonic Agents

The pharmacokinetics of ouabain have been studied in the dog and in man.[196] Plasma $t_{0.5}$ values from terminal portions of biphasic plasma-level curves following i.v. doses were 19 h and 18 h in dog and man, respectively. The $t_{0.5}$ in man is in reasonable agreement with the $t_{0.5}$ of the pharmacological effect.

The pharmacokinetics of amrinone, a new cardiotonic agent with significant inotropic activity, have been investigated in six male patients with moderate to severe congestive heart failure.[197] Orally administered amrinone was rapidly absorbed, with a mean peak time of 1.4 h. At the dose level of 1 to 1.5 mg kg^{-1}, the decline of serum amrinone concentrations was monoexponential, with a mean $t_{0.5}$ of 5.1 h. There was an apparent positive correlation between serum levels and percentage change in cardiac index. In that study, a four-fold interpatient variability in the area under curve was observed, which could be due to interpatient differences in either amrinone bioavailability or volume of distribution. The absorption, distribution, metabolism, and excretion of the cardiotonic agent heptaminol hydrochloride was studied in the rat after single p.o. and i.v. doses of the ^{14}C-labeled drug.[198]

Antiarrhythmic and Antianginal Agents

Procainamide

A number of reviews have discussed the pharmacokinetics of procainamide and its active metabolite N-acetylprocainamide (NAPA).[199,200] Biopharmaceutic aspects of procainamide therapy, particularly p.o. sustained-release formulations, have attracted considerable interest.

Early investigations showed that procainamide is efficiently absorbed from both fast- and slow-release p.o. formulations, with minimal first-pass metabolism.[201] However, slow-release formulations give rise to more satisfactory plasma profiles by reducing peak to trough drug fluctuations.[202,203] Three such formulations produced procainamide blood or plasma levels within the therapeutic range of 4-8 μg ml^{-1} with little or no evidence of toxicity.[204-206] Comparable blood levels of procainamide from q6h sustained-release tablets and from q3h conventional capsules are accompanied by comparable effects between the two formulations on blood pressure and heart rate.[207]

Considerable species differences have been observed in procainamide and also procainamide ethobromide disposition.[208,209] The ethobromide is cleared rapidly in the bile of rabbits and rats, but only slowly in dogs. Sixty-four percent of p.o. dosed procainamide is voided as unchanged drug in human urine, whereas in the rhesus monkey the drug is almost completely metabolized.

The pharmacokinetics of procainamide and NAPA have been studied extensively in the rat.[210] After i.v. administration of ^{14}C labeled compounds, procainamide plasma concentrations declined monoexponentially while NAPA levels suggested two-compartment disposition. Little differences were observed in the values of the volume of distribution, V_β, of either compound, which were 4-5 1 kg^{-1} in this study. The mean terminal $t_{0.5}$ and plasma clearance of procainamide were 0.66 h and 4.84 1 h^{-1} kg^{-1}, respectively, compared with 2.13 h and 1.24 1 h^{-1} kg^{-1} for NAPA. Urinary excretion of unchanged procainamide and NAPA accounted for 41.0 and 16.6%, respectively, of the i.v. dose of ^{14}C labeled procainamide. Less than 5%, and <u>ca</u>. 3%, of administered radioactivity were recovered in the 0-48 h feces of the rats receiving ^{14}C labeled procainamide and ^{14}C labeled NAPA, respectively, indicating that biliary excretion is of minor importance in the elimination of procainamide in this species. This observation was supported by the study of Basseches and DiGregorio,[211] who found that ligation of the common bile duct immediately prior to i.v. administration of 50 mg kg^{-1} procainamide in the rat did not alter plasma, saliva, or urine concentrations of the drug.

Procainamide undergoes both filtration and renal tubular secretion in man, and renal clearance may be altered by changes in urinary pH but not by increased urine flow.[212] Renal, cardiac, and hepatic impairment may cause prolonged procainamide levels in plasma and there is evidence that procainamide may inhibit its own metabolism.[213,214]

After i.v. infusion, procainamide blood levels indicated two-compartment model kinetics with alpha and beta $t_{0.5}$ values of 9 min and 3.4 h, respectively.[215] Three-compartment model kinetics have been used in a comparison of procainamide and NAPA in healthy individuals.[216] Both compounds had similar steady-state distribution volumes of <u>ca</u>. 1.4 1 kg^{-1}, but intercompartmental clearances of NAPA were slower than those of procainamide. In that study the average terminal elimination $t_{0.5}$ and plasma clearance of procainamide were

2.5 h and 590 ml min^{-1}, respectively, compared to 6.2 h and 234 ml min^{-1} for NAPA.

In renal insufficiency the $t_{0.5}$ of NAPA, and to a lesser extent procainamide, are prolonged.[217,218] Typically, plasma levels of NAPA were detected in a uraemic patient 38 d after dosing, indicating a biological $t_{0.5}$ of several days. In one patient who ingested <u>ca.</u> 7 g procainamide, the elimination $t_{0.5}$ of parent drug was prolonged to 10.5 h, and that of NAPA to 36 h.[218] Haemodialysis increased the rate of procainamide and NAPA elimination by twofold and fourfold, respectively.

The procainamide elimination $t_{0.5}$ has been shown also to be prolonged in patients with heart disease[219] and with chronic respiratory insufficiency.[220] Acetylation and hydrolysis of procainamide are both impaired in liver disease. Whereas the degree of impairment of hydrolysis is related to the severity of disease, no such relationship was demonstrable for acetylation. The acetylation of p-amino-benzoic acid increases in patients with liver disease, the degree of acetylation increasing with decreasing procainamide hydrolysis.[221] A cryptic note on procainamide pharmacokinetics and pharmacodynamics is provided by Galeazzi et al.[222] These authors showed that the kinetics of pharmacological effects, as indicated by QT interval prolongation, are indistinguishable from concentrations of drug in saliva, both of these being delayed with respect to plasma levels of drug, at least after bolus i.v. injection. Thus, although saliva levels of procainamide may not be used to predict plasma levels, drug levels in saliva may be the more clinically appropriate measure. On the other hand, saliva levels may not be useful for NAPA monitoring due to large interindividual variations in measured values.[223]

The rate of procainamide acetylation to form NAPA differs markedly among individuals and the degree of acetylation may vary from 6 to 50% of dosed procainamide.[224] Comparative studies in man showed that procainamide acetylation is polymorphically controlled and correlates well with rates of isoniazid acetylation.[225,226] There is some evidence that N-acetylation of procainamide may be a saturable process.[227] In this case, it should be possible to demonstrate polymorphism in the maximum rate of acetylation. Neither procainamide nor NAPA is significantly bound to plasma proteins at therapeutic concentrations.[228]

Observations that NAPA has similar antiarrhythmic activity to procainamide[229] have stimulated interest in the bioavailability and pharmacokinetics of this metabolite.[230] NAPA has a $t_{0.5}$ of about 6 h compared with <u>ca</u>. 3 h for procainamide. This contrasts with previous observations in monkeys that the two compounds have similar $t_{0.5}$ values.[230] As NAPA is excreted largely unchanged via the kidneys, appropriate dose adjustment is required if this drug, or procainamide, is administered to patients with renal insufficiency. NAPA has been shown by the use of a novel stable isotope method to be efficiently absorbed from p.o. doses.[231]

Approximately 14 to 18 h are required for steady-state plasma levels of procainamide to be reached during infusion[232] and methods are described to achieve steady-state levels rapidly, with minimum toxic effects, by the use of a two-stage infusion procedure.[233] A maximum serum level of 5.8 μg ml^{-1} procainamide was obtained with an initial 1 h infusion of 16.6 mg min^{-1} in both fast and slow acetylator phenotypes, and an average steady-state serum level of 5.1 μg ml^{-1} was obtained with a maintenance infusion of 222 mg h^{-1}. Although the metabolite NAPA is reported to have pharmacological effects comparable with the parent drug,[234] this premise has been challenged by Schröder et al.[235] who showed that the metabolite antagonized the action of procainamide in arrhythmic patients. The biological $t_{0.5}$ of NAPA is increased from a normal value of 6 h to 42 h in severe renal impairment,[236,237] but the plasma clearance of metabolite is increased 4-fold by haemodialysis.[236]

Procainamide elimination is impaired in the elderly.[238] Both the procainamide:creatinine clearance ratio and NAPA:creatinine clearance ratio have been shown to decline with age, which would imply that the glomerular filtration rate as well as the age-related variation in renal tubular secretion must be monitored in dosage individualization. However, in patients with good renal and hepatic function, initial procainamide infusion rate could be selected on the basis of body weight regardless of the initial presence of moderate heart failure.[239] The total body clearance of procainamide may be estimated using the regression line shown in Figure 1.7.

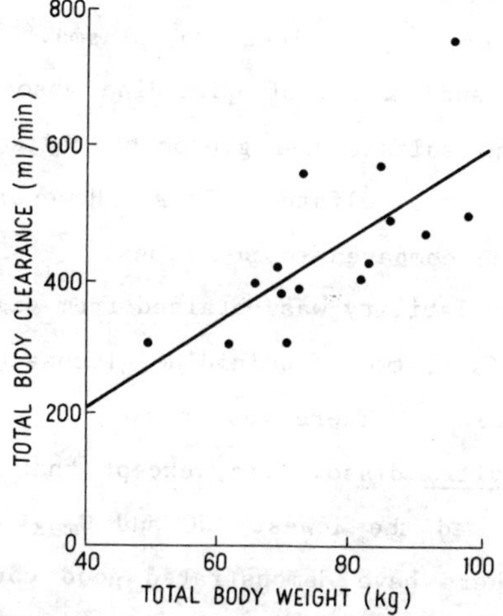

Figure 1.7 Relationship between total body clearance of procainamide in acute myocardial infarction patients and body weight of the patients. The equation which best fits these data is Cl_B = (6.27 x body weight) − 40, where body weight is given in kg and Cl_B is obtained in ml min^{-1}. Reproduced by permission from J. Clin. Pharmacol., 1981, 21, 20.

The elimination of procainamide appeared to be more rapid in pediatric patients than in adults.[240] In a group of children between 7 and 12 years of age, the $t_{0.5}$ and plasma clearance were 1.7 h and 19.4 ml min^{-1} kg^{-1}, respectively. Reduced renal clearance and prolonged $t_{0.5}$ of NAPA have been reported in patients with cardiomyopathy or coronary heart disease.[241,242] Various aspects of therapeutic drug monitoring of antiarrhythmic agents including procainamide,[243] and also the clinical pharmacokinetics of NAPA,[244] have been reviewed.

Quinidine

Various studies have examined the absorption of quinidine from conventional and sustained-release p.o. dosage forms.[245] The absorption of quinidine from conventional dosages may be dependent on the salt used and also the formulation, although some reports are somewhat contradictory. Some have claimed that quinidine sulfate is absorbed more rapidly but not necessarily more efficiently than the gluconate salt, giving rise to shorter t_{max} values in plasma.[246] Other reports claim that the rate and extent of quinidine absorption are similar from solutions of the sulfate and gluconate salts and also from different commercial quinidine sulfate tablets. However, tablets gave rise to slower absorption compared to solutions.[247] In another study similar quinidine bioavailability was obtained from eight tablet formulations of quinidine sulfate, two of quinidine gluconate, and one of quinidine polygalacturonate.[248] There was no correlation between quinidine absorption and *in vitro* dissolution, except that the slow-dissolving gluconate product had the lowest AUC and C_{max} values and the longest t_{max} value. Others have demonstrated good correlations between *in vitro* dissolution[249] and disintegration[250] rates and absorption rates of quinidine formulations.

Apart from reports on variable relative rate and efficiency of quinidine absorption from different oral dosages the absolute bioavailability of quinidine, at least from the gluconate salt, has been shown to be only moderately efficient. The relatively poor absorption of oral quinidine may be explained by first-pass metabolism.[251] Prediction of mean systemic availability of oral doses from i.v. data was 76% and mean actual availability of orally dosed quinidine gluconate in the same individuals was 72%.

The bioavailability of quinidine was 77% and 56% from two p.o. sustained-release formulations compared with a standard tablet, and the time taken to reach steady-state serum levels was longest for the least bioavailable formulation.[252]

Slow-release tablets of quinidine bisulfate yielded lower and more prolonged levels of drug in serum than conventional quinidine sulfate tablets, and approximately one-quarter of the drug from each dosage form was recovered in urine.[253] In this study, serum levels of quinidine after multiple dosing were higher than those predicted from single dose data, suggesting the possibility of saturation kinetics with increasing drug levels. However, this phenomenon was not observed in another study in which mean steady-state quinidine levels in plasma were consistent with values predicted from single i.v. doses.[254] Good correlation has been reported between plasma quinidine levels and dose size of sustained release quinidine bisulfate tablets.[255]

Inter-product variability has been demonstrated in the bioavailability of some slow-release preparations containing the same,[256] and different[257] salt forms of quinidine. One p.o. preparation containing quinidine bisulfate yielded 50% more drug to the circulation than another brand of the same salt. Quinidine arabogalactansulfate is claimed to be less efficiently absorbed than the polygalacturonate and sulfate salts, although this is not clearly evident from the data.[257]

Various other factors unrelated to the dosage forms may affect quinidine absorption. The absolute systemic bioavailability of quinidine from a 400 mg p.o. dose of quinidine gluconate solution was <u>ca</u>. 72% in cardiac patients with congestive heart failure, similar to that observed in control subjects.[258] However, the absorption rate appeared to be faster in the heart failure patients, with peak plasma quinidine concentration occurring at 2.4 h, compared to 1.0 h in the control cardiac patients. A second peak or shoulder in the mean plasma quinidine concentration profile observed at <u>ca</u>. 3 h, was explained in terms of the possible effect of food that was permitted after a standard fasting period following drug administration.[259] Stress conditions in rats significantly increased the gastrointestinal absorption of quinidine sulfate, but did not influence the absorption of sodium salicylate.[260] Observed differences may have been due to increased gastric emptying under stress conditions favoring absorption of the basic quinidine molecule while not markedly influencing absorption of salicylate ion. Absorption of i.m. quinidine lactate in human volunteers was erratic, and only 87% complete compared with an i.v. infusion.[246]

Guentert et al.[261] demonstrated considerable individual variation in quinidine disposition after p.o. doses, and used both two- and three-compartment models with zero-order input to describe quinidine plasma levels. The accuracy of pharmacokinetic analysis of quinidine data is a function also of assay specificity, and earlier estimates of appropriate therapeutic levels of quinidine may be erroneous due to metabolite interference in nonspecific assays.[262]

Theoretical considerations[263] have been used to predict plasma-protein binding characteristics of quinidine.[264] Free drug concentrations in plasma may vary from 11 to 26% of total circulating drug, depending on drug and protein concentrations. This variation may partially explain observed differences in quinidine kinetics and dose-response relationships in patients. Studies in rabbits have shown that the pharmacological, biological, and derived biophasic $t_{0.5}$ values of quinidine are similar following both rapid and slow i.v. infusions and that the biophase is located in tissues kinetically indistinguishable from plasma.[265] An assay method, relatively specific for unchanged drug, has indicated that kinetics of quinidine elimination are similar in normal subjects and in patients with renal impairment.[266] These observations are contrary to previous reports, based on nonspecific fluorimetric assays, of delayed quinidine elimination in uraemia. It is suggested that previous results were influenced by delayed excretion of fluorescing quinidine metabolites rather than impaired quinidine elimination.

Both the apparent volume of distribution and total body clearance of quinidine, but not the elimination rate constant, are linearly related to the free drug fraction in plasma.[267,268] Although the β-receptor antagonist propranolol alters hepatic blood flow and hepatic clearance, it does not affect quinidine disposition on concurrent administration.[269-270] Plasma levels of both quinidine[271] and dihydroquinidine are elevated in patients with congestive heart failure, but the elimination $t_{0.5}$ values of both compounds (<u>ca</u>. 6 h) in these patients are similar to those in patients without congestive heart failure. The elevated drug levels appear to be related to decreased extravascular distribution, probably resulting primarily from impaired tissue perfusion, and the increased levels of drug in the circulation may be related to the higher incidence of toxic reactions associated with quinidine in patients suffering from congestive heart failure.[272] Whereas NAPA:procainamide concentration ratios in plasma increase with renal failure, due to accumulation of the acetylated metabolite, the plasma concentration ratios of each of the active quinidine metabolites, 3-hydroxyquinidine and 2'-oxoquinidine, to parent drug are unchanged in azotaemic and dialysis patients.[273] However, circulating levels of unchanged drug and its metabolites are elevated under these conditions.

Similar to procainamide and NAPA, no significant correlation was found between quinidine concentrations in saliva and its total or free levels in serum.[274] Quinidine serum protein binding was not related to serum levels of albumin, cholesterol, urea, creatinine, or the adult patient's age. Kessler and Perez[275] suggested that quinidine binding may be directly related to α_1-acid glycoprotein concentrations. These investigators found that the percent of quinidine unbound in serum decreased from a normal value of 9.9% to 6.5% in haemodialysis patients, but increased to 12.2% after heparinization.

Heparin significantly increased the serum concentrations of free fatty acids which are known to compete with quinidine for protein binding sites. In pediatric patients, _in vitro_ serum protein binding increased with age, apparently due to increasing total serum proteins. The percentage of free quinidine was 39.2 in serum obtained at the time of delivery, 24.4 at 8–18 m, and 16.6 at 2 yr or older.[276] Experiments using rabbit plasma have shown that the serum protein binding of quinidine is concentration-independent; the fraction unbound was 0.11–0.14 within the total quinidine concentration range of 250–3000 ng ml^{-1}.[277]

Russo et al.[278] proposed that the elimination of quinidine may be dose-dependent, particularly its hydroxylation to form 3-hydroxyquinidine. However, the limited number of subjects and conflicting results in their study precluded any definitive conclusions. Quinidine clearance decreased with age, and this was reflected by the concentration of the active metabolite 3-hydroxyquinidine relative to the parent drug concentration in serum.[279] Average clearance of quinidine was 9.0 and 3.8 ml min^{-1} kg^{-1} in patient groups with metabolite: quinidine ratios greater and smaller than 0.50, respectively. The ratio of plasma 3-hydroxyquinidine to parent drug was also increased by phenytoin.[280] The elimination $t_{0.5}$ of orally administered quinidine in the dog decreased from 6.5 to 3.5 h after two weeks of phenytoin pretreatment. However, phenytoin also caused a decrease in the apparent volume of distribution of quinidine from 2.23 to 0.78 l kg^{-1}. Therefore, overall plasma clearance actually decreased in some animals. It was suggested that induction of hepatic microsomal enzymes by phenytoin alone may not account for the observed changes in quinidine kinetics.

Plasma quinidine levels in patients receiving i.v. infusion were described in terms of a two-compartment open model.[281] The mean volume of the central compartment and the overall steady-state distribution volume (V_{dss}) were 0.9 and 3 l kg^{-1}, indicating extensive extravascular distribution. The drug distributed into the body with a $t_{0.5}$ of 7 min, total body clearance ranged from 1.5 to 7.2 ml min^{-1} kg^{-1}, while mean renal clearance was only 0.8 ml min^{-1} kg^{-1}. As noted previously with $t_{0.5}$ values, there was considerable individual variation in quinidine disposition.

In rhesus monkeys, prolonged infusion of quinidine resulted in increased $t_{0.5}$ whereas drug clearance was unchanged.[282] This may be due to compensating increases in drug distribution volumes with prolonged dosing as discussed previously in the dog.[280] The percentage of free quinidine in plasma increased from 3 to 14% over a concentration range of 2-22 µg ml^{-1}.

Considerable species differences occur in quinidine pharmacokinetics, with plasma $t_{0.5}$ values varying from 0.85 h in goats to 5.59 h in dogs, and specific distribution volumes varying from 1.25 l kg^{-1} in pigs to 6.32 l kg^{-1} in ponies.[283]

Lidocaine

Lidocaine has a narrow therapeutic index and is frequently used in life-threatening situations. Detailed knowledge of its pharmacokinetic behavior is therefore important, and many publications have been devoted to resolving its pharmacokinetics and tissue distribution, and to examining the optimum dosage in therapy for cardiac arrhythmia and myocardial infarction.[284,285]

Oral absorption of lidocaine is limited, because of extensive first-pass metabolism, and only 30-40% of a p.o. dose reaches the systemic circulation.[286] Systemic availability of lidocaine may be decreased further to _ca_. 15%, if the patient has been receiving hepatic enzyme inducing agents, but may increase to 60-70% of the dose if administered rectally.[287] GI absorption of lidocaine is delayed in patients undergoing anesthesia, and plasma elimination $t_{0.5}$ values increase from 1.3 to 2.8 h.[288]

The systemic availability of lidocaine was approximately 7% from a p.o dose in the rat, but improved to over 83% when the same dose was administered rectally.[289] The rectal absorption of lidocaine could be further enhanced by the presence of salicylate in the rectal membrane, although the mechanism of this drug interaction is unclear.[290]

Absorption of p.o. dosed lidocaine is delayed by i.m. dosed atropine, presumably resulting from delayed gastric emptying,[291] but neither phenytoin nor procainamide influenced circulating lidocaine levels when this drug was administered by i.v. infusion.[292] A high incidence of c.n.s. side effects was obtained in man and dogs during combined lidocaine-phenytoin dosing, presumably because of a pharmacodynamic interaction.

Owing to poor p.o. bioavailability, lidocaine is generally given parenterally, whereas some reports have suggested that plateau therapeutic blood levels of lidocaine in man can be obtained shortly after commencing i.v. infusion, Bassan et al.[293] have shown that steady-state levels are not reached until after about 6-7 h. As the risk of cardiac arrhythmias is often extremely high during the early stage of lidocaine infusion, i.e. within a few hours following a myocardial infarction, loading doses are needed to achieve therapeutic circulating drug levels quickly. Shen and Gibaldi[294] have proposed, from pharmacokinetic considerations, that the most appropriate loading dose should be given by i.m. injection as i.v. bolus injections can produce instantaneous subtherapeutic or toxic circulating drug levels.

Considerable variation is observed in lidocaine blood levels after i.m. injection.[295] However, therapeutic blood levels were obtained for up to 90 min following an i.m. injection of a 300 mg, 10% solution into the lateral vastus muscle, and this may be the preferred dose and dose site for clinical efficacy.

Higher plasma levels of lidocaine were obtained in patients from an i.m. injection of a dilute solution than from a more concentrated solution.[296] This may be due to hypertonicity of more concentrated solutions, the volume of the solution injected, or precipitation of drug from concentrated solutions at the injection site. Other studies

provide the alternative explanation that limited absorption from concentrated solutions may result from a direct vasoactive property.[297]
Oltmanns et al.[298] used a 300 mg i.m. loading dose followed 1-2 h
later by infusion at 0.029-0.039 mg kg^{-1} min^{-1} to achieve safe and
antiarrhythmically effective plasma levels of lidocaine between 1.5
and 6 μg ml^{-1}.

Guidelines have been suggested for lidocaine therapy involving
initial administration of divided loading doses or a relatively rapid
infusion.[284] Although the guidelines are general in nature they may
not apply to the individual, nor in cases of altered lidocaine disposition in liver disease[299] and myocardial infarction[300,301].

Blood and tissue levels of lidocaine were examined in dogs after
a bolus injection, i.v. infusion, and a bolus injection followed by an
i.v. infusion.[302] By using the relationship bolus dose = k_0/k_1,
where k_0 and k_1 are the zero-order rate constant for absorption
and the first-order rate constant for elimination, almost instantaneous steady-state levels were achieved (Figure 1.8). Tissue levels

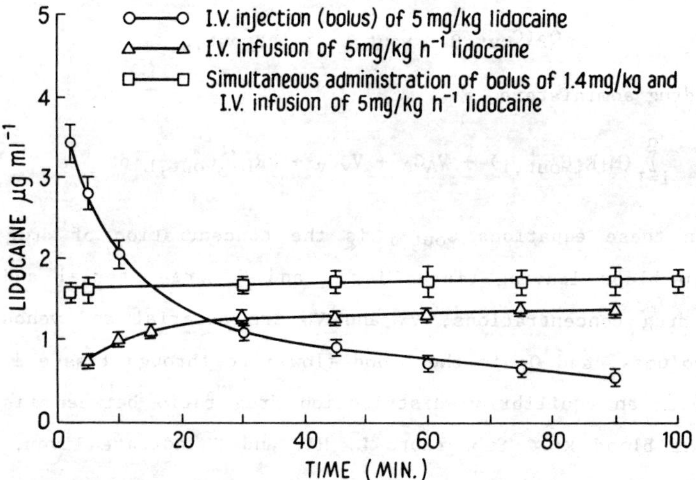

Figure 1.8 Concentration of lidocaine in blood of
dogs after a bolus injection, an i.v. infusion, and
after simultaneous administration of a bolus and i.v.
infusion. Each point is the mean ± SD of four dogs.
Reproduced by permission from <u>Res. Comm. Chem. Path.
Pharmacol.</u>, 1971, <u>2</u>, 813.

of unchanged drug varied, with highest concentrations occurring in the kidney, and lowest in the heart. Maximum tissue levels of ^{3}H-lidocaine and metabolites are obtained 30 min after i.v. or p.o. dosing to rats.[303] However, peak intestinal radioactivity was reached 2-4 h after each treatment. Little ^{3}H is voided in faeces, suggesting extensive enterohepatic circulation of lidocaine and its metabolites.

A perfusion model has been developed in monkeys and in man to investigate the role of regional circulation on the pharmacokinetics of lidocaine.[304] The model, comprising eight different tissues including the gut, is reproduced in Figure 1.9 while equations 1.9 to 1.11 typify those used to describe drug movement.

Rate of change of drug mass in noneliminating tissue =

$$M_i R_i \frac{dC_{out}}{dt} = Q_i (C_A - C_{out,i}) \qquad (1.9)$$

Rate of change in mass of drug in liver, L, =

$$M_L R_L \frac{dC_{out,L}}{dt} = Q_{HA} (C_A - C_{out,L}) +$$

$$Q_P (C_{out,P} - C_{out,L}) - k R_L C_{out,L} \qquad (1.10)$$

Total drug administered =

$$\sum_{i=1}^{n} (M_i R_i C_{out,i}) + V_A C_A + V_V C_V + k R_L \int_0^t C_{out,L} \cdot dt \qquad (1.11)$$

In these equations $C_{out,i}$ is the concentration of drug at any time in blood leaving tissue i, C_A and C_V are arterial and venous blood drug concentrations, V_A and V_V are arterial and venous blood pool volumes, and Q_i is the blood flow rate through tissue i of mass M_i having an equilibrium distribution drug ratio between tissue and emergent blood R_i. Subscripts L, HA, and P indicate liver, hepatic artery, and portal system, respectively.

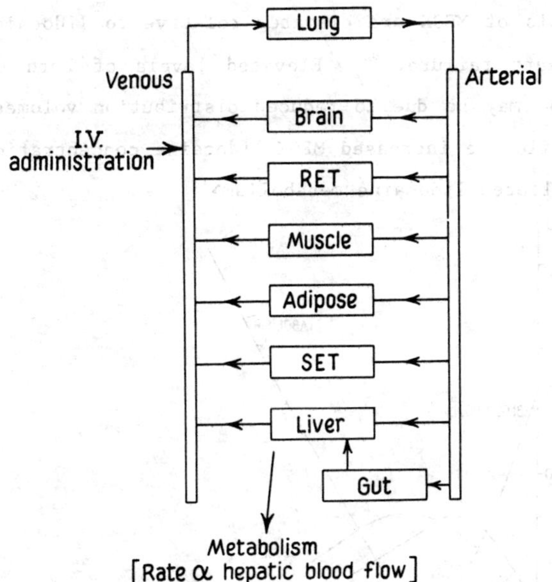

Figure 1.9   Blood perfusion model used to describe disposition kinetics of lidocaine in the monkey and man.   RET represents rapidly equilibrating tissue including heart and kidneys, SET represents slowly equilibrating tissue including skin and bone.   Boxes represent tissue capacitance, the product of mass and partition coefficients.   Arrows represent individual organ blood flows.   Arterial and venous blood represent one-third and two-thirds total blood volume, respectively.   Reproduced by permission from <u>Clin. Pharmacol. Ther.</u>, 1974, <u>16</u>, 87.

A typical simulation using this model system is given in Figure 1.10. This simulation suggests that lidocaine is sequestered first by the lungs and then by other rapidly perfused tissue after i.v. injection. Redistribution then occurs into muscle and adipose tissue. The model was further used to simulate perturbation of drug disposition in various pathological conditions in monkey and man.[305] Observed circulating drug levels, and also pharmacokinetic parameter values, were in good agreement with those predicted from the model. The kinetic profiles of the lidocaine and its metabolite, monoethylglycinexylidide (MEGX) were similar in uraemic and normal subjects.[306] However, the biological $t_{0.5}$ of the metabolite glycinexylidide (GX) was prolonged and accumulation of this active metabolite may occur in uraemia. Circulating levels of MEGX are elevated relative to lidocaine levels in congestive heart failure.[307] Elevated levels of both compounds in this condition may be due to reduced distribution volumes and plasma clearance, while the increased MEGX:lidocaine concentration ratio may result from altered lidocaine metabolism.

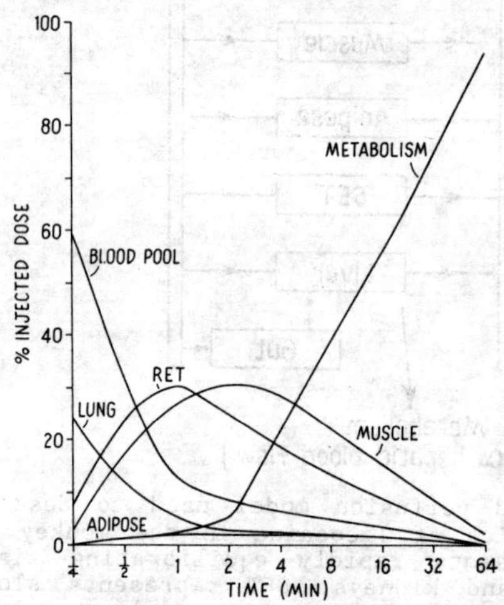

Figure 1.10   Perfusion model simulation of the distribution of lidocaine in rhesus monkey tissues, and its elimination following an i.v. bolus. Reproduced by permission from <u>Clin. Pharmacol. Ther.</u>, 1974, <u>16</u>, 87.

A profound increase in total plasma lidocaine concentrations was observed during a constant infusion in patients with myocardial infarction, which was attributed to enhanced plasma lidocaine binding.[308,309] Thus, the ratio of bound (B) to free (F) fractions of lidocaine in plasma increased with elevated plasma α_1-acid glycoprotein concentrations associated with the disease (Figure 1.11), while free lidocaine concentrations did not change significantly. Considerable interindividual variation in lidocaine binding was observed even in the plasma of normal subjects, with percent unbound lidocaine varying from 19.9 to 38.8.[310] While the binding ratio of lidocaine was directly related to the plasma α_1-acid glycoprotein concentration, it showed no significant relationship with the plasma level of albumin.

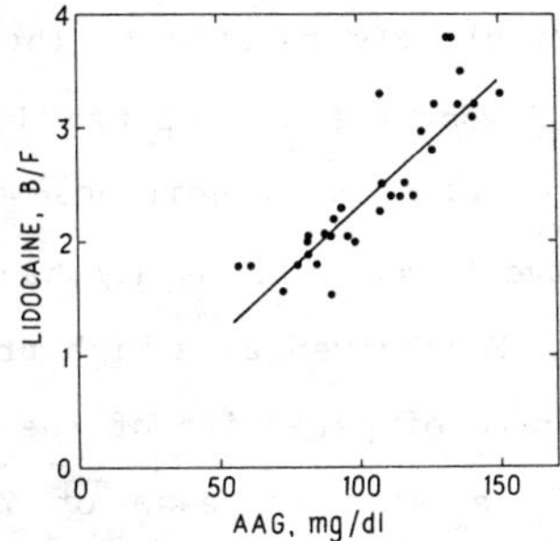

Figure 1.11   Relationship between the binding ratio (B/F) for lidocaine and plasma α_1-acid glycoprotein (AAG) concentration (r = 0.87).   Reproduced with permission from <u>Clin. Pharmacol. Ther.</u>, 1981, <u>30</u>, 154.

After crossing the placenta, lidocaine concentrates in the liver, heart, and brain of the guinea-pig foetus.[311]   High myocardial levels could account for the susceptibility of the foetal heart to lidocaine, administered to the mother.

While hepatic clearance of lidocaine is blood-flow related, and should be unaffected by enzyme induction, experiments in dogs suggest that the observed increases in hepatic clearance due to inducing agents may be caused by increased liver mass and proportionate increase in blood-flow.[312]   Other experiments in animals have shown that lidocaine may inhibit its own clearance following high dose infusion in the dog[313] and that lidocaine clearance is independent of age in sheep.[314]   In the latter study the $t_{0.5}$ values of lidocaine in non-pregnant ewes, neonatal lambs, and foetal lambs, were 31, 51, and 33 min, respectively, while total body clearance in the neonatal lamb and adult sheep were 53 and 41 ml min^{-1} kg^{-1}.   The unexpected capacity of the newborn to metabolize lidocaine effectively has been reported also in humans.[315]

A study in healthy subjects using stable isotope lidocaine labeled with two deuterium atoms showed that lidocaine kinetics may be nonlinear after long-term (30 h) infusion.[316]   The $t_{0.5}$ increased to 1.7 h and clearance decreased to 11 ml min^{-1} kg^{-1} from respective values of 1.2 h and 17 ml min^{-1} kg^{-1} obtained after a bolus i.v. dose, although the apparent volume of distribution remained constant.

The clearance of lidocaine was closely related to that of indo-cyanine green,[317] both compounds demonstrating hepatic blood flow-dependent elimination. Accordingly, clinical conditions which alter hepatic blood flow such as congestive heart failure may have signifi-cant effects on lidocaine kinetics. Food given as a high-protein meal caused a transient increase in the rate of perfusion of the splanchnic vascular system, which resulted in a mean increase of 21% in the hepatic clearance of i.v. lidocaine, from 1245 to 1477 ml min^{-1}.[318] Lidocaine serum protein binding was not influenced by the postprandial state. During continuous lidocaine infusion (2 mg min^{-1}) in eight healthy volunteers,[319] propranolol pretreatment decreased lidocaine clearance significantly by 14.7% in association with a 10-20% decrease in heart rate and cardiac output. Pindolol, which did not change cardiac output or heart rate significantly, produced no significant change in steady-state concentration or clearance of lidocaine. Typical plasma lidocaine concentrations representing these conditions are shown in Figure 1.12. Hepatic metabolism is accelerated by phenobarbital pretreatment.[320]

The hepatic clearance of lidocaine decreased in four, was un-changed in one, and increased in one of six subjects with acute viral hepatitis.[321] The distribution volume of lidocaine was also variable.

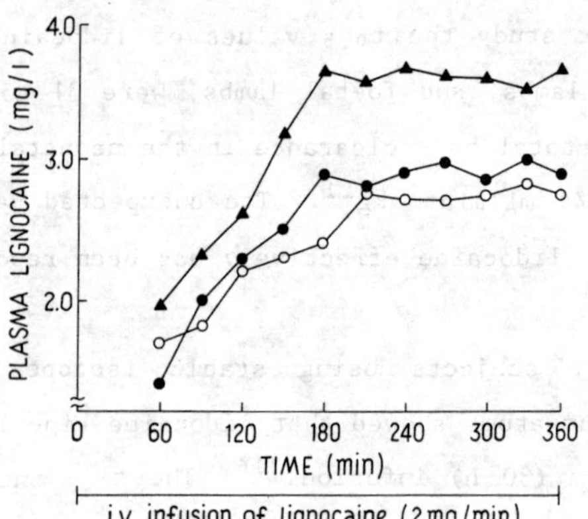

Figure 1.12   A typical example of plasma lignocaine concentrations when placebo (o), pindolol (●), and propranolol (▲) were coadministered. Reproduced by permission from Brit. J. Clin. Pharmacol., 1982, 13, 223S.

Both the distribution volume and elimination kinetics of lidocaine are influenced by age.[322] The average drug $t_{0.5}$ in elderly patients with a mean age of 65 yr was 140 min compared with 80 min in 24-yr-old subjects. The steady-state distribution volume of lidocaine was larger in the elderly subjects, however, so that drug clearances were similar in both groups. Neither the plasma clearance nor the distribution volume of lidocaine are affected by uraemia but both are significantly reduced in heart failure.[323] Both the plasma $t_{0.5}$ and distribution volume are significantly increased in liver disease.

Tocainide

The p.o. antiarrhythmic agent, tocainide, is quantitatively absorbed following p.o. doses to healthy subjects and exhibits dose-independent linear kinetics over a dosage range of 80-1000 mg.[324] Blood levels of drug after i.v. infusion obeyed two-compartment kinetics with a mean terminal $t_{0.5}$ of 11 h and a total body clearance of 166 ml min^{-1}. Giving the drug 5 min after a test meal reduced the peak blood level by 40% but did not influence the overall systemic bioavailability. For patients who respond to tocainide, antiarrthymic response was related to blood levels with an average of 70% suppression of premature ventricular contractions occurring at a drug level of 6 µg ml^{-1}; 90% at a drug level greater than 10 µg ml^{-1}.[325] In patients who received 400 mg tocainide every 8 h for 7 d following acute myocardial infarction the mean terminal plasma $t_{0.5}$ values of tocainide and its metabolites lactoxylidide and tocainide carbamoyl glucuronide were 13.6, 29.1, and 13 h, respectively.[326] Experiments in mice and rabbits showed that the metabolites had no antiarrhythmic, direct cardiac, or central nervous system effects.

Lorcainide

The new antiarrhythmic agent lorcainide was shown to obey two-compartment model kinetics after a single 10 mg kg^{-1} i.v. dose in the rat.[327] The drug was almost completely metabolized prior to excretion, with an average elimination $t_{0.5}$ of 3.3 h and total plasma clearance of 121.5 ml min^{-1} kg^{-1}. No tissue retention of the drug was detected.

Disopyramide

Characterization of disopyramide pharmacokinetics has been made difficult, but also interesting because of its concentration-dependent binding to plasma proteins. The proportion of drug that is bound decreases from 80% to 50% over the disopyramide concentration range of 2-8 μg ml^{-1} in plasma.[328,329] As only unbound disopyramide is cleared by the liver and kidney, the total body clearance is independent of the disopyramide concentration unbound to plasma proteins. This is illustrated in Figure 1.13 in which the observed steady-state concentration of disopyramide C_t^{ss} is equal to the value calculated

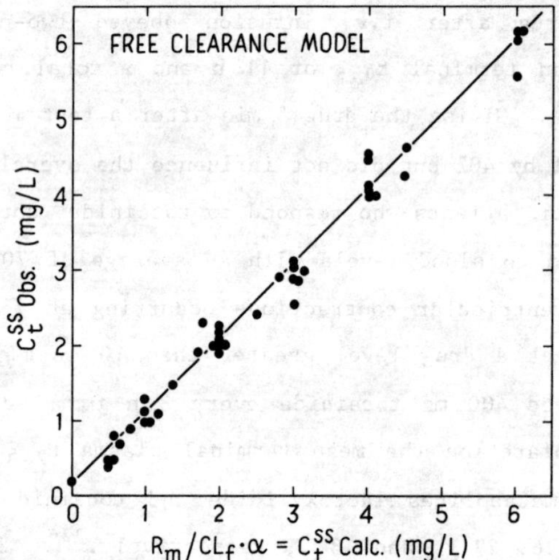

Figure 1.13 Total steady-state disopyramide plasma concentrations, calculated on the basis of a model which assumes that clearance is independent of the disopyramide concentration unbound to plasma proteins C_t^{ss} (calc) versus the mean observed concentration C_t^{ss} (obs). Mean observed concentrations were measured over periods of approximately 4 h. The slope and intercept are not significantly different from 1 and 0, respectively, and r^2 = 0.984, indicating that the free clearance model satisfactorily describes the data. Reproduced by permission from J. Pharmacokin. Biopharm., 1979, 7, 29.

from equation 1.12

$$C_t^{ss} \text{ (calc)} = Rm/Cl_f \cdot \alpha \qquad\qquad (1.12)$$

where Rm is the drug infusion rate, Cl_f is the clearance of unbound drug, and α is the free fraction at that particular plasma concentration. Dose proportionality has been demonstrated also for the concentration of free disopyramide, but not for total disopyramide, in plasma, and concentration dependent differences in disopyramide clearance following i.v. and p.o. doses can lead to erroneous conclusions regarding systemic availability of oral dosage forms.[330] However, in a comparison of p.o. disopyramide phosphate, p.o. disopyramide base, and i.v. disopyramide phosphate, based on total drug profiles in plasma, all three dosage forms were shown to be essentially bioequivalent, with apparently quantitative absorption of drug from the two p.o. dosage forms.[331] Systemic bioequivalence of disopyramide has been demonstrated also between conventional and sustained-release p.o. formulations. The bioavailability of disopyramide controlled-release tablets after multiple dosing, 300 mg every 12 h, was compared with that of the standard capsules, 150 mg every 6 h, in a crossover study using ten patients.[332] The two formulations were found to be bioequivalent based on the AUC values during one dosing interval and the percentage of dose excreted unchanged in the 0-12 h urine, 48.5 and 46.3% following capsules and controlled-release tablets, respectively.

Nonlinear binding to plasma proteins has been shown to influence disopyramide clearance, and also the predictive quality of this parameter in individuals with normal and also impaired renal function.[333,334] In one study,[333] the mean renal clearance of total disopyramide during 0-12 h after a single 1.5 mg kg^{-1} i.v. dose in eight healthy subjects was 0.62 ml min^{-1} kg^{-1} , which decreased to 0.37 ml min^{-1} kg^{-1} for the 12-36 h postdose interval. The renal clearance of unbound disopyramide on the other hand averaged <u>ca</u>. 3 ml

min^{-1} kg^{-1} and was not time-dependent. In another study,[334] six healthy volunteers received i.v. disopyramide at infusion rates of 2.5, 7.5, and 15 mg h^{-1} following bolus doses of 25, 75, and 150 mg, respectively, on separate occasions. The plasma clearance and renal clearance of total drug both increased markedly with increasing infusion rate and higher resulting plasma concentrations, from an average of 3.3 1 h^{-1} (infusion rate = 2.5 mg h^{-1}) to 6.7 1 h^{-1} (infusion rate = 15 mg h^{-1}) and 2.0 to 4.8 1 h^{-1}, respectively. Again, there was no significant difference in free disopyramide clearances between the different infusion rates. These results suggest that the clearance of unbound disopyramide is independent of the unbound fraction (α), while the clearance of total disopyramide is dependent on α. Although considerable interindividual variability in binding existed in these studies, the results provided direct explanation for the time-dependent change in total disopyramide renal clearance following bolus injection which was previously ascribed to a systematic error attributable to arterio-venous concentration differences.[335]

Impaired elimination of disopyramide was observed after an i.v. dose (2 mg kg^{-1}) of the drug in patients with varying degrees of renal insufficiency.[336] A linear relationship existed between the composite elimination rate constant (β) and creatinine clearance (Cl_{CR}) values below 40 ml min^{-1}, $\beta = 0.0310 + 0.00121$ Cl_{CR} ($r = 0.952$, $p < 0.001$). This would imply a $t_{0.5}$ of 22 h in anephric patients, compared with 5.1-8.5 h in normal individuals. Disopyramide plasma clearance also correlated directly with Cl_{CR}. Total urinary recovery of disopyramide and its mono-N-dealkylated metabolite in 72 h ranged from 70 to 81% of the dose in normal subjects but was less than 34% in patients with Cl_{CR} below 30 ml min^{-1}. Similar results were obtained after a 300 mg p.o. dose of disopyramide in 11 patients with reduced creatinine clearance values between 2.4 and 52.6 ml min^{-1}.[337] The mean disopyramide elimination $t_{0.5}$ in this group was 12.7 h. Following p.o. doses, serum disopyramide concentrations in patients with acute myocardial infarction tended to be lower than in the healthy state, as illustrated in Figure 1.14.[338] This phenomenon was explained in terms of reduced GI absorption in the patients, although a subsequent study showed no apparent effect of ischemic heart disease on oral disopyramide bioavailability.[339] In patients with cardiac failure, both disopyramide distribution and elimination appeared to be slower than in healthy subjects, with mean α and β phase $t_{0.5}$ values of 11.1 min and 9.7 h, respectively.[340] The absolute bioavailability of p.o. disopyramide in these patients averaged 97.5%. In another study in patients with confirmed infarction the β-phase $t_{0.5}$ was 38 and 21

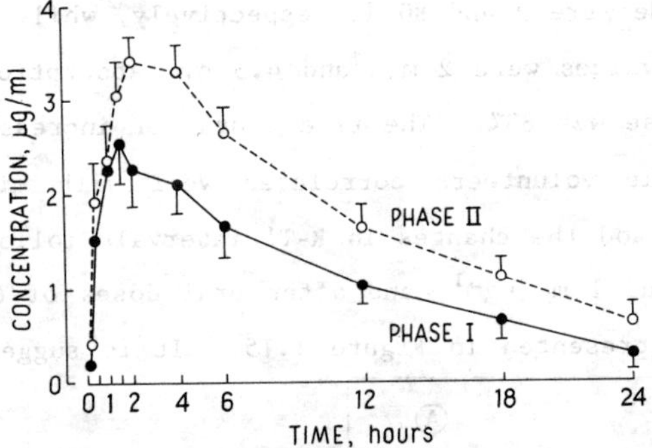

Figure 1.14 Mean ± SE serum levels of disopyramide obtained after administration of an oral dose of 200 mg disopyramide base to seven patients during the acute phase of myocardial infarction (phase I) and after the recovery 7-14 d later (phase II). Reproduced by permission from *Int. J. Clin. Pharmacol. Ther. Toxicol.*, 1982, <u>20</u>, 276.

h following repeated 100 mg and 200 mg doses, respectively. In patients with unconfirmed infarction the respective values were 24 h and 7 h.[341] The longer $t_{0.5}$ of disopyramide in infarct patients may be related to higher plasma protein binding.

Additional complications in the interpretation of disopyramide kinetics have been introduced by the observation that marked differences occur in the binding characteristics of this compound to dog and human plasma proteins.[342] Unlike the situation in humans, binding of disopyramide to dog plasma is constant at <u>ca</u>. 80% over a wide concentration range.

Apparent displacement from plasma proteins by rubber Vacutainer® stoppers has given rise to problems in disopyramide assays.[329] Exposure of blood to the stoppers caused a <u>ca</u>. 60% increase in disopyramide free fraction, apparently by competitive inhibition of disopyramide binding to α_1-acid glycoprotein. In contrast, heparin and EDTA had no effect on the plasma binding of disopyramide.

Studies by Hinderling and Garrett[343,344] and others have confirmed that the pharmacokinetics of disopyramide are linear when measured in terms of the free drug. Following i.v. doses to human volunteers the mean volumes of central and peripheral body compartments for disopyramide were 9 and 80 l, respectively, while the alpha and beta phase $t_{0.5}$ values were 2 min and 4.5 h. Absorption efficiency from an oral dose was 83%. The time course of increases in the R-T' interval in male volunteers correlated well with circulating disopyramide levels, and the changes in R-T' intervals following i.v. doses of 2 mg kg^{-1} and 1 mg kg^{-1}, and after oral doses of 6 mg kg^{-1} and 3 mg kg^{-1} are represented in Figure 1.15. It is suggested that

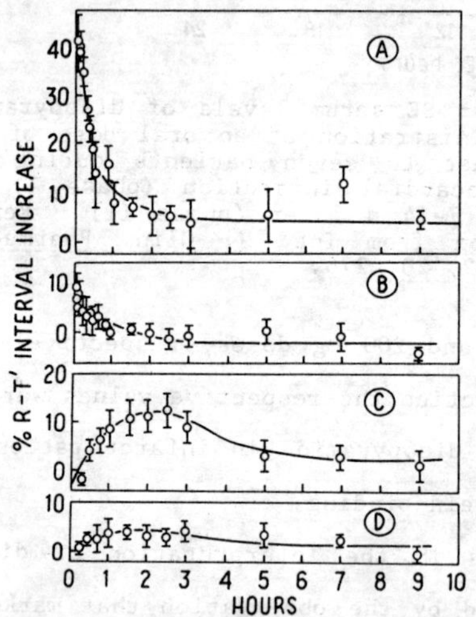

Figure 1.15   Plots of the mean R-T' [R-T interval/(R-R interval)$^{0.5}$] interval increases over control values against time after i.v. administration of 2 mg kg^{-1} (A, n = 5) and 1 mg kg^{-1} (B, n = 3) and after oral administration of 6 mg kg^{-1} (C, n = 3) and 3 mg kg^{-1} (D, n = 3) disopyramide phosphate. The bars indicated ± 1 SEM. Reproduced by permission from <u>J. Pharmacokin. Biopharm.</u>, 1976, <u>4</u>, 231.

this relationship may be of clinical use if antiarrhythmic potency of disopyramide and the length of the R-T' interval an be correlated in patients with rhythmic disorders.

Organic Nitrates

The absorption of the organic nitrates from a variety of dosage forms and dosage routes continues to be a subject of intense interest and activity.

Absorption rates and intensity of action of organic nitrates have been investigated by measuring peripheral vasodilation in man[345] and decreased pulse pressure in the dog.[346] Results obtained in the dog indicate that both standard and stabilized sublingual nitroglycerin and isosorbide dinitrate gave rise to a rapid onset of activity that lasted 5 to 10 min for nitroglycerin and up to 1 h for isosorbide dinitrate. The effects of p.o. dosed isosorbide dinitrate lasted up to 5 h after dosing. In man the maximum response to nitroglycerin occurred within 15 min of sublingual doses and 30 min of p.o. doses.

In order to prolong the duration of pharmacologic effect, sustained-release or percutaneous dosage forms of nitroglycerin have been developed. It was shown that a 30.4 mg ointment dose yielded serum concentrations approximately twice those obtained from a 2.5 mg sustained-release capsule, the peak values being 0.5 and 0.3 ng ml^{-1}, respectively, both achieved at 30 min postdose.[347] The absorption of nitroglycerin from an ointment was significantly influenced by the surface area of application.[348] In a study in the rhesus monkey using ^{14}C-labeled nitroglycerin ointment,[349] absorption increased significantly from 13.4% when applied to a 2-cm^2 surface area of the chest to 36.4% when applied to a 50-cm^2 area. However, the anatomical site of ointment application appeared to have no effect on absorption, the mean percent of radioactivity absorbed from the chest, arm, inner thigh, and the postauricular region being 13.4, 12.9, 14.8, and 8.9, respectively.

Imhof et al.[350] compared the plasma concentrations and hemodynamic effects of nitroglycerin during and after i.v. infusion at 3.4 and 7.5 µg min^{-1} for 30 min in normal volunteers. These authors reported that drug-induced postural increase in heart rate and the change in digital-pulse-wave morphology appeared to parallel the plasma concentration profile, whereas the systolic blood pressure in the upright position remained reduced at 15 min postinfusion when no measurable nitroglycerin was detected in plasma.

Nitroglycerin is rapidly eliminated from the body. After an intravenous infusion at a rate of 18 µg min^{-1} in healthy subjects, the mean plasma clearance of nitroglycerin was 0.7 l min^{-1} kg^{-1} while the volume of distribution and $t_{0.5}$ were 3.3 l kg^{-1} and 2.8 min, respectively.[351] Large intersubject variation was noted in the parameter values.

Comparisons of the _in vivo_ disappearance rates of organic nitrates in the rat, and also in perfused rat liver and blood _in vitro_ suggest that _in vivo_ disappearance of organic nitrates is due to distribution, nonhepatic metabolism, and hepatic metabolism, which is limited only by the rate at which drug is presented to the liver.[352]

Several reports have appeared on the bioavailability of isosorbide dinitrate (ISDN) from a variety of formulations. Some of the results obtained have been contradictory. For example, one study reported the overall bioavailability of p.o. ISDN from conventional tablets to be _ca_. 60%, while that from sustained release doses was _ca_. 50%.[353] Another study comparing 12.5 mg single p.o. solution doses and a 5 mg h^{-1} 150 min infusion concluded that systemic availability of p.o. ISDN was only 3%, indicating significant first-pass metabolism.[354] The infusion data showed an ISDN elimination $t_{0.5}$ of 9 to 10 min, a distribution volume of 2-4 l, and a systemic clearance of 0.16-0.32 l min^{-1}.

Morrison et al.[355] conducted a similar study by infusing ISDN to 11 angina patients at the same infusion rate (5 mg h^{-1}) for 2 h. While the terminal $t_{0.5}$ values (10-30 min) were similar to those observed in the previous study,[354] the mean steady-state plasma ISDN concentration (<u>ca.</u> 25 ng ml^{-1}) was approximately ten-fold lower, resulting in much higher clearance values ranging from 1.8 to 6.3 1 min^{-1}. The reasons for this discrepancy were not apparent. Although a substantial adsorptive loss of ISDN to plastic infusion bags or infusion sets has been reported,[356] it could not account for the differences observed in these studies.

Other studies have compared plasma levels of ISDN following conventional tablets and sustained-release doses, and also between different sustained-release products. In some cases considerable differences have been observed.[357]

Following sublingual doses of 5 mg, p.o. conventional tablets of 5 mg, and p.o. sustained-release tablets of 20 mg, mean peak ISDN levels of drug were considerably prolonged after the sustained-release dosage with levels being maintained above one-half of the mean peak level for 10 h.[358] The same dose of a different sustained-release formulation gave rise to peak drug levels in plasma of 3.2 ng ml^{-1} occurring at 2 to 4 h, and levels were still detectable in plasma 12 h after dosing.[353]

The plasma levels of ISDN and its pharmacologically active metabolites isosorbide 2-mononitrate (2-MN) and isosorbide 5-mononitrate (5-MN) were compared following administration of two p.o. sustained-release formulations, a capsule and a tablet, of ISDN in healthy volunteers.[359] Both products appeared to release the drug at a constant rate for about 5 h, although the capsule resulted in higher plasma concentrations of ISDN and the metabolites than the tablet. A high degree of intersubject variation in plasma levels was observed. The relative potencies of ISDN:2-MN:5-MN based on finger pulse plethysmography in these subjects were found to be 1:0.1:0.025.[360] In another study,[361] the bioavailability of 30 mg sustained-release ISDN and 7.5 mg standard-release pindolol were compared after administering these drugs alone and in combination to healthy adults. Neither drug showed a significant influence on the bioavailability of the other. The relative bioavailability of 30 mg sustained-release ISDN was similar to that of 5 mg standard-release ISDN alone, although the former showed prolonged release for approximately 6 h whereas the latter had a short terminal $t_{0.5}$ of 24 min and plasma ISDN levels below detection after 2 h. While isosorbide has a short biological $t_{0.5}$, high levels of unchanged drug may appear in plasma after chronic doses. This is probably due to saturation of hepatic biotransformation.

Absorption of ISDN from a topical ointment is approximately 30% of that from a sublingual tablet.[363] Plasma levels of drug resulting from the ointment are prolonged relative to the sublingual dose, and topical application may be useful to maintain ISDN in plasma over relatively long periods.

ISDN was not extensively bound to plasma proteins in both healthy individuals and in angina patients.[364] The free fraction averaged 0.72 in the ISDN concentration range of 1-100 ng ml^{-1}. After intravenous dosing in the rhesus monkey, cynomolgus monkey, and baboon, mean ISDN clearance values were 188, 200, and 169 ml min^{-1}, respectively, and the mean terminal $t_{0.5}$ values were 62, 23, and 24 minutes.[365]

Unlike the parent drug, isosorbide 5-mononitrate (5-MN) was completely bioavailable after p.o. administration.[366,367] The compound was distributed throughout total body water. Its half-life after i.v. and p.o. administration was 4 to 5 h, and its systemic clearance was ca. 120-130 ml min^{-1}. The $t_{0.5}$ reported here is similar to but somewhat shorter than the previously reported[368] $t_{0.5}$ of 7.6 h for 5-MN after a sublingual dose of ISDN. The $t_{0.5}$ of the other active metabolite isosorbide 2-mononitrate was 1.75 h after sublingual ISDN. The pharmacokinetics of ISDN and the mononitrates in patients with renal failure (creatinine clearance from 6 to 15 ml min^{-1}) were similar to those observed in subjects with normal renal function.[369]

Rapid de-esterification of pentaerythritol tetranitrate (PETN) after p.o. dosing to man resulted in measurable serum levels of pentaerythritol (PE), pentaerythritol mononitrate (PEMN), and small amounts of the dinitrate, but no unchanged drug.[370,371] The kinetics of urinary excretion of PE were first-order and apparently dose-independent whereas those of PEMN were first-order and dose-dependent. The ratio of PEMN to PE excreted in the urine was 3:1 from a 40 mg dose and 1:1 from a 20 mg dose, suggesting a limited capacity for conversion of PEMN into PE. Similar kinetics of these metabolites were observed after doses of pentaerythritol trinitrate. However, urinary excretion of PE was biphasic, with the rapid initial rate coinciding with maximum PE blood levels. This was not observed after PETN doses, probably due to prolonged absorption.[372]

Mexiletine

The absorption of mexiletine was rapid and complete from intramuscular injection sites, and was proportional to the dose within a tested range of 50-400 mg.[373] In normal subjects, the drug had an elimination $t_{0.5}$ of 8 to 15 h and an overall clearance of approximately 10 ml min^{-1} kg^{-1}. A 200 mg p.o. capsule dose of mexiletine combined with a 200 mg i.m. loading dose as a 25 mg ml^{-1} or 100 mg ml^{-1} solution provided therapeutically effective plasma levels above 0.75 µg ml^{-1} within 43 min. The elimination of mexiletine occurred mainly by metabolism, and was enhanced by the enzyme inducer rifampicin.[374] Pretreatment with rifampicin 300 mg twice daily for 10 d had no effect on GI absorption, distribution, or renal clearance of mexiletine, but significantly increased the total and nonrenal clearances of the latter. The mean mexiletine $t_{0.5}$ values before and after rifampicin were 8.5 and 5.0 h, respectively, as indicated by the serum data in Figure 1.16. The amount of unchanged mexiletine excreted in the 0-48 h urine decreased from 9.7 to 5.4% of the dose due to rifampicin pretreatment.

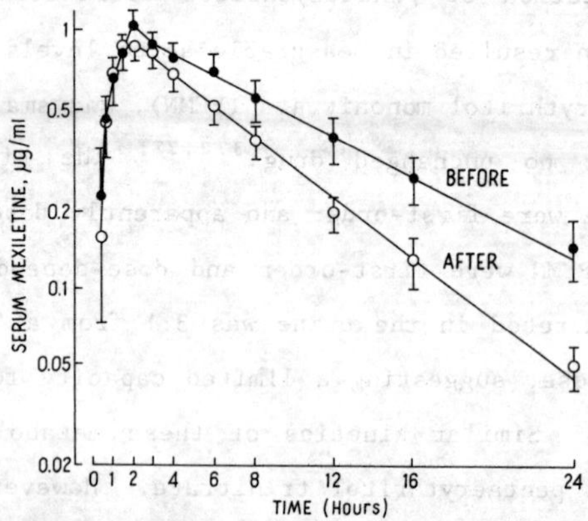

Figure 1.16   Serum concentrations of mexiletine following an oral dose of mexiletine hydrochloride 400 mg
in eight healthy volunteers before and after treatment
with rifampicin 300 mg b.i.d. for 10 d.   Mean ± SE.
Reproduced by permission from Eur. J. Clin. Pharmacol.,
1982, 23, 261.

Verapamil

The antianginal and antiarrhythmic agent verapamil was completely
absorbed after p.o. administration, but had a relatively low bioavailability of ca. 22% due to extensive first-pass metabolism.[375,376]
Intravenous dosing experiments revealed a terminal $t_{0.5}$ of 2 to 4 h
and mean plasma clearance of 1.26 1 min^{-1}, which approached liver
blood flow.   The PR interval on ECG recordings correlated significantly with the log plasma level of verapamil (r = 0.732, p < 0.001) but
not with that of the metabolite norverapamil (r = 0.078, p > 0.7),
which was detectable in plasma only after p.o. doses.[376]   Verapamil
was approximately 90% bound to plasma proteins over the usual therapeutic concentration range.[377]   The binding was not affected by the
presence of norverapamil, warfarin, end-stage renal failure, or the
postoperative state in coronary bypass graft patients.   In children,
the elimination of verapamil appeared to be slower than in adults,
with a mean total clearance and elimination $t_{0.5}$ of 0.5 1 min^{-1} and
9.2 h.[378]

Compared to that in healthy young subjects, the elimination of verapamil in patients with atrial fibrillation was decreased; the $t_{0.5}$ and plasma clearance were 6 h and 0.26 l h^{-1} kg^{-1}.[379] The oral bioavailability in these patients was also lower than in normal subjects, with a mean value of 10.5%, which agreed with the reported mean hepatic extraction of verapamil of 0.86 in patients with organic heart disease.[380] In contrast, Kates et al.[381] observed an enhanced bioavailability of 35% in their patients with chronic atrial fibrillation, though with considerable interindividual variability ranging from 13% to 64%. Similar discrepancies were observed in patients with liver cirrhosis whose bioavailability could be reduced, unchanged,[382] or increased,[383] probably depending on the severity of the disease.[384] Liver disease patients also had a reduced systemic verapamil clearance, and a prolonged $t_{0.5}$ of 14 h.[382,383]

Diltiazem

The pharmacokinetics of the calcium antagonist diltiazem have been described after p.o. administration in normal volunteers in terms of a one-compartment open model.[385] Diltiazem bioavailability appeared to be dose independent. The mean peak plasma concentrations were 72, 117, and 151 ng ml^{-1} after 60, 90, and 120 mg doses, respectively, each achieved within 3 to 4 h postdose. The $t_{0.5}$ of p.o. diltiazem was 4 to 5 h.

Amiodarone

Amiodarone is another antiarrhythmic agent which shows considerable interpatient variability in pharmacokinetic characteristics. After a single i.v. dose, plasma amiodarone declined biexponentially, with a mean $t_{0.5}$ of 4.3 h and a total clearance of 125-288 ml min^{-1}.[386] Secondary concentration peaks were observed after 2 to 4 h, and were attributed to enterohepatic circulation.[387] Following a single p.o. dose in the 200-400 mg range, peak plasma or serum concentrations were obtained between 3 and 7 h.[386,387] Systemic availability was estimated to be less than 50%. The elimination $t_{0.5}$ for the single p.o. dose was _ca_. 17 h,[386] but chronic dosing resulted in much slower elimination of amiodarone.[387] In patients maintained on three times daily amiodarone therapy, the trough serum concentration continued to rise for over one month (Figure 1.17). Amiodarone $t_{0.5}$ after discontinuation of eight months of therapy in one patient was 13.7 d. Kannan et al.[388] reported the same phenomenon in patients receiving 400-800 mg daily p.o. doses whose mean amiodarone $t_{0.5}$ increased from 7.2 h to 29 d after therapy for 39 d.

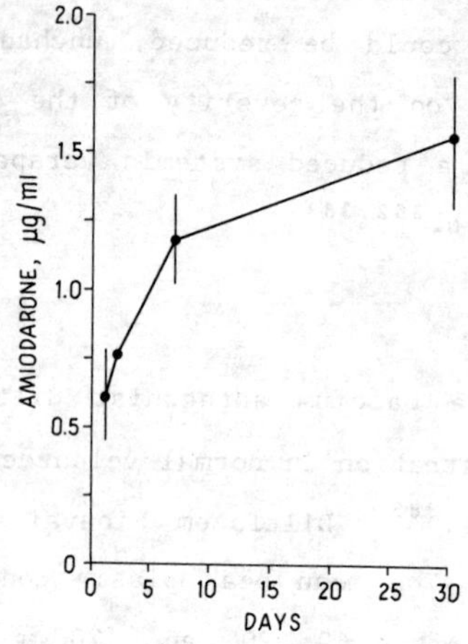

Figure 1.17 Trough (morning) concentration of serum amiodarone during prolonged oral therapy with 200 mg three times daily. Average values (± SD) from six or seven patients. Reproduced by permission from _Eur. J. Clin. Pharmacol._, 1981, _19_, 293.

Bretylium Tosylate

Garrett et al.[389] conducted a comprehensive study on the pharmacokinetics of bretylium tosylate. Single doses between 100 and 400 mg were administered to nine healthy, young, male adults by i.v. infusion, i.m. injection, and p.o. as a solution or tablet. Following an i.v. dose, plasma bretylium declined triexponentially, with a mean terminal $t_{0.5}$ of 9 h. Total clearance and apparent volume of distribution averaged 735 ml min^{-1} and 589 l, respectively, while the urinary recovery of unchanged drug was 74% of the dose. Intramuscularly administered bretylium was completely bioavailable, with an absorption $t_{0.5}$ of 1.3 h. The elimination kinetics were similar to those observed after i.v. dosing; the $t_{0.5}$ was 7.3 h and the plasma clearance was 686 ml min^{-1}. However, the urinary recovery of bretylium increased to 95.4% with the i.m. route, the reasons for which are unclear. Bretylium bioavailability from the p.o. solution and tablet averaged 22 and 27%, respectively, with a wide intersubject range of 14-36%. The solution had a shorter lag time but a longer absorption $t_{0.5}$, 17 min and 3.9 h, respectively, compared with 56 min and 1.5 h for the tablet dose. The terminal $t_{0.5}$ for the p.o. doses, 9.9 h, was similar to those observed after parenteral drug administration. In general, bretylium pharmacokinetics appeared to be independent of dose, regardless of the mode of administration. Additional i.v. dosing experiments in the dog revealed a terminal $t_{0.5}$ similar to that in humans, <u>ca</u>. 8.7 h.

Carnitine

l-Carnitine obeys apparent two-compartment kinetics in man following i.v. infusion, distributing initially into a volume comprising 20% of body weight, and equilibrating into a volume of 28% body weight.[390] The α- and β-phase of the biphasic drug elimination curve have $t_{0.5}$ values of 0.6 and 3 h. Dog studies indicate that d-carnitine does not affect plasma levels of the l-isomer,[391] but no information is available regarding the interactions of the isomers at the cellular level. Plasma levels of l-carnitine are seriously depleted during dialysis, with total (free and bound) concentrations dropping from 40-50 to 20 μmol 1^{-1} during 6 h dialysis.[392] This transient fall in l-carnitine levels has been associated with muscular weakness and cramp. Although plasma levels of l-carnitine return to normal values by 6 h postdialysis, due to equilibration with body stores, any fall in l-carnitine levels during dialysis may be prevented by addition of l-carnitine to the dialysate.

Beta-Adrenergic Receptor Antagonists

The appearance of an increasing number of this class of anti-hypertensive agents during recent years, and the associated proliferation of related literature, prevents more than a superficial coverage of this area. Reviews have been published on the clinical pharmacokinetics of β-adrenergic receptor blocking agents,[393] and particularly on propranolol.[394] Various aspects of pharmacokinetic differences between the β-receptor blocking agents, and their clinical implications, have been reviewed by Meier[395] and others. The β-adrenergic receptor blocking agents have been reviewed also in terms of relationships between pharmacokinetic properties and their wide range of therapeutic doses.[396] The greatest dose variation occurs with propranolol, alprenolol, and oxprenolol, all of which have short biological $t_{0.5}$ values and high hepatic clearances, and may be subject to variable first-pass clearance after p.o. doses.[397,398] In this brief and necessarily incomplete review compounds will be discussed alphabetically.

Acebutolol

It is well established that acebutolol is extensively metabolized in the body, and undergoes extensive first-pass metabolism after p.o. doses. However, there are divergent reports on its rate of metabolism. Following i.v. injection to human subjects acebutolol was reported to obey two-compartment model kinetics with fast and slow $t_{0.5}$ values of 6 min and 2 h, respectively.[399]

After a single 400 mg p.o. dose, however, the decline in plasma levels following peak values was again biphasic but the fast and slow $t_{0.5}$ values were extended to 3.1 and 11 h, respectively.[400] It is claimed by these authors that the previously claimed $t_{0.5}$ of ca. 2 h is based on combined distribution and elimination rather than elimination alone.[401] The major metabolite of acebutolol, diacetolol reaches

higher plasma levels compared to parent drug after p.o. doses and is
more slowly eliminated.[400,402]   Typical mean plasma levels of
acebutolol and diacetolol following a p.o. dose are shown in Figure
1.18.

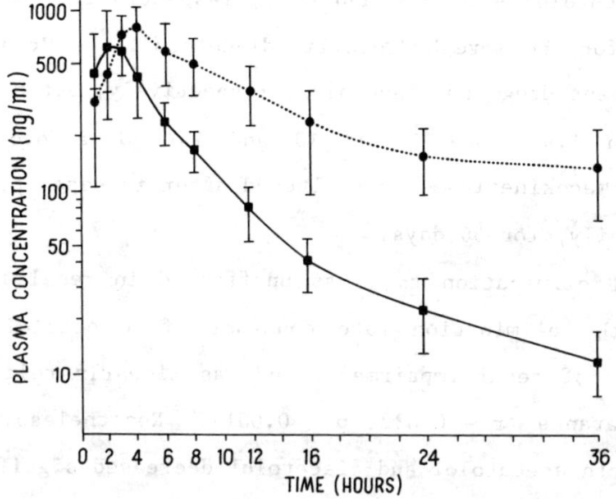

Figure 1.18   Mean plasma concentrations of acebutolol
(■——■) and diacetolol (●---●) in 8 male volunteers,
after a single 400 mg oral dose of acebutolol.   Error
bars indicate ± S.D.   Reproduced by permission from
Biopharm. Drug Dispos., 1981, 2, 103.

After i.v. infusion, metabolite levels are lower than those of
parent drug,[403] a pattern that is consistent with first-pass metabolism after p.o. doses.   The relatively long elimination $t_{0.5}$ of
the metabolites compared to parent drug causes greater accumulation of
metabolites with repeated dosing.[404]   While both drug and metabolite
plasma levels correlate well with pharmacological effect, correlations
are generally higher for unchanged drug.

Dose dependency has been demonstrated for acebutolol following
single and repeated doses.[405]   Dose-corrected AUC values after a 10 mg
kg^{-1} p.o. dose increase 87% compared with AUC values after a 1 mg
kg^{-1} dose, while circulating drug levels also increase dispropor-
tionately during repeated doses.   Increased availability from higher
p.o. doses of acebutolol may be due to saturation of hepatic uptake
and this, together with possible metabolite inhibition, may be responsible for drug accumulation after chronic doses.

Acebutolol and diacetolol were weakly bound to plasma proteins, about 11-19% and 6-9%, respectively.[406] However, their hydrophilic nature restricts the distribution of these compounds into extravascular spaces. The mean saliva:plasma and cerebrospinal fluid:plasma ratios for acebutolol were 2.6 and 0.11, respectively, compared with 0.72 and 0.04 for the more hydrophilic diacetolol.[407] Urinary excretion of the parent drug and diacetolol, respectively, accounted for 31 and 18% of an i.v. dose[401] and 10 and 14% of a p.o. dose.[400] Acebutolol pharmacokinetics were unaltered after repeated p.o. dosing, 400 mg twice daily, for 56 days.

Acebutolol elimination $t_{0.5}$ was unaffected in renal failure.[408] In contrast, the elimination rate constant of diacetolol decreased with the degree of renal impairment, and was linearly related to the creatinine clearance ($r = 0.832$, $p < 0.001$). Nonetheless, the renal clearance of both acebutolol and diacetolol decreased significantly in renal insufficiency; the urinary recovery of unchanged drug and metabolite accounted for only 5 and 17% of the acebutolol dose compared with 14 and 26% in subjects with normal renal function in the same study. Since the metabolite also exhibit cardiac β-adrenoceptor blocking activity that is directly related to plasma concentration,[409,410] it is necessary to adjust the dose of acebutolol according to the degree of renal function impairment.

Alprenolol

Alprenolol is rapidly absorbed from the GI tract, but first-pass metabolism reduces absorption efficiency.[411,412] Poor bioavailability is partly compensated for by formation of the active metabolite 4-hydroxyalprenolol. The considerable variation that may occur in alprenolol plasma levels after p.o. doses was indicated by Rawlins et al.,[413] who observed a 25-fold difference in steady-state drug levels in patients receiving identical multiple-dose therapy.

The absorption efficiency of orally dosed alprenolol as unchanged drug varies from 1 to 15% of a 200 mg dose and, as with metoprolol, availability of the drug increases nonlinearly with increasing doses.[414] The availability of p.o. alprenolol is also markedly decreased by pentobarbital pretreatment, but the elimination rate is unchanged.[415,416] These phenomena may be reconcilable if the hepatic metabolism of alprenolol is saturable and also capable of induction, and if the changes in liver metabolic capacity are not reflected directly in elimination rate changes.[417]

The percentage binding of alprenolol in plasma is related to the plasma concentration of α_1-acid glycoprotein rather than to that of albumin. Changes in the concentration of α_1-acid glycoprotein in disease have been shown to correlate with correspondingly large variations in the binding of both alprenolol and propranolol.[418]

Other studies, related to β-blocking agents, describe serum levels and pharmacological effects of alprenolol in man.[419] Linear relationships have been demonstrated between the degree of hypotensive activity and the logarithms of steady-state plasma alprenolol levels in responding patients.[420-423] As a result of this relationship the decline of pharmacologic effect occurs at a zero-order rate with respect to time. However, poor correlations were observed between the degree of beta blockade, or of plasma drug levels, with the prescribed dose of alprenolol.

<u>Atenolol</u>

The bioavailability of atenolol from p.o. doses is <u>ca.</u> 50%,[424] and this value is constant from 25, 50, and 100 mg doses.[425] Other kinetic parameters for atenolol, including plasma clearance (9 l h^{-1}) and elimination $t_{0.5}$ (7 h) are also independent of dose size, while C_{max} and AUC values are dose proportional.

Atenolol is extensively distributed into body tissues giving rise to low plasma levels. Typically after p.o. solution doses of 100 mg atenolol, a mean peak blood level of 0.9 µg ml^{-1} was obtained at 2 h and the elimination $t_{0.5}$ was 9 h.[426]

In another study, mean peak blood levels of 0.51-0.65 µg ml^{-1} were obtained at 3 h from 100 mg doses of tablet and solution formulations.[427] Urinary excretion of atenolol averaged 42-47% of the dose.

The absorption and disposition of atenolol were not significantly affected by concomitant administration of 25 mg[428] or 50 mg[429] of the diuretic chlorthalidone. Coadministration of an antacid reduced the systemic availability of atenolol by an average of 33% (Figure 1.19) while increasing that of metoprolol by approximately 11%, though it

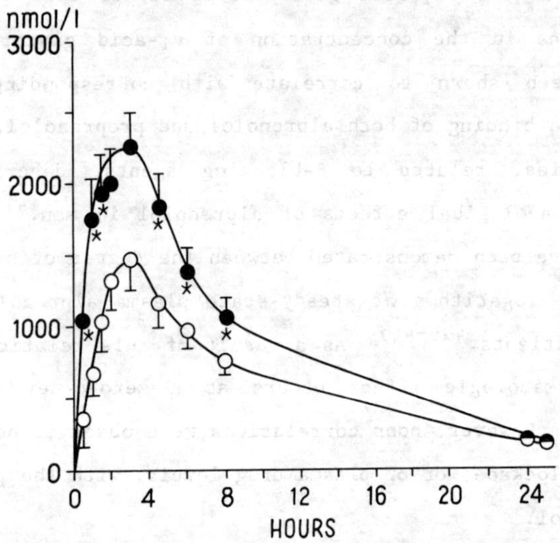

Figure 1.19   The effect of concomitant administration of antacid on the plasma levels of atenolol.   (●) atenolol alone; (o) atenolol + antacid.   Mean values ± SEM are indicated.   n = 6.   (*) p < 0.05.   Reproduced by permission from Biopharm. Drug Dispos., 1981, 2, 79.

had no apparent effect on the rate of absorption and elimination of the two β-blockers.[430] The negative effect of the antacid on atenolol bioavailability was due to a reduction in the *in vivo* dissolution rate of atenolol secondary to increased gastric pH. Metoclopramide, which increases the rate of gastric emptying, had no effect on the plasma concentration-time profile of atenolol. In contrast, pretreatment with propantheline, which decreases gastric emptying rate, caused a significant decrease in the absorption rate of atenolol, delaying the mean time of peak plasma concentration from 2.1 to 4.5 h. However, the prolonged residence time in the stomach also enhanced atenolol dissolution and increased its bioavailability by 36%.

The ocular penetration and systemic availability of ^{14}C-atenolol solution instilled into the rabbit eye were relatively poor compared with ^{14}C-labeled metoprolol, timolol, and propranolol which were 100, 160, and 2600 times more lipophilic, respectively, than atenolol.[431] Atenolol readily crosses the human placenta, and similar levels of drug have been demonstrated in maternal and umbilical cord serum.[432]

Atenolol elimination is variably affected by disease conditions. In patients with angina pectoris atenolol elimination $t_{0.5}$ was increased to <u>ca</u>. 11 h.[433] Hyperthyroidism, a disease state which increases the general metabolic rate and, therefore, the presystemic clearance of the β-blockers propranolol and metoprolol, had no effect on the pharmacokinetics of atenolol, which is excreted primarily unchanged in the urine.[434] On the other hand, exercise caused an approximately 8% decrease in the renal clearance of atenolol, probably due to redistribution of total cardiac output during exercise which resulted in reduced renal blood flow.[435] As would be expected, the excretion of atenolol is retarded in patients with compromised kidney function, the distribution volume may be slightly reduced, while the bioavailability of the drug is unaffected.[436-440] McAinsh et al.[438] reported a direct linear relationship between atenolol elimination rate constant and creatinine clearance from 0 to 122 ml min^{-1} 1.73 m^{-2} (Figure 1.20), with the $t_{0.5}$ increasing from <u>ca</u>. 6 h to more than 100 h with progressive renal failure. In patients undergoing hemodialysis, the mean plasma atenolol $t_{0.5}$ decreased from 73.4 h to 7.5 h during dialysis but returned to 51.2 h after dialysis.[439] In individuals with normal renal function, atenolol pharmacokinetics were not influenced by age.[441]

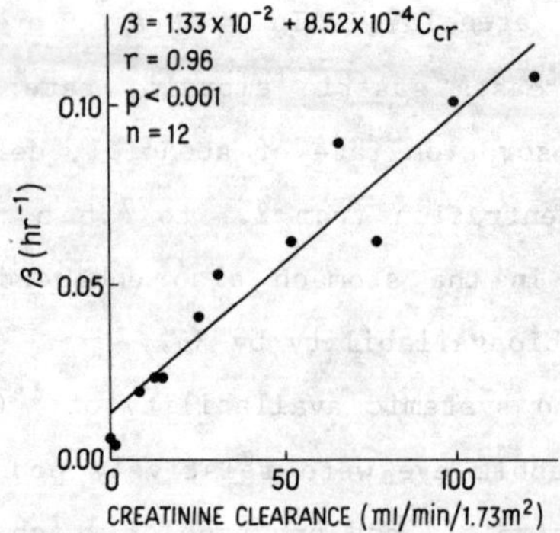

Figure 1.20 Relationship between atenolol elimination rate constant and creatinine clearance after a single 100-mg oral dose to subjects with varying degrees of renal impairment. Reproduced by permission from Clin. Pharmacol. Ther., 1980, <u>28</u>, 302.

The clinical significance of changes in atenolol levels, due to renal impairment or other pathological conditions is uncertain, as poor correlations have been reported between blood levels of drug and hypotensive effect.[442]

Bevantolol

The new β-adrenergic antagonist bevantolol is rapidly absorbed after p.o. administration reaching peak concentrations in 1 to 2 h.[443] With single doses ranging from 100 to 400 mg, bevantolol produces plasma levels that are directly proportional to the administered dose; mean peak plasma levels range from 800 to 3400 ng ml^{-1} (depending on dose) and decline with a $t_{0.5}$ of <u>ca</u>. 2-3 h.

Bioavailability of bevantolol tablets is equivalent to bioavailability of the drug from a p.o. solution. However, like propranolol, about one-half of the administered dose may be metabolized by the liver before it enters the systemic circulation. Bioavailability of the tablet is only 52 to 58% compared to when the drug is administered as an i.v. solution.

The presence of food in the GI tract decreases the rate but not the extent of bevantolol absorption. When the drug is taken after

a meal, the time to peak drug concentration is increased, but there is
no effect on peak concentration, area under the curve, elimination
rate constant, or $t_{0.5}$. Typical mean plasma levels of bevantolol
obtained in fasted and nonfasted subjects are shown in Figure 1.21.
There is no evidence of significant drug accumulation, or of change in
pharmacokinetic behavior when the drug is given in multiple doses.
Steady-state is reached by the second day of dosing.

Approximately 87% of administered radioactive dose is recovered
in the urine and feces in five days (72 and 15%, respectively),
confirming availability. Most of bevantolol is excreted in urine as
the carboxyl derivative. The remainder is excreted as phenolic and
alcohol metabolites. All are excreted mainly as conjugates.[443]

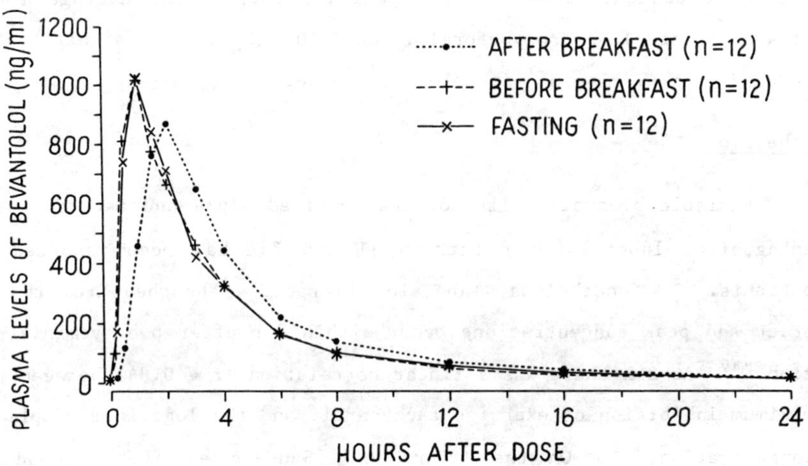

Figure 1.21 Mean plasma levels of bevantolol following a single 100-mg dose of bevantolol given fasting
or before or after breakfast. Reproduced by permission from Ref. 443.

Bufuralol

The lipophilic drug bufuralol has a low renal clearance and is
eliminated mainly by biotransformation in the liver. For reasons yet
to be determined, renal failure caused a decrease in the hepatic
metabolism of bufuralol.[444] The systemic availability of a 20 mg

p.o. dose of bufuralol increased from 67% in normal adults to 84% in patients with creatinine clearances below 30 ml min^{-1}, due to diminished first-pass effect. Compared with normal subjects, uraemic patients showed an increase in the 24 h urinary excretion of the parent drug, from 0.6 to 0.9% of a p.o. dose, but a 3- to 5-fold decrease in the excretion of three major metabolites, including the pharmacologically active 1'-hydroxybufuralol. The mean intrinsic clearance of bufuralol decreased from 54 1 h^{-1} in healthy subjects to 15 1 h^{-1} in patients with renal insufficiency. However, the $t_{0.5}$ values of the drug in the two groups were similar, about 3 to 6 h, suggesting a decrease in bufuralol distribution volume in renal patients. The net result was a significant increase in plasma bufuralol concentrations in the patient group. The average renal clearance of 1'-hydroxybufuralol was 10 ml min^{-1}, significantly reduced from 67 ml min^{-1} in normal volunteers.

Labetalol

Variable bioavailability of the combined alpha and beta receptor antagonist, labetalol, of between 11 and 76% has been reported in patients.[445] Nonetheless, labetalol is rapidly absorbed from the GI tract and peak concentrations occur within 2 h after p.o. administration.[446] At 2 h there was a linear correlation (r = 0.84) between the maximum inhibition of exercise tachycardia and the logarithm of plasma concentration.[446] On the other hand, Sanders et al.[447] found no correlation between β-adrenoceptor blockade or antihypertensive effect and steady-state plasma concentration of labetalol in hypertensive patients.

The bioavailability of labetalol tended to be less from noncoated or coated tablets compared to a p.o. solution, although the differences were not statistically significant. Food delayed the time of peak plasma concentration from 0.5 h to ca. 1.3 h, but increased the bioavailability of a 200 mg coated labetalol tablet by approximately

20% according to area under curve values.[448] The greater bioavailability of labetalol after food intake was explained in terms of reduced first-pass metabolism secondary to a food-induced increase in the splanchnic blood flow.

Plasma levels of labetalol declined biexponentially after i.v. dosing, with mean distribution and elimination phase $t_{0.5}$ values of 5.9 min and 4.9 h, respectively, and a steady-state distribution volume of 9.4 l kg^{-1}.[449] Labetalol pharmacokinetics were unaffected by renal function impairment.[450]

Mepindolol

Mepindolol sulphate, a new nonselective β-receptor blocker, is well absorbed orally, being 82% bioavailable from a 20 mg p.o. dose.[451] The drug has an elimination $t_{0.5}$ of <u>ca</u>. 4 h. During a 2.5 mg twice daily regimen, steady-state for both mepindolol plasma concentrations and also its effect on heart rate was reached on the second day of dosing.

Metipranolol

Metipranolol is rapidly and completely metabolized to the active species deacetyl metipranolol during absorption from the gastro-intestinal tract. Abshagen et al.[452] reported an absolute bioavailability of deacetyl metipranolol of approximately 50% from a 40 mg p.o. dose of metipranolol. Serum concentrations of deacetyl metipranolol peaked within 1 h of metipranolol administration, and declined with a terminal $t_{0.5}$ of <u>ca</u>. 3 h, similar to that observed after i.v. doses. The kinetics of deacetyl metipranolol were linear after i.v. infusion doses between 6 and 25 mg; the total clearance was about 1200 ml min^{-1}. Approximately 12.3% of the i.v. dose of deacetyl metipranolol was excreted unchanged in 0-24 h urine. Deacetyl metipranolol was moderately bound to serum proteins, <u>ca</u>. 70% in the concentration range 70-200 μg l^{-1}.

<u>Metoprolol</u>

The pharmacokinetics and pharmacodynamics of metoprolol have been reviewed.[453] Biopharmaceutic aspects of metoprolol therapy, particularly regarding optimal drug delivery, continue to generate interest. Approximately 40% of a p.o. dose of metoprolol reaches the circulation, and the drug distributes extensively into extravascular tissues with a distribution $t_{0.5}$ of about 12 min.[454] The elimination $t_{0.5}$ of unchanged metoprolol, and also of total metabolites, is about 3 h.[455] After i.v. doses, however, the $t_{0.5}$ of metoprolol is increased to 5 h and it is suggested that the metabolic pathways may be a function of the route of administration.

Although the relationship between areas under metoprolol plasma concentration versus time curves and doses ranging from 20 to 200 mg is statistically compatible with a linear function in man, there is some evidence of increased systemic bioavailability at higher doses.[456] This is consistent with previous observations,[457] and with saturable first-pass metabolism. ^{3}H-Metoprolol was rapidly absorbed, underwent extensive distribution, and was rapidly eliminated after p.o. doses to the rat and dog, with 70-100% of dosed ^{3}H appearing in the 24 h urine.[458] The drug elimination $t_{0.5}$ was 0.6 h and 1.5 h in the rat and dog, respectively, and drug kinetics did not change in either species after repeated dosing.

Several sustained-release formulations of 200 mg metoprolol have been shown to produce plasma metoprolol concentrations and cardio-vascular effects after a single daily dose comparable to those obtained from conventional 100 mg tablets given twice daily.[459-462]

Mean plasma levels and reduction in exercised heart rate for sustained and conventional oral metoprolol dosage forms are shown in Figures 1.22 and 1.23.[463] Included also in the figures are data obtained during the 12-24 h period following an evening dose of metoprolol. While peak plasma levels were considerably reduced following the sustained release formulation, areas under plasma curves were similar for the two dosage forms.

Similar results to these have been obtained with repeated dose regimens.[464] However, increased area under curve values on day 8 of treatment relative to day 1, and the emergence of an effect on resting pulse rate and blood pressure not observed on day 1, suggested changing metoprolol kinetics upon repeated dosing. This phenomenon has been reported also by others.[465,466] Myers and Thiessen[466]

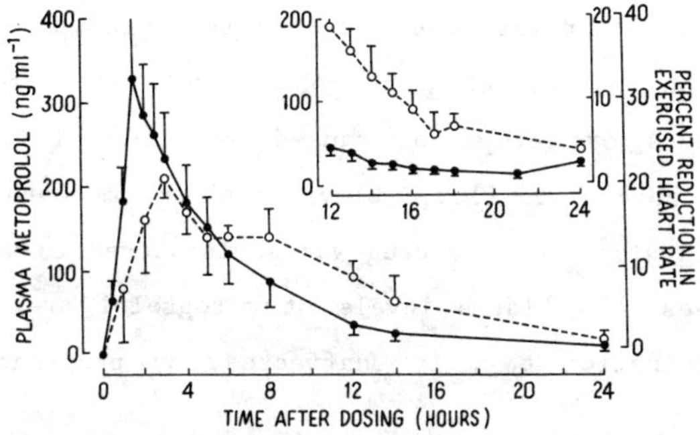

Figure 1.22 Plasma metoprolol levels and percent reduction in exercise-induced heart rate following a single morning dose of 200 mg conventional metoprolol. Equivalent values obtained during 12-24 h following a single evening dose of 200 mg conventional metoprolol are shown in the inset. Reproduced by permission from Eur. J. Clin. Pharmacol., 1979, 15, 97.

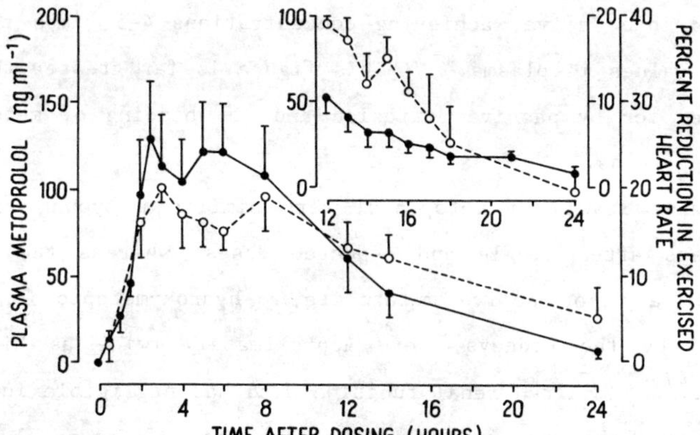

Figure 1.23 Plasma metoprolol levels and percent reduction in exercise-induced heart rate following a single morning dose of 200 mg slow-release metoprolol. Equivalent values obtained during 12-24 h following a single evening dose of 200 mg slow-release metoprolol are shown in the inset. Reproduced by permission from Eur. J. Clin. Pharmacol., 1979, 15, 97.

noted an increase in the mean metoprolol elimination $t_{0.5}$ in 14 hypertensive patients from 4.1 h after a single 100 mg dose to 5.6 h after 6 to 12 weeks of therapy. Thus pharmacokinetic data from a single metoprolol dose may be a poor predictor of steady-state kinetics.

The peak plasma concentration and area under curve of metoprolol after a 100 mg p.o. dose were significantly increased by concomitant administration of 50 mg hydralazine, while the elimination $t_{0.5}$ and the percentage of metoprolol dose excreted unchanged in urine were unaffected.[467] The observed changes probably reflect a reduction in the first-pass loss of metoprolol caused by a hydralazine-induced increase in splanchnic blood flow. Elevated plasma metoprolol levels have been observed also when the drug was administered to women using oral contraceptives.[468] Plasma levels of metoprolol are decreased, although the elimination $t_{0.5}$ is unaffected, by pretreatment with pentobarbital.[469]

Previous reports of good c.n.s. penetration by metroprolol in animals have been confirmed in man, in whom the concentration of drug in c.s.f. is approximately equal to that of the free drug in plasma.[470] Unlike oxprenolol, metoprolol appears to be actively secreted into saliva, achieving concentrations 4-5 times the corresponding values in plasma.[471] This figure is far greater than can be accounted for by passive diffusion and low binding of metoprolol to plasma proteins.

Plasma levels of metoprolol were similar in young and elderly volunteers after single and repeated doses, whereas the concentrations of a major active metabolite, α-hydroxymetoprolol, which is excreted by the kidneys, were approximately twice as high in the elderly.[472] Impaired renal function also had negligible influence on the bioavailability and elimination rate of metoprolol,[473] but affected the excretion of those metabolites that were cleared via the kidneys.[474] In these studies, employing 6 healthy male volunteers and

6 hypertensive patients with chronic renal failure, the bioavailability of a 50 mg p.o. dose of metoprolol in both groups was 55-60%, and the total body clearance was <u>ca.</u> 1 l min^{-1}. Mean elimination $t_{0.5}$ values were 4.1 and 4.6 h, respectively, in the healthy subjects and renal patients. On the other hand, a reduction in glomerular filtration rate by 70-80% caused a nearly 3-fold increase in the elimination $t_{0.5}$ of total metabolites and α-hydroxymetoprolol. The metabolites were dialysable and approximately 50% of them were removed in anephric patients during a 5 h dialysis.[475]

Hepatic cirrhosis increased the systemic availability of metoprolol to 84% as it decreased the total body clearance of the drug to 0.6 l min^{-1}, compared to 0.8 l min^{-1} in control subjects.[476] Metoprolol elimination $t_{0.5}$ was doubled in patients with impaired liver function, as shown in Figure 1.24.

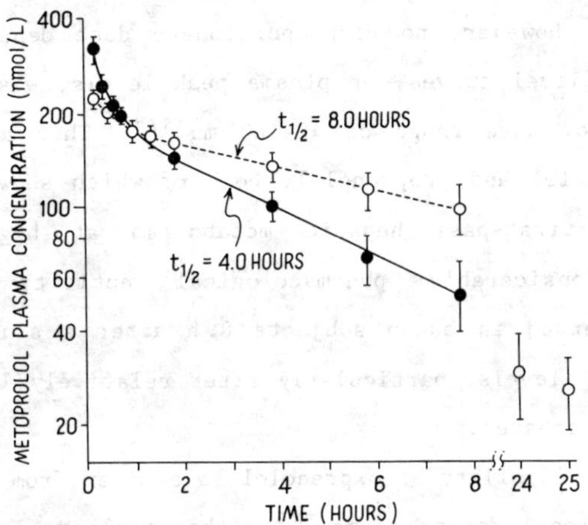

Figure 1.24   Plasma concentrations of metoprolol in patients with cirrhosis (n=10) [o] and in healthy subjects (n=6) [●] following administration of 20 mg (58.4 μmol) intravenously.   Values given are mean ± SEM.   Reproduced by permission from <u>Clin. Pharmacokin.</u>, 1981, <u>6</u>, 375.

<u>Nadolol</u>

Considerable species differences have been demonstrated in the absorption efficiency of ^{14}C-nadolol.[477]   While this agent is almost completely (88-104%) absorbed in dogs, absorption is generally not greater than 30% in other animal species, and in man. The reason for the high absorption in dogs in not known, but it throws doubt on the use of this species for pharmacokinetic or dose-response studies.

In 12 lactating women who received 80 mg nadolol once daily for a period of 5 d, milk concentrations of the drug exceeded serum levels on day 3 and continued to be 2-8 times higher than mean serum concentrations throughout the remainder of the study.[478] However, the mean $t_{0.5}$ of elimination of nadolol from milk was identical to that from serum, _ca_. 22 h. Furthermore, serum concentrations of nadolol in these lactating normotensive subjects were similar to those observed in hypertensive patients.

Oxprenolol

Oxprenolol is eliminated from the body largely by metabolism and has a short $t_{0.5}$. However, no disproportionate dose dependency of areas under plasma level curves, or plasma peak levels, was observed in man within a p.o. dose range of 40-160 mg.[479] This agent thus differs from alprenolol and propranolol, both of which show evidence of saturation of first-pass hepatic metabolism at higher p.o. doses.[480,481] Considerable pharmacological activity due to oxprenolol was observed in human subjects 8 h after a single dose, although plasma drug levels, particularly after relatively low doses, had essentially disappeared.

The systemic availability of oxprenolol is similar from sustained release and conventional dosage forms,[482] although plasma levels from the sustained release forms are lower and more prolonged, and the absorption profile of neither dosage form is significantly affected by food.

Penbutolol

This nonselective beta-adrenergic blocking agent is rapidly absorbed after p.o. doses, with little evidence of first-pass metabolism, and plasma levels peak at _ca_. 1 h.[484] After reaching the peak, plasma levels decline biexponentially with alpha and beta $t_{0.5}$ values of 2.5 and 27 h, respectively.[484] The absorption of penbutolol appears to be consistent and dose related.[485] Reliable absorption, with little evidence of first-pass clearance, is consistent with the long $t_{0.5}$ of this extensively metabolized compound.

In contrast to propranolol, there is only a poor correlation between peak penbutolol plasma levels, <u>ca</u>. 1 h postdose, and peak biological activity, <u>ca</u>. 2 h postdose.[486] Also, for an equal degree of cardiac beta-adrenergic receptor inhibition (16% at 1 and 7 h post-dose) corresponding plasma levels of penbutolol varied 1- to 6-fold. This is due to penbutolol giving rise to several active metabolites including 4-hydroxypenbutolol. This metabolite accounts for more than 50% of total metabolites in 12 h urine following p.o. administration of penbutolol.[486]

Peak serum concentrations and areas under serum curves, from a 25 mg penbutolol capsule administered with 200 ml water, were not affected by food, which merely delayed the mean peak time from 1.0 h to 2.3 h.[487] The mean $t_{0.5}$ values after the fasting and postprandial treatments were 1.6 and 2.6 h, respectively; the difference was not statistically significant.

<u>Pindolol</u>

Like many other agents in this group, pindolol is rapidly absorbed after p.o. doses, achieving peak plasma levels within 1 h.[488] Although only 40% of oral drug is eliminated unchanged in urine, only 10-15% of the dose is cleared by first-pass metabolism,[489] despite a relatively short biological $t_{0.5}$ of <u>ca</u>. 3-4 h.

The decline in plasma levels of pindolol is biphasic in man after i.v. doses, and the mean α- and β-phase $t_{0.5}$ values are 0.13 and 3 h, respectively.[490] Following single p.o. doses of 5, 10, and 20 mg pindolol, plasma levels of drug are dose proportional and bioavailability is approximately 80%. Steady-state circulating levels of pindolol can be predicted from single-dose data, and there is no evidence that pindolol induces or inhibits its own metabolism with repeated dosing.[491] A study in hypertensive Africans has shown that both the pharmacokinetics and the β-blocking effects of pindolol in that population are similar to published data in other races.[492]

The availability of orally dosed pindolol appears not to be significantly different in fasted and nonfasted normal individuals,[493] but is reduced from 86 to 52% in patients with impaired renal function.[494,495] Decreased drug availability appears to be due to reduced absorption rather than to increased first-pass metabolism.

Although approximately 35% of a dose is excreted unchanged in urine of normal subjects, the elimination $t_{0.5}$ does not change or increases only slightly[494,495] with declining renal function.[496] This appears to be due to a compensating increase in pindolol metabolism. In uraemic patients dosed with ^{14}C-pindolol, the $t_{0.5}$ of total radioactivity was 48 h, indicating impaired elimination of metabolites.

In patients with various liver diseases, a significant correlation was found between antipyrine clearance and the nonrenal clearance of pindolol.[497] Increased pindolol metabolism was observed in patients with acute hepatitis, probably due to increased liver blood flow. In contrast, metabolism of pindolol decreased in patients suffering from hepatic cirrhosis, although some patients compensated by increasing the urinary excretion of the intact drug, up to 65% of the administered dose compared with the usual 30-40% in normal individuals. In patients with severe renal impairment (creatinine clearance below 5 ml min^{-1}), a single 5 mg p.o. dose of ^{14}C-pindolol yielded plasma pindolol levels similar to those observed in healthy volunteers.[498] However, the elimination $t_{0.5}$ appeared to be longer in renal patients, leading to steady-state plasma concentrations, after dosing 5 mg three times a day for 5 d, almost twice as high as those in healthy subjects.

As with alprenolol and metoprolol, a linear relationship was observed between the β-blockade and plasma levels of pindolol in patients.[499] However, owing to considerable individual differences the authors concluded that drug plasma levels could not be used as a general guide to pharmacological effect, and hence to pindolol dosage.

Johansson et al.[500] examined the duration of action and the adequacy of once-daily administration for a series of β-blockers. The daily dose, given for at least 1 week, ranged from 10 mg for pindolol to 400 mg for alprenolol. The reduction of exercise tachycardia at 24 h after the last dose of pindolol was found to be similar to the effects obtained from β-blockers with longer $t_{0.5}$ values and those given as slow-release formulations.

Administration of a single dose of pindolol significantly reduced both the glomerular filtration rate and also the effective renal plasma flow in normal individuals, but caused no such changes in patients with renal impairment.[501]

Practolol

Practolol behaves differently to most other β-adrenergic blocking agents in that it is excreted almost entirely as unchanged drug by glomerular filtration and has a relatively long $t_{0.5}$ of 9-12 h.[502] Linear correlations have been demonstrated between pharmacological effect and the logarithm of plasma levels of this drug. However, its pharmacological $t_{0.5}$ is 4 times longer than its plasma $t_{0.5}$.[503] Whereas the circulating concentration of propranolol required to elicit a certain pharmacologic response after an i.v. dose was almost double that after a p.o. dose, there was no such disparity between p.o. and i.v. blood levels of practolol.[504] This observation is consistent with the absence of practolol metabolism in man. Practolol undergoes enterohepatic cycling, but probably not to a sufficient extent to influence circulating drug level versus time profiles.[505]

Practolol rapidly distributed into tissues after p.o., i.v., or i.p. doses to rats, mice, and dogs[506,507] and after i.v. doses to man.[508] Elimination from blood and tissues was biphasic, and $t_{0.5}$ values for the slow phase of blood elimination curves were 12 h in man and 6-8 h in the dog and rat. The very short $t_{0.5}$ in the rat reported in one study may be due to insufficient blood samples being taken.[506] At least 85% of p.o. and i.p. administered doses were excreted unchanged in the urine of the dog and rat. Unlike propranolol, the urinary excretion of practolol is independent of pH over the pH range 4.68-8.54.[509]

Propranolol

There has been intense interest and considerable literature on propranolol during the review period. Much of this has been related to propranolol's unusual absorption and metabolism characteristics.

Propranolol is extensively metabolized, with at least one of the metabolites, 4-hydroxypropranolol (HO-P), being pharmacologically active. Studies in man and experimental animals indicate that rapid hepatic clearance is responsible for the appearance of only trace amounts of unmetabolized propranolol in the blood after small p.o. doses.[510] With larger doses blood levels are linearly related to dose, suggesting saturation of the hepatic metabolizing system. Saturation of metabolism and drug binding in the liver results, not only in increased bioavailability at high doses and after chronic administration, but also in decreased systemic clearance and a longer drug $t_{0.5}$.[511,512]

The increased cardiac β-blocking activity of propranolol after p.o. dosing compared with i.v. dosing may be due to HO-P, which is produced in the liver only after enteral drug absorption.[513-516] Paterson et al.[517] have proposed that hydroxylation in the 4-position may be a secondary metabolic pathway, which occurs only if propranolol reaches the liver in high concentrations. An alternative hypothesis, put forward by Hayes and Cooper,[518] is that further metabolism of HO-P may be overloaded at high liver concentrations after p.o. dosing but not after i.v. dosing. Shand et al.[519] reported 7-fold variations in plasma propranolol levels in man after p.o. doses but only 2-fold variations after i.v. doses. Prolonged plasma $t_{0.5}$ values after p.o. doses were attributed to continued absorption. Although the matter is still in some doubt,[520] some recent studies have challenged the concept that unchanged propranolol does not appear in the systemic circulation below a minimum, threshold dose.[521] Following single 10 mg doses to healthy adults, peak plasma propranolol levels, measured using a sensitive fluorimetric assay, were 6-8 ng ml^{-1} and the elimination $t_{0.5}$ was 2.5-5.6 h, a range similar to that reported from higher doses.

Several studies in patients and in healthy subjects have demonstrated direct dose-bioavailability proportionality within p.o. propranolol dose ranges of 40-120 mg,[523] 5-40 mg, and 20-640 mg d^{-1}.[524] In these studies, the apparent distribution volume of propranolol was <u>ca</u>. 6 1 kg^{-1}, the terminal $t_{0.5}$ averaged 3-6 h, and the systemic bioavailability compared to i.v. reference doses was approximately 25%, with no indication of a threshold dose or saturable hepatic extraction from the portal circulation.

In patients with essential hypertension as well as healthy volunteers, multiple oral dosing with propranolol, 120 mg daily[523] or 80 mg twice daily[525,526] for up to 6 weeks resulted in no significant change in the bioavailability or clearance of the drug. Nevertheless, large intersubject variations in plasma propranolol concentrations are common, presumably due to differences in the extent of presystemic biotransformation.[527]

The rate of propranolol absorption is delayed somewhat by propantheline, and accelerated by metoclopramide,[528] but these changes were not significant in the small subject population studied. Reduced, but more sustained, plasma levels of propranolol are obtained from a sustained-release formulation compared to conventional dosage forms.[529] The area under the plasma curve was reduced following the sustained-release dosage form, but it is not known whether this is due to incomplete absorption across the gut wall or to greater first-pass metabolism accompanying the slower absorption. Studies in dogs have shown that p.o. doses of the hemisuccinate ester of propranolol give rise to plasma propranolol levels that are 8-fold higher than those from an equivalent dose of propranolol hydrochloride.[530] The hemisuccinate is absorbed rapidly and decomposes to form propranolol with a $t_{0.5}$ of 0.5 h *in vivo*.

Plasma levels of p.o. dosed propranolol are increased by concomitant administration of chlorpromazine[531] and furosemide.[532] While the increases due to chlorpromazine are attributed to reduced presystemic clearance, the effect of furosemide may be related to increased absorption or a reduction in extracellular fluid in the presence of the diuretic agent. In any event, the increased plasma levels of propranolol in the presence of furosemide are accompanied by simultaneous increase in β-adrenoreceptor blockade.

The release rate of propranolol from a polyvinyl chloride matrix in the dog GI tract is reduced by the presence of food.[533] This could produce additional variation in propranolol bioavailability from this type of formulation. The availability of p.o. propranolol is decreased by the presence of aluminium hydroxide, the mean peak plasma level of drug being reduced to one-half normal values,[534] whereas the absorption of both propranolol and metoprolol from conventional formulations is increased by food.[535]

A protein-lipid meal nearly doubled the peak plasma concentration and AUC of propranolol after a 1 mg kg^{-1} p.o. dose of ^{14}C-propranolol in normal volunteers, but had no effect on the urinary recovery of ^{14}C label.[536] Furthermore, food did not alter the systemic clearance of i.v. dosed propranolol, about 20-30 ml kg^{-1} min^{-1}. Similar observations were made by Walle et al.,[537] who showed a linear correlation

between the meal-induced increase in propranolol bioavailability and
the protein content in the meal, with an apparent threshold protein
content of 7.2 g, as shown in Figure 1.25. No significant food effect
was found on the plasma levels of 5 metabolites of propranolol, including the pharmacologically active HO-P. Summarizing the above
information, one can conclude that the food-induced increase in p.o.
propranolol bioavailability is not due to increased absorption or
decreased systemic clearance, but probably reflects reduced first
pass-metabolism secondary to an increase in hepatic blood flow.

The bioavailability of a 1 mg kg^{-1} p.o. dose of propranolol was
enhanced by the concomitant administration of 25, 50, or 100 mg

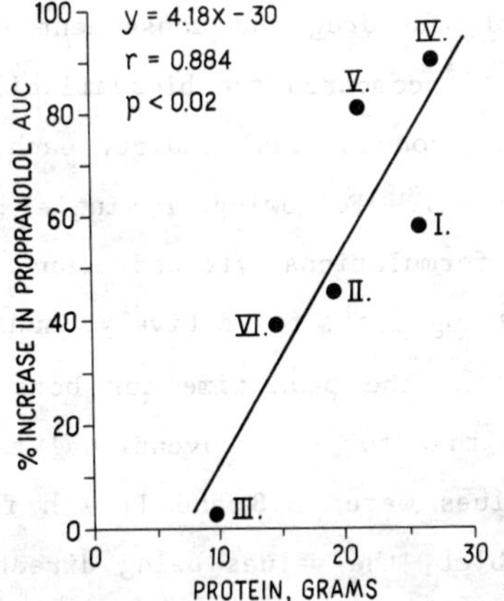

Figure 1.25 Relationship between the protein content
of the meal and the meal-induced increase in the AUC
of propranolol in six normal subjects. Reproduced by
permission from <u>Clin. Pharmacol. Ther.</u>, 1981, <u>30</u>, 790.

hydralazine.[538] Peak plasma propranolol concentrations nearly doubled
and the AUC increased by 60-80%, regardless of the dose of hydralazine. No change was observed in the total absorption or systemic
clearance of propranolol, suggesting that enhanced bioavailability was
a result of reduced first-pass clearance, probably due to either competitive inhibition of metabolism by hydralazine, or hydralazine-
induced transient increase in splanchnic blood flow. The blood level
profile of propranolol was not affected by bendrofluazide, whether the

two drugs were administered as a free combination of 80 mg and 2.5 mg film-coated tablets, respectively, or as a fixed combination in a hard gelatin capsule.[539] There was no kinetic interaction between quinidine and propranolol after simultaneous administration of 200 and 80 mg of the two drugs, respectively, every 6 h for 3 d.[540] Acute alcohol administration appeared to enhance the overall bioavailability of propranolol.[541]

In situ experiments using the rat GI tract showed that, while propranolol was not absorbed from the stomach, first-order absorption was equally effective throughout the small and large intestines.[542] Hence, sustained-release formulations of propranolol would be useful in extending the absorption of the drug and consequent duration of drug activity. McAinsh et al.[543] compared the bioavailability of two sustained-release capsules and a conventional tablet, each containing 160 mg propranolol hydrochloride. Following a single dose in 12 healthy subjects, the three formulations yielded mean peak blood concentrations of 9, 14, and 94 ng ml^{-1}, respectively, and AUC values of 175, 264, and 595 ng h ml^{-1}. The peak time for both sustained-release capsules was 5 h while that for the conventional tablet was 2 h. Mean propranolol $t_{0.5}$ values were 18.8 and 11.0 h for the two capsules and 3.6 h for the tablet, the values being directly related to respective dissolution times. Thus, the longer $t_{0.5}$ values of the sustained-release forms evidently reflected the rate of drug absorption. The decrease in propranolol bioavailability with increasing dissolution time was attributed to an increase in first-pass effect when the drug was more slowly presented to the liver. Upon repeated daily administration, a sustained-release capsule yielded much smaller peak to trough fluctuations in plasma propranolol concentrations as well as cardiac effects than the conventional tablet,[544] as shown in Figure 1.26. Thus, once-a-day administration of the sustained-release capsule would provide adequate pharmacologic effect over the dose interval without a high initial risk of toxicity.

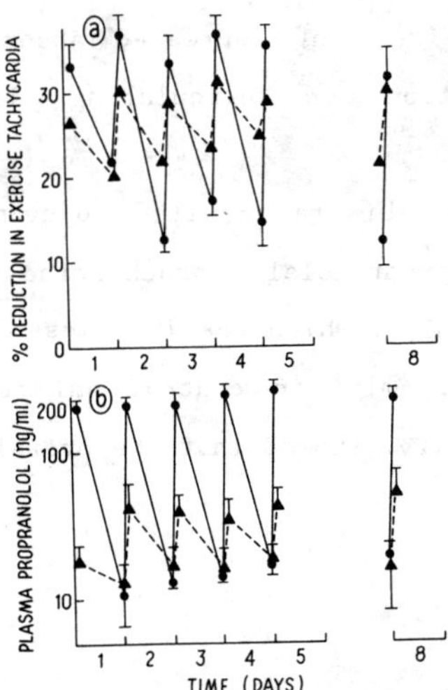

Figure 1.26   (a) The mean (± s.e. mean) percentage reductions of an exercise tachycardia and (b) the mean (± s.e. mean) plasma propranolol concentrations before and 3 h after the daily oral administration of 160 mg propranolol (●) and 160 mg S.R. propranolol (▲) to five subjects for 8 days.   Reproduced by permission from Brit. J. Clin. Pharmacol., 1980, 9, 33.

Increased circulating levels of propranolol observed in patients with Crohn's disease[545] have been interpreted as indicating increased drug absorption.[546,547]   However, it is uncertain whether the changes in circulating levels of propranolol, and also some other drugs in Crohn's disease, coeliac disease, and other pathological conditions, are due to changes in GI absorption, reduction in first-pass metabolism, altered drug distribution, or a combination of these. While increased absorption may be partially responsible for the increased levels in Crohn's disease, this is unlikely in patients with rheumatoid arthritis, where the main contributing factor appears to be a marked increase in plasma α_1-acid glycoprotein.[548]   Increased circulating levels of this acute phase protein, which binds cationic drugs, may cause increased binding of propranolol resulting in higher levels of total circulating drug in plasma.   Recent studies in rats with adjuvant induced arthritis, which received both p.o. and i.v. propran-

olol, have confirmed the dual effect of increased absorption and
reduced extravascular distribution on circulating levels of
propranolol.[549,550]

These authors showed that in rats with adjuvant-induced
arthritis, a 2 mg p.o. dose of propranolol hydrochloride yielded a
mean peak plasma level of 855 ng ml^{-1}, which was 10 times higher than
the peak concentration of 80.2 ng ml^{-1} in control animals (Figure
1.27).[549] Additional doses given i.v. showed that the overall distri-

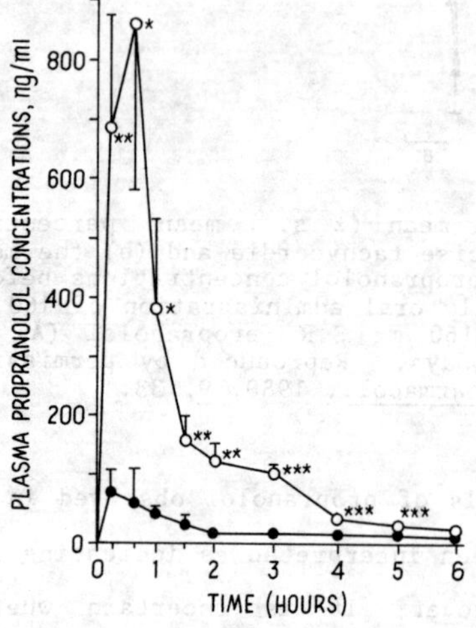

Figure 1.27   Mean plasma propranolol concentration (±
S.E.M.) in normal rats (●) and in rats with adjuvant-
induced arthritis (o) after a 2 mg oral dose. *** p <
0.001; **p < 0.01; *p < 0.05.   Reproduced by permission from Biopharm. Drug Dispos., 1981, 2, 291.

bution volume of propranolol in arthritic animals was approximately
one-half that in controls, thus indicating a 5-fold increase in the
p.o. bioavailability of unchanged propranolol in arthritic rats, since
the elimination $t_{0.5}$ values in control and arthritic rats were
similar. The decrease in the apparent volume of distribution of propranolol in arthritic rats could be related to an increase in drug
protein binding whereas the enhanced systemic bioavailability was
explained in terms of a decline in first-pass hepatic clearance in
these animals. Increases in propranolol binding to plasma proteins,

probably due to elevated α_1-acid glycoprotein levels, were observed following myocardial infarction.[551]

Repeated administration of propranolol, 40 mg 3 times a day for 3 d, reduced the mean antipyrine clearance in 13 normal subjects from 41.3 ml min^{-1} to 35.0 ml min^{-1}, suggesting that propranolol may be a microsomal enzyme inhibitor.[552] In another study the bioavailability of p.o. dosed propranolol increased after repeated administration to man because of a decreased hepatic extraction ratio.[553] The mean bioavailability of unchanged drug increased from 22% on the first day, to 34% on the seventh day of repeated dosing. Although the drug elimination $t_{0.5}$ also increased somewhat with repeated dosing, the difference between initial and steady-state values was not significant.

In patients receiving chronic propranolol therapy, steady-state peak plasma levels are linearly related to doses between 160 and 960 mg d^{-1} (divided doses), but not at doses below that range.[554] The individual variation of propranolol plasma levels was 3-fold at doses of 40 mg d^{-1}, this value decreasing to 1.3-fold at doses exceeding 600 mg d^{-1}. However, other workers have reported somewhat larger variation in circulating levels of both free and total propranolol after oral doses.[555]

Propranolol penetrates into the c.s.f. and may act directly on the central nervous system. Taylor et al.[556] reported that the c.s.f. concentrations of propranolol and pindolol were proportional to plasma concentrations of unbound drug, while the c.s.f. concentration of the poorly lipid-soluble drug atenolol was independent of its plasma concentration.

The disposition of propranolol before, during, and immediately after cardiopulmonary bypass (CPB) was examined in patients who had been on long-term p.o. propranolol therapy, some of whom received an additional i.v. dose approximately 100 min before CPB began.[557] With the onset of CPB, plasma propranolol levels decreased abruptly by <u>ca</u>. 50%, probably caused by haemodilution due to the added volume of pump prime, and also by a decrease in drug binding to plasma proteins. Wood et al.[558] reported that following administration of heparin and establishment of CPB, the free fraction of plasma propranolol doubled from 6.6 to 13.5%, apparently because of an increase in the concentration of free fatty acid (from 649 to 1967 μmol l^{-1}) which displaced propranolol from its protein binding sites. Plasma propranolol levels declined slowly and insignificantly during CPB.[557] Immediately after CPB ended, plasma propranolol levels increased by as much as 57%, and continued to rise slowly during the 4 h postoperative period. The cause of this phenomenon is unknown although the authors suggested redistribution of propranolol from tissues, particularly the lungs, to plasma as a possible explanation.

Experiments in a dog showed that heparin in doses needed to maintain the patency of indwelling catheters (130 U over 500 min) had no effect on either plasma protein binding or disposition of propranolol.[559] On the other hand, cigarette smoking tended to increase propranolol clearance and reduce its serum levels.[560]

The role of the metabolite HO-P in the cardiovascular effects of propranolol has created considerable interest. Walle et al.[561] first detected measurable levels of the active metabolite HO-P in plasma after single 4 mg i.v. doses of propranolol, the mean AUC of the metabolite being 12% that of the parent drug. Much higher plasma concentrations of HO-P were found after p.o. doses, indicating the contribution of presystemic metabolism to its formation. The peak HO-P:propranolol plasma level ratio decreased with increasing doses of propranolol, from an average of 1.07 at 40 mg daily to only 0.09 at 640 mg daily. Therefore, it appears that the pathway of HO-P formation is saturated at elevated doses.

The major metabolites of propranolol found in the urine are naphthoxylactic acid (NLA) and the conjugates of propranolol and HO-P. After single p.o. doses of propranolol in normal subjects, the plasma NLA:propranolol concentration ratio varied from 6 to 25 while the

HO-P:propranolol ratio was approximately unity at 0.5 h but declined rapidly with time after dose.[562] Increasing the propranolol p.o. dose from 20 to 320 mg reduced the mean intrinsic plasma clearance from 425 to 200 l h^{-1}, accompanied by a decreased HO-P recovery and an increased NLA recovery in the urine. It was suggested that ring hydrolysis of propranolol represents a high-affinity low-capacity enzyme pathway whereas N-dealkylation represents a low-affinity high-capacity enzymatic pathway. Thus increasing propranolol concentration in the liver after progressively larger doses would saturate ring hydroxylation and enhance conjugation and N-dealkylation to form NLA.

Metabolic clearance of propranolol is not restricted to circulating free drug. Binding of drug to plasma proteins accelerates elimination by providing a carrier system from tissues to the site of elimination. Drug $t_{0.5}$ in plasma is actually a function of two independent variables: clearance, which is independent of free-drug concentration, and the distribution volume, which is free-drug dependent. As a consequence, differences in drug $t_{0.5}$ values may not necessarily be reflected in steady-state drug concentrations.[563,564] Hepatic extraction of propranolol is influenced by the combined effects of saturable metabolism and high-affinity protein binding,[565,566] and is sensitive to hepatic blood flow rate.[567,568] Rapid hepatic clearance of propranolol has also been demonstrated after infusion of drug into the portal vein of the rat[569,570] and the dog.[571]

In a study using patients with fatty liver, hepatitis, or cirrhosis, plasma clearance of propranolol was significantly related to liver enzyme activity as represented by antipyrine clearance and hepatic cytochrome P-450 content.[572] Propranolol clearance was also affected by liver blood flow, as shown in Figure 1.28.

No statistically significant difference was found in plasma propranolol concentrations in the hyperthyroid or euthyroid state, the plasma clearance was <u>ca</u>. 50 ml min^{-1} kg^{-1} in both cases.[573] Feely

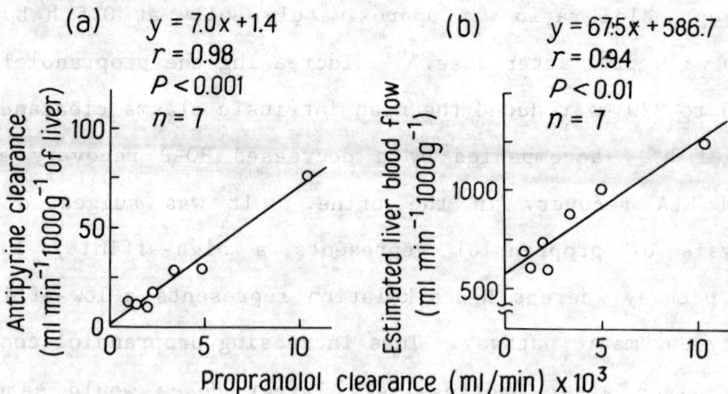

Figure 1.28   Relationship of propranolol clearance to (a) antipyrine clearance and (b) estimated liver flow. Reproduced by permission from <u>Brit. J. Clin. Pharmacol.</u>, 1980, <u>9</u>, 399.

et al.[574] studied the influence of surgery on plasma propranolol levels in patients undergoing thyroidectomy. Compared with preoperative levels, there was a 2- to 3-fold rise in total and free propranolol concentrations 24 h after surgery, suggesting decreased hepatic clearance of drug due to reduced hepatic drug-metabolizing enzyme activity. The degree of plasma protein binding of propranolol also increased to <u>ca</u>. 90% 24 h after surgery compared to 85% before surgery.

Previous reports that the blood:plasma propranolol concentration ratio is less than unity have been disputed by Sawchuk et al.[575] who obtained a mean ratio of 1.33 ± 0.28 (SD) in 29 patients. These data suggest a selective, but variable uptake of propranolol by red cells in most patients. Various problems associated with interpretations of propranolol plasma levels have been discussed by Cotham and Shand.[576]

Comparison of the effects of propranolol, practolol, and metoprolol on exercise-induced tachycardia showed different plasma level:response ratios. A 30% reduction in tachycardia was achieved by plasma levels of 50-60 ng ml^{-1} for propranolol, 1050-1100 ng ml^{-1} practolol, and 140-150 ng ml^{-1} for metoprolol.[577] Reduction of 70-80% in tachycardia was achieved with plasma propranolol levels > 100 ng ml^{-1}.[578] Although reduction in blood pressure is also more pronounced with increasing propranolol doses, correlations between mean decreases in blood pressure and either the mean dose or plasma levels of propranolol are poor.[579] Considerable interindividual variation was observed in circulating propranolol levels, while other studies have reported wide variations in both interindividual and intraindividual values.[580] Propranolol therapy is further complicated by individual differences in the affinity of propranolol to the receptor and its binding to plasma proteins.[581] In 23 hypertensive male patients receiving 40-320 mg of propranolol daily, there was a 20-fold variation in steady-state propranolol plasma levels.[582] Hypotensive response to propranolol appears to be biphasic, as patients with high sympathetic activity and high plasma renin activity exhibited substantial falls in blood pressure at propranolol levels of less than 30 ng ml^{-1}.

Observations that fast metabolizers of propranolol are more sensitive to the drug than slow metabolizers have been rationalized by Perrier and Gibaldi[583] from a pharmacokinetic viewpoint. By assuming that the site of action for propranolol resides in the tissue compartment of a two-compartment model, changes in drug sensitivity in fast and slow metabolizers could be predicted from changing relative drug levels in this compartment with varying elimination rates.[584] Different reactions of the two patient populations were thus explained without the need to postulate different intrinsic sensitivities to propranolol.

Intensity of β-blockade in man is linearly related to plasma concentrations of unchanged propranolol.[585] However, the distribution of the degree of β-blockade in patients is bimodal, and is related to the ability of the patient to form the active metabolite. Although β-blockade is greater after single p.o. doses of propranolol than after the i.v. doses, no difference is observed after multiple doses.[586] This may be due to an enzyme saturation effect after p.o. doses, enhanced metabolism of HO-P, an alternative metabolic pathway, or decreased metabolism resulting from elevation of plasma growth hormone.[587,588]

Several factors have been shown to affect the elimination of propranolol. Propranolol is effectively cleared by the liver and hepatic extraction amounts to 69-92% during one circulation after i.v. doses to dogs.[589] However, release of unchanged drug from the liver subsequent to hepatic extraction indicates the possibility of either saturation of metabolism or rapid redistribution of unchanged drug from liver when drug concentrations in blood are decreased.

Although the plasma $t_{0.5}$ of propranolol was essentially unchanged in renal failure, first-pass hepatic clearance was reduced, resulting in elevated plasma drug levels.[590] Propranolol clearance was also reduced in chronic liver disease,[591] and in aged patients.[592] Practolol plasma levels were also increased in aged patients, but to a lesser extent than propranolol.

Changes in the disposition of propranolol, and also of other drugs, in liver disease have been described in terms of "intact hepatocyte theory," which suggests that reduced liver function may be caused by a reduction in the number of normal functional cells and the development of portosystemic vascular shunts.[593] Reduced hepatic clearance of propranolol, and greater systemic availability of the drug after p.o. doses, have been reported for patients with terminal uraemia.[594] Typical blood levels of propranolol observed in five healthy volunteers, six patients on dialysis, and five patients not on dialysis, are summarized in Figure 1.29. Analysis of the data indicated that the fraction of dose available to the circulation was significantly increased to 62% in uraemia compared with 19% in normal controls. The elimination $t_{0.5}$ was also increased somewhat in uraemic patients, although the mechanism of decreased hepatic clearance of propranolol in uraemia is unknown.

Changes in hepatic clearance with age appear to occur more in smokers than in nonsmokers.[595] In the latter group, although liver

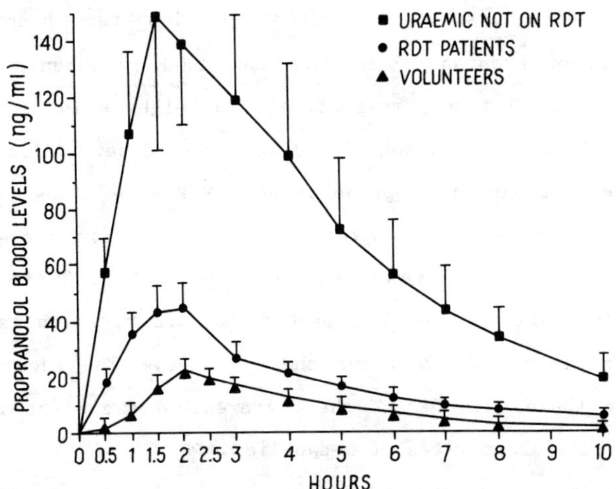

Figure 1.29   Average blood levels of propranolol in healthy volunteers (▲), uraemic patients not on regular dialysis (■), and patients on regular dialysis treatment (●) after a single p.o. dose of 40 mg propranolol.   Bars indicate 1 SEM.   Reproduced by permission from Clin. Pharmacokin., 1976, 1, 373.

blood flow decreases with age, intrinsic total clearance of propranolol approaches a constant value.   Propranolol kinetics are markedly altered in conditions of hypothermia.[596]   In hypothermic dogs, the apparent distribution volume of propranolol was reduced from a normal value of 6.8 l kg^{-1} to 2.1 l kg^{-1}, and the total clearance was reduced from 64 to 32 ml kg^{-1} min^{-1}.   These changes give plasma levels significantly higher than those predicted from normothermic conditions. Plasma levels of propranolol are increased in cirrhosis due to increased systemic availability, decreased systemic clearance, and an increased free drug fraction in plasma.[597]   As a consequence of both clearance and distribution changes, the plasma $t_{0.5}$ of propranolol is increased from a normal value of 4 h to 11 h in cirrhosis.   In contrast to the effect of cirrhosis, the free fraction of propranolol in plasma is not influenced by changes in thyroid function.[598]

Significant accumulation of the acid metabolites of propranolol occurred in patients with severe renal impairment.   These compounds are eliminated only by renal mechanisms and are not efficiently removed by haemodialysis. In patients on long-term haemodialysis, plasma levels of propranolol glucuronide, OH-P glucuronide, and NLA were 18, 20, and 29 times, respectively, as high as in patients with normal renal function, and correlated well with dose.[599] In contrast, plasma concentrations of propranolol and OH-P were almost unaffected by severe renal disease. Propranolol $t_{0.5}$ values in these patients were similar to those in normal subjects, ca. 3-5 h. The plasma $t_{0.5}$ of pharmacologically active l-propanolol is 3.2 h, which is signifi-cantly longer than 2.0-2.4 h for the d-isomer. The racemate has a $t_{0.5}$ between these values, and the difference between the isomers is due to their different rates of metabolism.[600]

Propranolol is excreted in breast milk, although the milk:plasma concentration ratio is less than would be expected from pH considera-tions.[601] Propranolol readily crosses the human placenta, giving rise to cord drug levels similar to maternal levels at parturition.[602] After birth, however, redistribution of the drug may occur giving rise to higher and possibly more toxic foetal blood levels.

Sotalol

Sotalol is similar to atenolol and pindolol in that it is meta-bolized to only a negligible extent, does not undergo first-pass metabolism, and is cleared predominantly by renal excretion as unchanged drug. Sotalol is also bound to only a negligible extent by plasma proteins. The p.o. availability of sotalol is superior to that of atenolol and pindolol, and is also unaffected by co-administered hydrochlorothiazide.[603] Absorption of sotalol is decreased by food however, particularly by milk, and interactions with Ca^{2+} may be responsible.[604]

The absorption of sotalol, like that of many other compounds, is unaffected by age. In a typical study, the drug was absorbed with equal efficiency from 80 or 160 mg p.o. doses to a group of elderly hypertensive patients (60-74 yr) and a group of healthy young subjects (19-35 yr).[605]

Despite its relatively uncomplicated pharmacokinetics, the elimination $t_{0.5}$ of sotalol varies widely with reported values in normal individuals ranging from 5 h to 17 h.[603,606-609] The elimination $t_{0.5}$ of sotalol is not affected by overdose of 2.4 and 8.0 g.[610] Whereas the pharmacological action of a drug generally disappears linearly following zero-order kinetics as the drug concentration in plasma decreases in first-order fashion, the effect of sotalol on the QT-interval in overdose patients appears to follow an exponential rather than a linear type decline.

As it is cleared from the body almost entirely by renal excretion sotalol elimination is markedly dependent on renal function. Typically a $t_{0.5}$ of 42 h has been reported in end-stage renal failure.[606] In this study haemodialysis reduced the mean plasma $t_{0.5}$ of sotalol to 7 h. Berglund et al.[611] also observed significant correlations between sotalol hybrid elimination rate constant (β) and glomerular filtration rate (GFR), as well as sotalol plasma clearance and GFR in hypertensive patients with moderate to severe impairment of renal function. The data projected a serum $t_{0.5}$ of 69 h and plasma clearance of 19.2 ml min^{-1} in anuric patients.

Sotalol elimination is also significantly impaired in the elderly, with renal clearance and plasma clearance values of 1.9 and 3.3 ml min^{-1} kg^{-1}, respectively, compared with 4.1 and 5.9 ml min^{-1} kg^{-1} in the young subjects.[605] The mean terminal $t_{0.5}$ increased from 7.1 to 11.4 h while the apparent distribution volume decreased from 3.6 to 2.2 l kg^{-1} with age. The altered elimination rate was apparently due to age-related diminution in renal function. A direct relationship was shown between sotalol renal clearance and creatinine clearance which averaged 118 ml min^{-1} in young subjects and 67.4 ml min^{-1} in elderly, hypertensive patients. The degree of β-blockade, especially as determined by the reduction in exercise heart rate, correlated well with log plasma drug concentration while the antihypertensive effect did not.[611]

Sulfinalol

After a single 0.5 mg kg^{-1} i.v. dose of sulfinalol hydrochloride
in the dog, plasma drug levels declined biexponentially, with mean α
and β phase $t_{0.5}$ values of 1.3 min and 1.3 h, respectively.[612] The
mean plasma clearance was 2.3 1 h^{-1} kg^{-1}, while the overall distribution volume averaged 3.9 1 kg^{-1}. Approximately 7.5% of the dose was
excreted as free sulfinalol in the urine, with a mean renal clearance
of 0.16 1 h^{-1} kg^{-1} which is similar to the normal glomerular filtration rate in the dog.   Although there was no correlation between
plasma sulfinalol levels and antihypertensive effect, the latter
appeared to correlate positively with the amount of sulfinalol in the
peripheral compartment calculated by equation 1.13

$$\text{Amount} = \frac{(k_{12})(\text{Dose})}{(\alpha - \beta)} \ (e^{-\beta t} - e^{-\alpha t}) \qquad (1.13)$$

where k_{12} is the first-order rate constant governing drug transfer
from central to peripheral compartment and α and β are hybrid rate
constants.

Timolol

Timolol appears to obey simple first-order kinetics in the body,
is only 10% bound to plasma protein and, like propranolol, is cleared
predominantly by hepatic metabolism.[613] However, unlike propranolol,
timolol does not appear to undergo extensive first-pass metabolism
after p.o. dosing.[614] Comparisons of plasma profiles following i.v.
and p.o. doses indicate that systemic availability of p.o. doses is
75% and that plasma levels are dose-proportional. After i.v. administration, the elimination $t_{0.5}$ and plasma clearance of timolol in
healthy subjects averaged 3.3-4.1 h and 0.45-0.52 1 h^{-1} kg^{-1}, respectively, and were independent of dose within the 1.25-5 mg range.[615]
The disposition kinetics were unaltered in patients with acute
myocardial infarction.

Following a single 20 mg p.o. dose of timolol maleate, the drug was rapidly absorbed, achieving a mean peak plasma concentration of 82.6 ng ml^{-1} at 1.55 h postdose.[616] Approximately 15% of the dose was recovered intact in 0-24 h urine. Timolol was absorbed systemically after administering a 0.8 mg dose of timolol maleate to the eyes as an ophthalmic solution.[617] Although plasma drug concentrations were below or near the detection limit of 1-2 ng ml^{-1}, measurable levels of timolol were found in the urine.

Using equation 1.14, El-Rashidy[618] estimated the systemic bio-availability, F, of a p.o. dose of timolol (<u>ca</u>. 0.2 mg kg^{-1}) to be about 0.6 in normal volunteers and in uraemic patients.

$$F = \frac{F_{abs} \cdot Q}{Q + CL_{int} (1 - F_k)} \qquad (1.14)$$

In equation 1.14, F_{abs} is the fraction of dose absorbed, Q is the hepatic blood flow rate, CL_{int} is the intrinsic clearance, and F_k is the fraction of dose eliminated via extrahepatic routes.

In control subjects and in patients with coronary disease wide interindividual variation in steady-state plasma timolol levels (2.6- to 13.8-fold) was observed for p.o. timolol doses between 5 and 25 mg thrice daily.[619] The degree of β-blockade, as determined by the inhibition of exercise-induced tachycardia, showed a weak correlation with plasma timolol levels (r = 0.45, p < 0.05), but a strong correlation with timolol dose (y = 3.87x + 6.50, r=0.98, p < 0.001). This observation could indicate the formation of pharmacologically active timolol metabolites.

Ishizaki and Tawara[620] have presented evidence that the clearance of timolol is reduced, and the $t_{0.5}$ significantly prolonged, after chronic dosing, but this has not been supported by other studies. There is no significant impairment in elimination of timolol in patients with chronic mild or severe renal insufficiency.[621] However, there is little information available on the nature of timolol metabolites that may contribute to the pharmacological activity attributed to timolol.

Diuretics

Diuretic agents play an important role in the reduction of edoema and they effectively reduce mild hypertension when taken alone or with other agents. The thiazides represent the largest single group of diuretic agents and they will be considered first in this section.

Thiazide Diuretics

Chlorothiazide

Early reports on chlorothiazide pharmacokinetics were hindered by inadequate assay procedures. Following reports from the US Food and Drug Administration[622,623] that individual variation in chloro-thiazide bioavailability may be due to interference by urine consti-tuents in colorimetric analysis, a comparison was made of a colori-metric procedure and a specific liquid chromatographic assay for chlorothiazide in dogs.[624] Although there was apparently a linear relationship between the results obtained from the two methods, only one-third of the paired assays agreed within 10%. The authors con-cluded that interference can cause appreciable errors in bioavail-ability estimates using the colorimetric procedure. Severe bioavail-ability problems with chlorothiazide were demonstrated in a subsequent study in which 250 and 500 mg doses of six products were administered to humans.[625] Mean 24 h urinary recovery from three different 250 mg tablets was 39, 37, and 49 mg, while recovery from three different 500 mg tablets was 4, 54, and 66 mg.

Application of a specific and sensitive HPLC assay method for chlorothiazide in plasma and urine showed that both the plasma levels and urinary excretion rate of chlorothiazide peaked at 1-2 h following a 500 mg p.o. dose, and subsequently declined irregularly.[626] Typical plasma profiles and urinary excretion rates are shown in Figure 1.30.

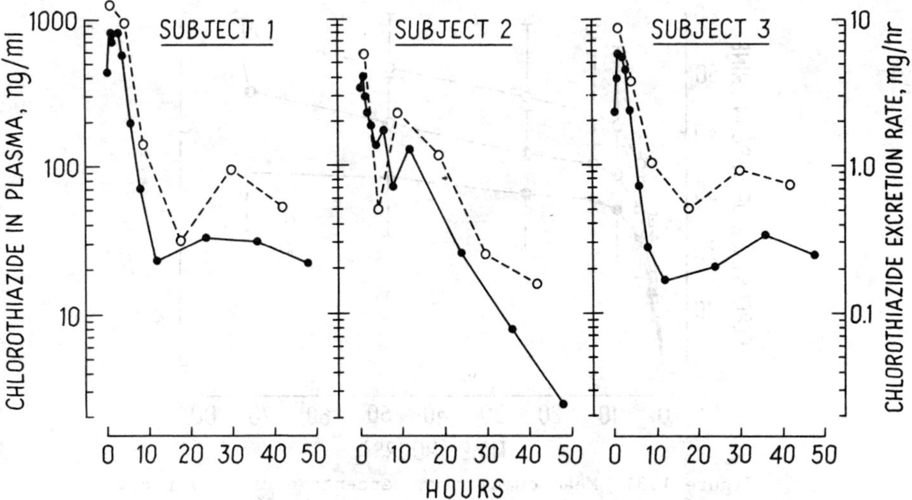

Figure 1.30   Plasma levels (●) and urinary excretion rates (o) for chlorothiazide in three subjects following a single 500-mg oral dose.   Reproduced by permission from J. Pharm. Sci., 1981, 70, 291.

The absorption of p.o. administered chlorothiazide is dose-dependent and saturable.[627] In 8 healthy male subjects who received 50, 100, and 250 mg solution doses of chlorothiazide, the recovery of intact drug in 72 h urine averaged 56.4, 47.0, and 33.3% of the dose, respectively (Figure 1.31).   Cumulative urinary excretion data are considered adequate as a bioavailability index for thiazide diuretics due to the erratic nature of circulating levels of these compounds after p.o. doses.[628]

In a study comparing various chlorothiazide tablet and solution doses, both the plasma[629] and urine[630] data indicated dose-related but not dose-proportional absorption. The area under the plasma curve and also 72 h urinary excretion following a 500 mg solution dose were approximately twice those obtained from a 125 mg dose. However, the observed diuresis and electrolyte excretion were consistent with the extent of chlorothiazide elimination in urine.

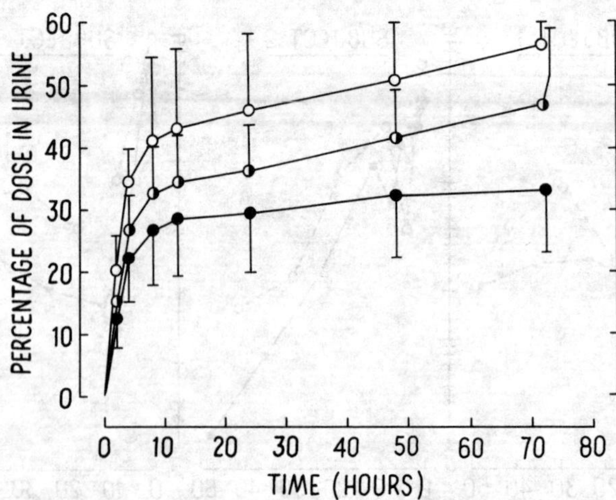

Figure 1.31 Mean cumulative percentage urinary recovery of chlorothiazide following single 50 mg (o), 100
mg (◑), and 250 mg (●) oral solution doses to healthy
male volunteers. Error bars indicate 1 standard deviation. Reproduced by permission from Biopharm. Drug
Dispos., 1982, 3, 89.

Various commercial tablets of 250 and 500 mg chlorothiazide were
shown to be bioequivalent, but again gave rise to incomplete and
saturable absorption of chlorothiazide.[631,632] The mean urinary
excretion during 72 h postdose ranged from 42 to 54 mg. Based on the
results of these studies, it was established that a dissolution speci-
fication of not less than 75% dissolved in 60 min in pH 7.4 phosphate
buffer, and a stirring rate of 75 rpm using the USP XX paddle method,
was consistent with in vivo absorption characteristics of chlorothiazide.

Welling and Barbhaiya[633] studied the influence of food and fluid
volume on chlorothiazide bioavailability. Nine healthy subjects received a 2 x 250 mg tablet dose with 20 or 250 ml of water on an empty
stomach and also with 250 ml of water immediately after a standard
breakfast. The plasma AUC, C_{max}, and 0-48 h urinary recovery showed
that chlorothiazide absorption was not influenced by the accompanying
fluid volume when taken in the fasting state, but was doubled when

taken with a meal. The increased and also delayed absorption in the presence of food is consistent with delayed stomach emptying and saturable or dissolution rate-controlled absorption.

The results of these studies culminated in a recommendation that both chlorothiazide and hydrochlorothiazide will exhibit similar potency in the 25-100 mg dosage range, and that greater therapeutic response to chlorothiazide is unlikely to be achieved by increasing the dose size from 250 to 500 mg.[634] In the same article the FDA encouraged dose response studies for chlorothiazide doses in the 50 to 250 mg range.

No statistically significant difference was found in the bio-availability of chlorothiazide from 500 mg doses of various tablets and an aqueous solution in the dog.[635] Mean urinary recovery of unchanged drug was between 15.7 and 22.0% of the dose.

The disposition of i.v. administered ^{14}C-chlorothiazde has been described in the rhesus monkey.[636] Apparent $t_{0.5}$ values ranged from 19 to 25 min, but increased to <u>ca</u>. 1 h when drug was given concurrently with probenecid. Although substantial interindividual differences existed among the three monkeys used in the study, plasma and renal clearances at low doses (6-8 mg kg^{-1}) were 20 to 50% higher than those observed after higher doses (up to 30 mg kg^{-1}), suggesting saturable elimination. Chlorothiazide was bound to monkey plasma proteins in a dose-dependent manner, the percent bound decreasing from 95.7% at a drug concentration of 3 μg ml^{-1} to 87.9% at 300 μg ml^{-1}.

<u>Hydrochlorothiazide</u>

Application of a specific and sensitive HPLC assay method in plasma and urine showed that hydrochlorothiazide is similar to chlorothiazide in that its plasma profiles are similar to its urinary excretion rates. However, it differs from chlorothiazide in that, after reaching peak values at 2-3 h following a 500 mg p.o. dose, plasma levels and urinary excretion rates decline in a regular, biphasic fashion, the slower elimination phase commencing at <u>ca</u>. 12 h post-dose.[626] Typical plasma profiles and urinary excretion rates in 3 subjects are shown in Figure 1.32. In another study, plasma levels of hydrochlorothiazide following single 50 mg p.o. doses were described in terms of a triexponential function and the mean $t_{0.5}$ values of the 3 components were 1.0, 2.2, and 9.0 h.[637] Changing the accom-

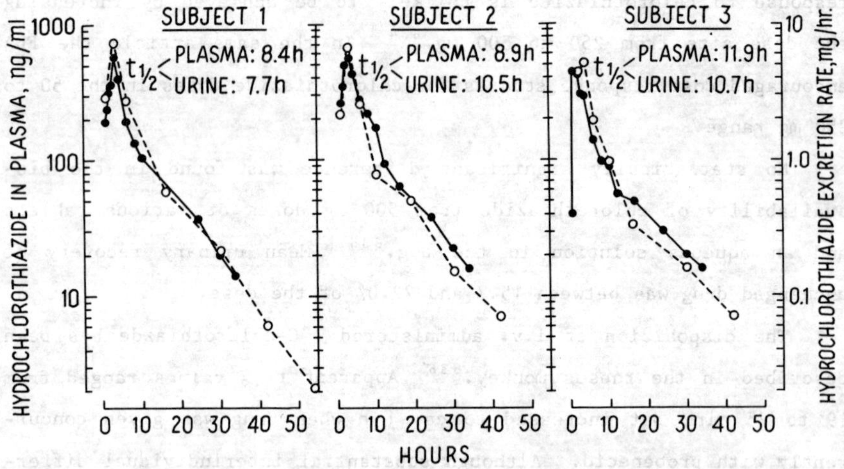

Figure 1.32 Plasma levels (●) and urinary excretion rates (o) for hydrochlorothiazide in three subjects following a single 50 mg oral dose. Reproduced by permission from <u>J. Pharm. Sci</u>., 1981, <u>70</u>, 291.

panying fluid volume had no effect on hydrochlorothiazide absorption but, unlike chlorothiazide, plasma levels of hydrochlorothiazide were significantly reduced by concomitant food intake. Mean urinary recovery of unchanged drug was 70.5% in fasted subjects, and 73.5% and 75.0% in fasted subjects administered with 20 and 250 ml of water, respectively. Another study reported increased hydrochlorothiazide availability with food, but the different results obtained in the two studies may have been due to procedural differences.[637,638]

The systemic availability of p.o. hydrochlorothiazide, unlike that of chlorothiazide, is dose proportional.[639] After p.o. doses of 12.5, 25, 50, and 75 mg hydrochlorothiazide, average peak plasma levels were 70, 142, 260, and 376 ng ml^{-1} and elimination $t_{0.5}$ values and plasma clearances were dose independent. Elimination of drug in this study was reported to be biphasic and the terminal $t_{0.5}$ varied between 5.6 and 14.8 h.

Considerable variation has been demonstrated in the bioavailability of commercial hydrochlorothiazide products.[640] Products from 10 out of 39 suppliers failed to meet USP dissolution requirements. Correlations between dissolution tests and bioavailability were generally poor. However, poor availability correlations between different hydrochlorothiazide products is not always the case. After a 50 mg tablet dose of two commercial products, similar plasma profiles were obtained, with peak levels of <u>ca</u>. 300 ng ml^{-1} occurring at 2.1-2.5 h, and biphasic elimination with a terminal $t_{0.5}$ of 9-10 h.[641] The bioequivalence of the two products was further established by the similarity between their respective AUC, mean residence time (MRT), and variance of residence time (VRT) values, as well as cumulative urinary excretion of intact drug. The MRT and VRT values, which are respectively, the first and second moments of the plasma drug profile, are defined by equations 1.15 and 1.16.

$$MRT = \int_0^\infty t \cdot C \cdot dt / AUC \tag{1.15}$$

$$VRT = \int_0^\infty (t - MRT)^2 \cdot C \cdot dt / AUC \tag{1.16}$$

In the equations, C is the plasma drug concentration at time t after dosing. The MRT and VRT are pharmacokinetic model independent, and reflect not only the extent of absorption but also the rate of transit of drug molecules through the body.

Administration of a 100 mg p.o. dose of hydrochlorothiazide yielded AUC and C_{max} values which <u>ca</u>. twofold greater than those obtained from a 50 mg dose, while T_{max} did not differ significantly between the two doses.[642] The percentage of dose excreted unchanged in urine and renal clearance were also similar for the 50 and 100 mg doses, 54-63% and 315-355 ml min^{-1}, respectively. In contrast, the pharmacologic effect of hydrochlorothiazide was not dose-proportional, with no major differences in diuretic or natriuretic response to the two doses. In this study using 10 healthy subjects, the pharmacokinetics and the pharmacologic effect of hydrochlorothiazide were not significantly influenced by concurrent administration of indomethacin.

The absorption of p.o. dosed hydrochlorothiazide is delayed by propantheline.[643] Delayed absorption due to propantheline indicates minimal drug absorption from the stomach. The haemodynamic effects associated with metoprolol therapy have no apparent influence on the rate or extent of hydrochlorothiazide absorption when these compounds are administered together,[644] but absorption of hydrochlorothiazide is reduced to one-half normal values after intestinal shunt surgery.[645] Following a single 75 mg dose to these patients, urinary recovery of unchanged hydrochlorothiazide was 31% of the dose, compared with 65% in normal controls. Renal clearance of hydrochlorothiazide in the patients was similar to that in normal subjects.

Hydrochlorothiazide accumulates in red cells to a lesser degree than chlorthalidone. In healthy individuals receiving p.o. ^{14}C-hydrochlorothiazide, the ratio of ^{14}C between red cells and plasma was 3.5.[646]

Other Thiazide Diuretics

Only a limited number of studies have examined the pharmacokinetics of other thiazide diuretics. Following single 100 mg p.o. doses to healthy volunteers peak plasma levels of 0.3 µg ml^{-1} hydroflumethiazide were obtained at 2 h, and 47 ± 20 (SD)% of the administered dose was recovered in 24 h urine.[647] Similar urinary recovery of hydroflumethiazide was obtained in cardiac patients.[648] The drug appears to have a prolonged distribution phase of 2 h in plasma and a β-phase $t_{0.5}$ ranging from 12.4 to 26.9 h in healthy subjects, and 6.3 to 13.8 h in patients. Small quantities of the metabolite 2,4-

disulphamyl-5-trifluoromethylaniline (DTA) were recovered in urine, and the metabolite has a longer plasma $t_{0.5}$ than the parent drug. Following repeated daily doses of 100 mg hydroflumethiazide, DTA accumulates to a greater extent than the parent drug, and the accumulation factor R for DTA, calculated from equation 1.17:

$$R = \frac{E_{dose\ 7}}{E_{dose\ 1}} \qquad\qquad (1.17)$$

where E is the urinary excretion rate in the 12-24 h period after doses, was 2.28 compared with 1.15 for parent drug.[649] Evidence has been presented that the absorption of hydroflumethiazide from p.o. tablets is zero-order, rather than first-order in nature.[650] The use of three criteria, correlation coefficients, standard deviations of parameter estimates, and visual fitting, showed that a model incorporating zero-order absorption is consistent with a saturable dissolution step in the limited volume of GI fluids. Following i.v. infusion of hydroflumethiazide, levels in plasma declined triexponentially, with average γ, α, and β $t_{0.5}$ values of 0.26, 0.85, and 5.2 h, respectively.[651] Slow diffusion of hydroflumethiazide into red cells is suggested, as plasma levels exceeded those in red blood cells after infusion. Longer elimination $t_{0.5}$ values of hydroflumethiazide after high (2 mg kg^{-1}) compared to low (0.6 mg kg^{-1}) p.o. doses suggests the possibility of dose-dependent kinetics for this compound. Very small amounts of hydroflumethiazide and no DTA were detected in the bile of patients with T-tube drainage.[652]

The pharmacokinetics of bendroflumethiazide are reported to be linear after p.o. tablet or capsule doses in the 1.25-10 mg range.[653,654] Peak plasma levels were reached at 2-3 h postdose, C_{max} and AUC values were dose-proportional and the elimination $t_{0.5}$ was <u>ca</u>. 3 h.[655]

Although peak plasma levels of bendroflumethiazide were dose-related in one study over the dosage range 2.5-5.0 mg, renal clearance from the higher dose was only one-half that from the lower dose.[656] Urinary recovery of unchanged drug was almost identical from the two doses, and represented only 18% of the higher dose. Concomitant administration of propranolol and hydralazine had no significant effect on the kinetic parameters of bendroflumethiazide.[649]

While bendroflumethiazide appears to have a relatively short elimination $t_{0.5}$, the $t_{0.5}$ of polythiazide is 26 h and detectable levels of this drug are present in plasma 48 h after a single 1 mg dose.[657] The prolonged plasma $t_{0.5}$ of polythiazide differs from most other thiazide diuretics, and is consistent with its relatively long duration of action.

Nonthiazide Diuretics

Furosemide

Reviews have been published on the clinical pharmacokinetics and pharmacodynamics of furosemide.[658-660] Furosemide is rapidly absorbed after p.o. doses, peak plasma drug levels occurring at ca. 1 h postdose.[661] The rate of absorption was reduced in the presence of food, but overall absorption efficiency was similar in fasted and non-fasted subjects. The drug has a short biological $t_{0.5}$ of about 30 min and it is eliminated predominantly in unchanged form via the kidneys. A 40 mg dose given orally as a tablet and as a solution yielded respective absolute bioavailabilities of 66% and 61%.[662] A mean peak plasma concentration of 1.7-1.8 µg ml^{-1} was achieved 50 min after the solution dose, and 1.5 h after the tablet dose.

Although equivalent bioavailability of furosemide has been demonstrated from different formulations,[663] marked differences in furosemide absorption have been obtained using different binding agents.[664] Tablets containing starch or stearic acid resulted in lower drug availability than those containing methylhydroxyethylcellulose or polyvinylpyrrolidone. These results were consistent with in vitro dissolution, but not disintegration, characteristics.

In another study, a sustained release preparation containing 60 mg furosemide yielded a maximum plasma concentration of 107 ng ml^{-1} at 4 h postdose, compared with 672 ng ml^{-1} at 1.5 h after a 40 mg conventional tablet.[665] The overall bioavailability from the sustained release product averaged 73% of that from the conventional tablet. The diuresis during the first 24 h after a single dose was also lower with the sustained release product than with the conventional tablet, although the cumulative effects during 48 h were similar. It was suggested that the conventional tablet could have yielded urinary furosemide concentrations exceeding those that induce maximal effect, thus resulting in some waste of drug.

After a 40 mg i.v. dose, plasma levels of furosemide declined biexponentially, with a mean terminal $t_{0.5}$ of 78 min.[662] The average steady-state volume of distribution was 0.13 l kg^{-1}, and the plasma and renal clearances were 118 and 89 ml min^{-1}, respectively. An 80 mg i.v. dose of furosemide resulted in a mean $t_{0.5}$ of 70 min,[666] similar to that for the 40 mg dose.

The distribution and plasma protein binding of furosemide are unaffected by severe arterial hypertension but serum clearance (mean 130 ml min^{-1}) is significantly reduced compared with normal (mean 219 ml min^{-1}) values.[667] The reduction in furosemide clearance may be due to a reduction in renal plasma flow, and consequently renal tubular secretion.

Both indomethacin[668] and probenecid[669,670] prolonged the biological $t_{0.5}$ of furosemide giving rise to elevated plasma levels in man. However, the pharmacodynamic effect associated with these changes is difficult to interpret. Indomethacin attenuates the natriuretic and diuretic effects of furosemide to a greater extent than can be accounted for by kinetic factors alone, while probenecid causes an increased overall response rather than a decrease.[671] The mechanisms of these reactions, possibly involving changes in prostaglandin transport, need further study. In another study increased circulating furosemide levels due to probenecid were accompanied by a reduction in diuretic action leading the authors to suggest that the concentration of furosemide in kidney tubules rather than in plasma may be the major determinant of its diuretic activity.[672]

The urinary excretion of unchanged furosemide is reduced by probenecid, which competes with furosemide for active tubular secretion.[673] In 4 healthy male subjects who received 40 mg of furosemide intravenously, pretreatment with probenecid increased the mean furosemide $t_{0.5}$ from 82 to 175 min and decreased the renal and plasma clearances from 118 to 23.1 ml min^{-1} and 160 to 51.4 ml min^{-1}, respectively. However, no significant changes in nonrenal clearance or steady-state volume of distribution were observed.

The plasma levels and relevant pharmacokinetic parameters of a 40 mg p.o. dose of furosemide and its effects on urinary water and electrolyte excretion were not affected by concurrent administration of 400 mg cimetidine, or by pretreatment with 1 g cimetidine daily for 5 days.[674] The pharmacokinetics of furosemide are similar in pregnant and nonpregnant women,[675] but the biological $t_{0.5}$ may be somewhat prolonged in pregnancy.[676] Furosemide crosses the human placenta readily, and drug levels in umbilical cord plasma and maternal plasma are similar at 8-10 h after drug administration to the mother.[677] The apparent volume of distribution is 4 times greater, the plasma clearance one-half, and the biological $t_{0.5}$ of furosemide 8 times longer in neonates than that in adults. Apparent changes in furosemide distribution in the neonate may be related to decreased binding to plasma proteins, and slow elimination in the neonate possibly explains the prolonged effects of furosemide in these patients.

In newborns who received furosemide transplacentally, the apparent $t_{0.5}$ in plasma was inversely related to the gestational age (Figure 1.33), ranging from 96 h at 32 wks to 6.8 h at 42 wks. A similar relationship was observed in neonates who received i.v. furosemide postnatally, but only after repeated dosing. In children with chronic renal failure undergoing regular haemodialysis, furosemide

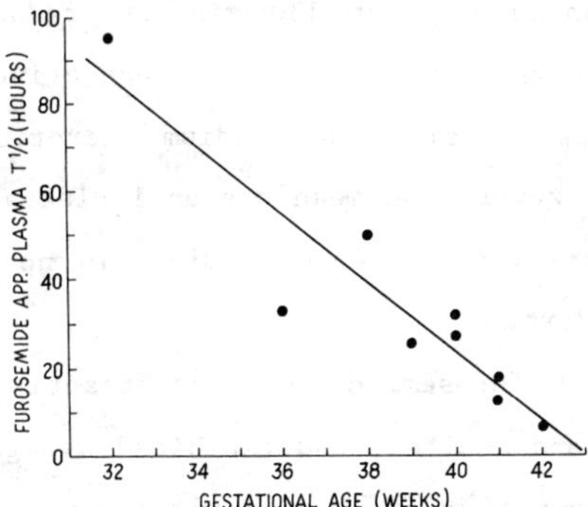

Figure 1.33   Relationship between gestational age and apparent half-life of furosemide in a group of new-borns who received the drug transplacentally. (r=0.926; df=7; p < 0.01). Reproduced by permission from Eur. J. Clin. Pharmacol., 1982, 22, 39.

$t_{0.5}$ averaged 250 min, which was much longer than that observed in adults.[678] Haemodialysis contributed to less than 10% of the systemic clearance of 0.6-0.8 ml min^{-1} kg^{-1}, probably due to extensive protein binding of furosemide. In adult patients with severe nephrotic syndrome, the free fraction of furosemide in plasma increased to 0.028 compared to 0.014 in healthy subjects, due to diminished plasma albumin levels.[679] Consequently, average nonrenal and total clearance values were higher in the nephrotic patients, 154 and 251 ml min^{-1} compared with 56 and 174 ml min^{-1} in normal subjects. Reduced diuretic and natriuretic response from a 40 mg i.v. dose of furosemide was observed in nephrotic syndrome, apparently due to impaired renal excretion.

Furosemide is useful for the treatment of volume overload after kidney transplant.   Smith et al.[680] classified those transplant patients as responders who showed adequate natriuretic and diuretic response to relatively low (40-80 mg) doses of furosemide, and non-responders who required 120 mg or more of furosemide to elicit an adequate response.   While both groups absorbed orally administered furosemide to a similar extent (ca. 50%) to healthy subjects, the nonresponders yielded a prolonged $t_{0.5}$ of 130 min and reduced plasma and renal clearances of 64 and 18.4 ml min^{-1}, respectively. These patients also had reduced urine volume and sodium excretion after a p.o. dose of furosemide. However, the mean nonrenal clearance values for the 2 patient groups were similar, 45.6 ml min^{-1} in nonresponders and 57.8 ml min^{-1} in responders.

The elimination $t_{0.5}$ of furosemide was significantly prolonged in patients with cirrhosis and ascites, and exhibited a high correlation with the apparent volume of distribution which was also higher than in normal subjects.[681-684] The increased distribution volume was due to reduced plasma protein binding secondary to depressed plasma albumin concentrations in liver disease. In one study, the mean unbound fraction of furosemide in plasma increased by 250%, from 4.0% in healthy subjects to 10.2% in cirrhotic patients.[681] In general, the renal and nonrenal clearances of furosemide were unaffected by cirrhosis, and similar quantities of parent drug were recovered in the 24 h urine of healthy subjects and patients, ca. 55% of an i.v. dose.[681] No significant amount of furosemide was found in ascitic fluid.[684]

The binding of furosemide to plasma proteins was also saturable in the rat;[685] the free fraction ranged from 0.92 to 9.1% of total drug concentrations between 11 and 425 µg ml^{-1}. Consequently, the apparent volume of distribution and the elimination $t_{0.5}$ both increased with increasing dose. While the total plasma clearance of furosemide did not change significantly as the i.v. dose increased from 10 to 40 mg kg^{-1} renal excretion, which depends on the free fraction of plasma furosemide, increased (Figure 1.34) and nonrenal clearance decreased, suggesting saturable furosemide metabolism. However, experiments in the dog have shown that, although nonrenal clearance accounted for about 50% of the elimination of furosemide, the liver did not play a significant role in this process.[686] No significant differences were found in the renal and nonrenal clearances,

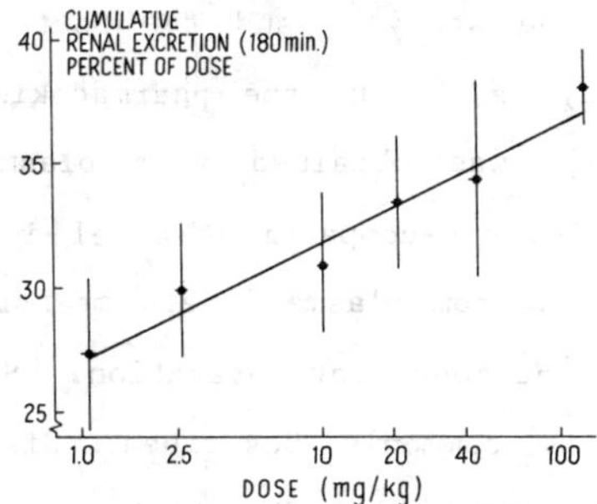

Figure 1.34   The cumulative excretion of unchanged furosemide into the urine up to 180 min expressed as a percentage of the dose. Mean values ± S.E.M. Reproduced by permission from <u>Biopharm. Drug Dispos.</u>, 1982, <u>3</u>, 345.

plasma protein binding, and urinary excretion of furosemide and its glucuronide between dogs with total devascularization of the liver and sham-operated animals.

Biliary excretion is a major elimination route for furosemide in the dog.[687] Following 5 mg kg^{-1} i.v. doses of ^{35}S-furosemide to 2 dogs, 41.9 and 49.5% of dosed radioactivity was recovered in urine while 52.4% and 50.4% was recovered in faeces. Analysis of urinary excretion data indicated that 50% of an orally dosed solution of ^{35}S-furosemide was absorbed into the systemic circulation.

In patients with advanced congestive heart failure, furosemide elimination $t_{0.5}$ was longer and the plasma clearance less compared to patients with moderate failure, probably due to reduced renal blood flow.[688] On the other hand, concurrent administration of i.v. hydralazine, which appeared to enhance renal blood flow in these patients, increased mean furosemide renal clearance from 45.4 to 60.9 ml min^{-1} and plasma clearance from 72.6 to 88.1 ml min^{-1}, despite unchanged creatinine clearance. The hydralazine effect was reflected also in a decrease in mean furosemide $t_{0.5}$ from 96 to 81 min.

Information regarding changes in furosemide elimination kinetics in renal failure is conflicting. The biological $t_{0.5}$ was reported to be increased to 80 min in one study[689] and to about 9.6 h in another.[690] The discrepancy may be due to the pharmacokinetic approaches used. The short $t_{0.5}$ was obtained from plasma levels measured to 4 h postdose and with one-compartment model interpretation. The long $t_{0.5}$ was obtained from plasma levels measured to 24 h postdose and with two-compartment model interpretation. Similarly, while reduced drug clearance is commonly described, distribution volumes (both V_1 and V_{dss}) are reported to decrease[691] and also to increase.[692] The binding of furosemide to plasma proteins is reported to decrease,[691,693] and also to be essentially unchanged[694] in renal failure, although the absolute binding percentages vary between these reports. Binding appears to be influenced by the serum albumin concentration. While both renal and extrarenal clearance of furosemide are significantly reduced in uraemia, extrarenal clearance is unaffected by the nephrotic syndrome.[693]

Renal clearance of furosemide is markedly depressed in azotaemia.[695] Linear regressions between furosemide renal clearance, Cl_R, and blood urea nitrogen, BUN, serum creatinine, C_{CR}, and creatinine clearance, Cl_{CR}, are given in equations 1.18-1.20. The plasma furosemide $t_{0.5}$ ranged from 0.8 h in healthy subjects to

$$Cl_R = 111.6 - 1.26(BUN), \ r = -0.81, \ p < 0.005 \qquad (1.18)$$

$$Cl_R = 127.6 - 33.9(C_{CR}), \ r = -0.81, \ p < 0.005 \qquad (1.19)$$

$$Cl_R = 1.32(Cl_{CR}) - 6.71, \ r = 0.93, \ p < 0.001 \qquad (1.20)$$

24.0 h in kidney disease, although some individuals with renal failure may have a furosemide $t_{0.5}$ approaching normal values.[696] The apparent distribution volume and also the nonrenal clearance of furosemide were unaffected by renal failure in this study.

Chennavasin et al.[697] commented on the reported variability in derived pharmacokinetic parameters of furosemide, which they attribute to the use of different methods of data analysis. Lee et al.[698]

showed that the actual time lapse between blood collection and centrifugation might also significantly affect measured plasma levels and pharmacokinetic interpretation of furosemide.

Spironolactone

Studies of metabolism and disposition of spironolactone in the dog have demonstrated that this diuretic agent is rapidly cleared from plasma ($t_{0.5} < 10$ min), and it is partially converted into canrenone, which equilibrates with the γ-hydroxylic acid canrenoate.[699] Disappearance of canrenone from plasma is biphasic, whereas that of canrenoate is triphasic. Typical plasma-level curves obtained after i.v. doses of all three compounds to dogs are given in Figure 1.35. With its extremely short biological $t_{0.5}$ spironolactone is unlikely to contribute to diuretic activity per se.[700]

Karim et al.[701] showed that plasma loss of radioactivity after i.v. doses of potassium ^{3}H-canrenoate to man was triphasic, with $t_{0.5}$ values of 0.073 h, 0.85 h, and 43.3 h. The first two elimination phases were due to excretion of canrenone and the hydroxy-acid derivative, whereas the third phase was a function of excretion of conjugated metabolite. Higher ratios of free to conjugated metabolite in urine than in plasma are attributed to a hydrolysis step during transfer of the conjugate from plasma to urine. However, relatively slow plasma clearance of the conjugate may be an alternative explanation. Studies in man revealed a similar pharmacokinetic and metabolic pattern to that in the dog.[702]

Spironolactone is a relatively water-insoluble drug, and as such its bioavailability from p.o. dosage forms is of interest. The mean bioavailability of spironolactone from 25 mg and 100 mg tablet formulations, expressed in terms of circulating levels of its major metabolite canrenone, were 100 and 92%, respectively, compared with an orally dosed solution.[703] Urinary excretion of canrenone constitutes less than 5% of administered spironolactone and is not a useful parameter for assessing bioavailability. Other studies have shown that

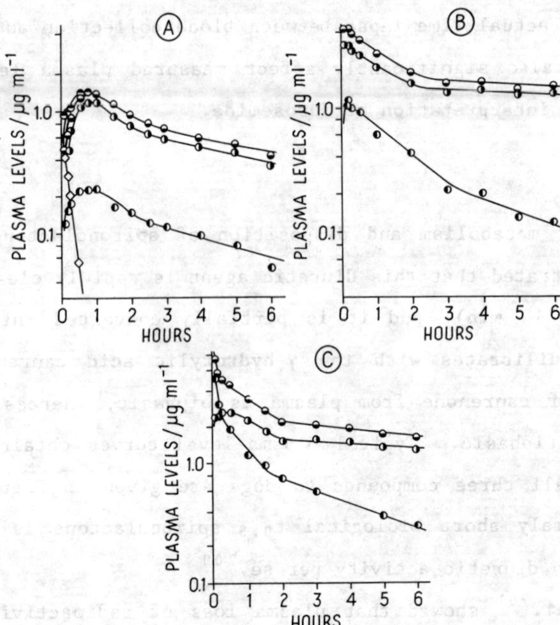

Figure 1.35 Plasma levels after i.v. doses of 100 mg spironolactone (A), 82 mg canrenone (B), and 95 mg potassium canrenoate (C). Key: ◊, spironolactone; ◑, canrenone; ◒, canrenoate; ◓, sum of canrenone + canrenoate; ◕, total fluorescence concentration. Reproduced by permission from J. Pharm. Sci., 1972, 61, 1129.

spironolactone is absorbed more rapidly, but not more efficiently, from a suspension than from tablets,[704] and that the bioavailability of spironolactone may vary markedly between different tablet formulations.[705] In the latter study areas under 96 h canrenone plasma level curves from 100 mg doses of ten commercial formulations varied from 267 to 478 µg 100 ml^{-1} h, while peak canrenone plasma levels varied from 13.1 to 29.0 µg 100 ml^{-1}. In all but two formulations good correlations were obtained between in vitro dissolution and bioavailability parameters.

The bioavailability of spironolactone from tablets made with micronized spironolactone (median particle size 2.21 µm) was compared with that from tablets containing standard spironolactone substance (median particle size 78.8 μm).[706] Due to extensive presystemic biotransformation of spironolactone, circulating levels and cumulative urinary excretion of canrenone were used as bioavailability indices. After single 200 mg doses to healthy men under fasting conditions, the micronized and standard spironolactone tablets yielded peak plasma canrenone concentrations of 0.55 and 0.43 μg ml^{-1}, respectively, both at approximately 3 h postdose. The overall bioavailability of the micronized tablets was greater than that of the standard tablets, the respective mean AUC values being 7.6 and 6.6 μg h ml^{-1}. The micronized tablets also tended to result in higher urinary excretion of canrenone, and significantly higher renal antimineralcorticoid activity compared to the standard tablets.

When spironolactone and hydrochlorothiazide were given in a combination preparation, the bioavailability of neither drug was significantly altered compared to the simultaneous administration of separate spironolactone and hydrochlorothiazide tablets.[707] While the bioavailability of spironolactone is not affected by hydrochlorothiazide,[708] it is increased by the presence of food.[709] Representative canrenone plasma profiles demonstrating this in one subject are shown in Figure 1.36. Enhanced absorption may be due to greater dissolution of tablets caused by delayed gastric emptying and to greater solubility of spironolactone through stimulated bile fluids.

After p.o. doses of 200 mg ^{3}H-spironolactone, mean peak canrenone serum levels of 415 ng ml^{-1} were obtained within 3 h, which then declined biphasically with a fast and slow $t_{0.5}$ of 4.4 and 16.8 h, respectively.[710] After repeated p.o. doses of spironolactone in tablets steady-state levels were reached within 4 days.[711] The plasma canrenone $t_{0.5}$ following repeated daily 100 mg doses of spironolactone was 19.2 h, which is indistinguishable from the single dose value. After repeated doses of 25 mg q.i.d. however, the mean plasma canrenone $t_{0.5}$ was reduced to 12.5 h. This is unexpected as the mean steady-state plasma levels of canrenone were similar from the two

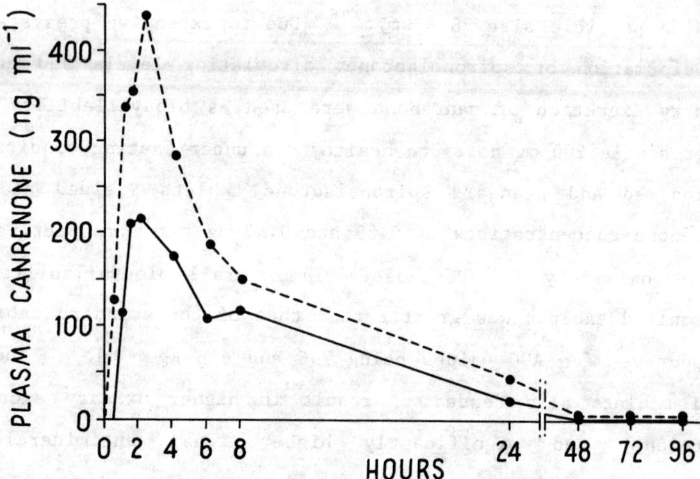

Figure 1.36   Plasma levels of canrenone in a healthy
volunteer after a single oral dose (4 x 25 mg) of
spironolactone given on a fasting stomach ●——● and
together with a standardized breakfast ●---●. Reproduced by permission from Clin. Pharmacol. Ther., 1977,
22, 100.

dosage regimens and plasma $t_{0.5}$ values were determined during 72 h
of the last dose, thus excluding the possible influence of absorption
effects. The rate of elimination of ^{3}H from plasma increased markedly
in four of six patients, suggesting induction of drug metabolism.[712]

Bell et al.[713] compared the effectiveness of single and divided
daily doses of spironolactone in the control of hypertensive patients
receiving 300 or 400 mg spironolactone daily as a single dose, or as
divided 100 mg doses for 21 days. No indication of improved blood
pressure control from the divided doses was observed compared with the
once daily regimen. Similarly, little or no significant differences
were noted in plasma canrenone levels and urinary canrenone excretion
between the two dosage regimens.

Reduction of canrenone excretion into urine by acetylsalicylic
acid is attributed to inhibition of active secretion in the proximal
renal tubules,[714] and this mechanism may account for the previously
reported reduction of spironolactone activity in the presence of ace-

tylsalicylic acid. Acetylsalicylic acid may also reduce the clinical
effectiveness of spironolactone by reducing the sodium output (dog) or
by increasing potassium excretion (rat), and spironolactone doses may
need to be increased in patients who chronically ingest aspirin.[715]

Chlorthalidone

The remarkable affinity of chlorthalidone for erythrocytes and
the influence of this on chlorthalidone pharmacokinetics provide the
basis of several reports on this drug. Collste et al.[716] showed that
after repeated doses at least 30% of the body load of chlorthalidone
is concentrated in erythrocytes. Concentrations of chlorthalidone in
plasma and whole blood in 6 individuals receiving repeated doses are
shown in Figure 1.37,[717] the average drug concentration in plasma
being 1.4% of that in whole blood. After repeated doses, the mean
elimination $t_{0.5}$ of chlorthalidone was 50 h in blood and 49 h in

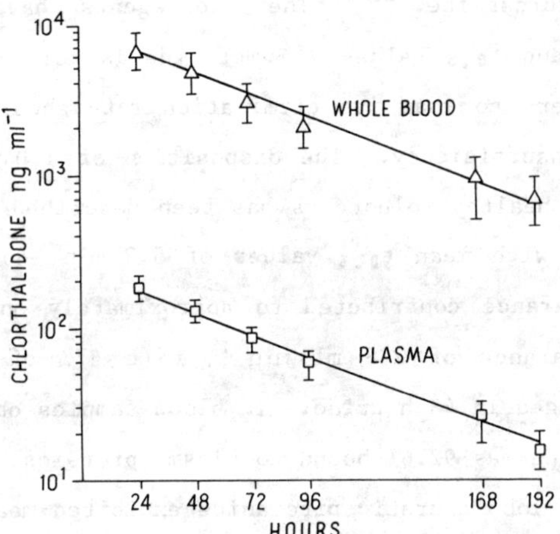

Figure 1.37   Concentrations of chlorthalidone in
plasma - □ - and in whole blood -Δ- measured following
50 mg per day for 14 days to human volunteers. Bars
represent 1 SEM. Reproduced by permission from <u>Eur. J.
Clin. Pharmacol</u>., 1977, <u>12</u>, 375.

plasma. Fleuren and van Rossum[718] reported a longer $t_{0.5}$ of chlorthalidone in red cells (60 h) than in plasma (40 h), and described a

pharmacokinetic model, including nonlinear binding of drug to red cells, which accounted for the observed time course of drug in plasma and erythrocytes.

Oral doses of chlorthalidone are slowly absorbed. The peak drug concentration in blood from two 25 mg chlorthalidone tablets averaged 4.0 µg ml^{-1} at 13.3 h while that from a 5 mg 100 ml^{-1} solution in 10% water-polyethylene glycol 4000 was 3.0 µg ml^{-1} at 18.2 h.[719] The elimination $t_{0.5}$ was approximately 35 h. Comparison of the respective AUC (322 and 272 µg h ml^{-1}) and cumulative urinary excretion (20.2 and 15.7 mg) data showed that, although polyethylene glycol 4000 enhanced the solubility of chlorthalidone in water, it caused a significant reduction in the bioavailability.

Other Diuretic Agents

Despite its smaller dose, bumetanide has similar pharmacokinetic characteristics to furosemide.[720] The two agents have similar distribution volumes and $t_{0.5}$ values. Bumetanide is more extensively metabolized, however, so that its elimination rate should be less influenced by renal insufficiency. The disposition of a 0.5 mg i.v. dose of bumetanide in healthy volunteers has been described by a triexponential function, with mean $t_{0.5}$ values of 5.9 min, 46 min, and 3.1 h.[721] Renal clearance contributed to approximately one-half of the total plasma clearance of 228 ml min^{-1}, with 47% of the dose being recovered unchanged in 48 h urine. In blood samples obtained 15 min postdose, bumetanide was 92.6% bound to plasma proteins. Similarly, the relatively new loop diuretic piretanide exhibited mean protein binding of 94.2% in normal serum at 1 mM piretanide concentration.[722] Tests at piretanide concentrations of 0.5 to 4.5 mM showed reduced protein binding in serum from uraemic patients, apparently due to depressed serum albumin levels.

The mean bioavailability of bemetizide from a combination tablet containing 25 mg bemetizide and 50 mg triamterene was 69% of that from a tablet of 25 mg bemetizide alone, based on the relative plasma AUC values as well as 24 h urinary recovery of intact drug.[723] While both products yielded plasma levels that peaked at <u>ca</u>. 4 h, the C_{max} from the combination tablet was 68.3 ng ml^{-1}, significantly lower than that after bemetizide alone, 87.9 ng ml^{-1} (Figure 1.38). Nevertheless, the pharmacologic effects of the two products, as measured by the increase in electrolyte excretion, were not significantly different. In this study, the mean $t_{0.5}$ of bemetizide was 8.4–11.2 h.

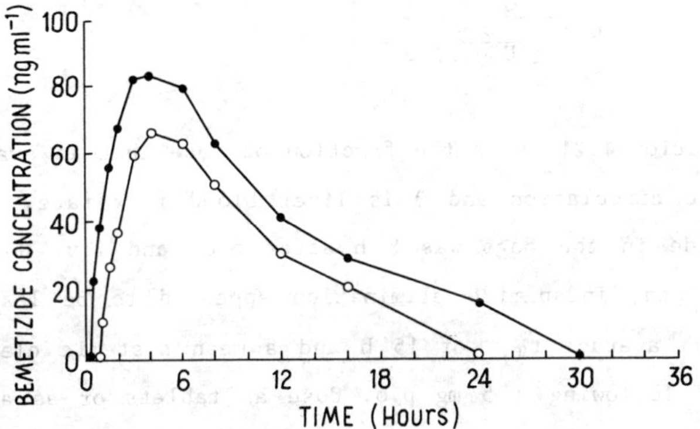

Figure 1.38   Mean plasma concentrations of bemetizide after single oral doses of 25 mg alone (Formulation A. ●-●) and 25 mg bemetizide and 50 mg triamterene in combination (Formulation B. o-o). Reproduced by permission from <u>Biopharm. Drug Dispos.</u>, 1982, <u>3</u>, 361.

Fleuren et al.[724] studied the pharmacokinetics of mefruside after single p.o. 25 or 50 mg doses to 8 young male volunteers. The drug was readily absorbed, reaching peak plasma levels of <u>ca</u>. 80 ng ml^{-1} and 68-128 ng ml^{-1} at approximately 2.5 h after administering the 25 and 50 mg doses, respectively. Mefruside distributed instantaneously between plasma and red cells, its concentration in red cells being <u>ca</u>. 30-fold higher than in plasma. The mean cumulative urinary excretion of unchanged drug accounted for only 0.49% of the dose, while that of the lactone metabolite (5-oxo-mefruside) and open acid metabolite amounted to 13.1% and 46.2%, respectively, of the dose. An additional 5-15% of the dose was recovered in urine as a conjugate of the open acid metabolite. Large interindividual variations in mefruside $t_{0.5}$ and plasma clearance were observed, the respective values being 2.9-12.5 h and 22.5-129 1 h^{-1}. The mean $t_{0.5}$ values of the lactone and open acid metabolites were 11.9 and 10.5 h, respectively, and these appeared to correlate well with duration of diuretic effect.

The bioavailability of the new antihypertensive agent indapamide was estimated to be virtually complete, using equation 1.21 and the relevant data in dogs[725] or humans.[726]

$$F = \frac{Q}{Q + \dfrac{Dose}{(AUC_{0-\infty})po}} \qquad (1.21)$$

In equation 1.21, F is the fraction of dose that is available to the systemic circulation and Q is liver blood flow rate. The $t_{0.5}$ of indapamide in the dogs was 8 h after p.o. and i.v. doses (1 mg kg^{-1}). In man, indapamide elimination appeared to be less efficient, with an average $t_{0.5}$ of 15 h and a mean systemic clearance of 20 ml min^{-1} following a 5 mg p.o. dose as tablets or as an aqueous solution in 20% polyethylene glycol 400.[726]

The bioavailability and distribution kinetics of amiloride were similar from two different formulations in man.[727] The relatively long $t_{0.5}$ of this drug, 9-10 h, is associated with prolonged diuretic activity.[728] Isosorbide, which like amiloride is not metabolized, has a biological $t_{0.5}$ of 7-8 h in man, and has a distribution volume similar to body water.[729] Isosorbide-induced diuresis has been associated with increased creatinine clearance, but the mechanism of this is uncertain.

The diuretic agent metozalone is excreted by glomerular filtration and tubular secretion in dogs, although the drug:creatinine clearance ratio is lower than most other diuretics.[730] The $t_{0.5}$ in dogs of 5-6 h is influenced by extensive binding to erythrocytes and plasma proteins, and possibly also to tissue proteins.[731]

Other Antihypertensive Agents

Hydralazine

The peripheral vasodilator hydralazine is commonly used in combination with other antihypertensive agents in the treatment of moderate to severe hypertension. The clinical pharmacokinetics of hydralazine have been reviewed recently by Ludden et al.[732] These and other investigators showed that hydralazine is subject to polymorphic N-acetylation.[733-737] After single (1 mg kg^{-1}) and multiple (1 mg kg^{-1} every 12 h x 5 doses) p.o. administration, hydralazine underwent extensive acetylator phenotype-dependent first-pass metabolism.[734] The mean bioavailability was 7-10% in the fast acetylators and 31-39% in the slow acetylators, with large interpatient variations in hydralazine C_{max} and AUC values. Quantitative analysis of hydralazine and two of its acetylated metabolites, methyltriazolophthalazine (MTP) and 3-hydroxymethyltriazolophthalazine (HOMTP), in the 0-24 h urine following a p.o. dose showed that slow acetylators excreted more hydralazine, similar amounts of MTP, and less HOMTP than rapid acetylators.[738,739] The respective urinary recoveries were 2.6, 3.5, and 4.0% of the hydralazine dose in slow acetylators, compared with 1.0, 3.5, and 14.6% of the dose in rapid acetylators.

Food has been reported to have no effect,[740] or to increase[741] the systemic availability of hydralazine. In the latter study, the quantity of drug entering the circulation increased 2- to 3-fold when drug was given after a standard meal compared to the fasting state.

The fraction of hydralazine absorbed increases at high doses in both fast and slow acetylator phenotypes and this appears to be due to saturation of N-acetylation at high doses.[742] Acetylator phenotype appears not to influence the elimination $t_{0.5}$ of hydralazine which is _ca._ 1 h after both p.o. and i.v. doses.[733-734] This phenomenon may reflect rapid conversion of systemic hydralazine to the major plasma metabolite, hydralazine pyruvic acid hydrazone (HPH). This is an extrahepatic elimination pathway which is probably not phenotype dependent. The elimination $t_{0.5}$ of HPH averaged 4-6 h and was not significantly different between rapid and slow acetylators. Other investigators have confirmed that acetylator phenotype is an important determinant of hydralazine plasma levels in normal individuals only after oral administration, as illustrated in Figures 1.39 and 1.40.[743-744]

A significant correlation exists between reduction in mean arterial pressure from baseline (ΔMAP) and the plasma concentration of intact hydralazine.[745] Accordingly, ΔMAP following single and repeated oral doses of hydralazine was inversely related ($p < 0.05$) to the acetylator index, as shown in Figure 1.41.

The hydralazine $t_{0.5}$ increased to 15.8 h in a patient with a glomerular filtration rate of 16 ml min^{-1}.[746] As hydralazine is

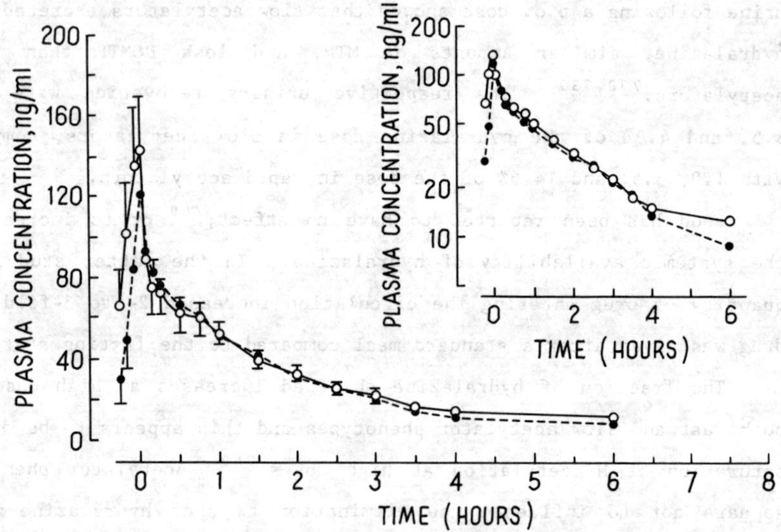

Figure 1.39   Time course of plasma drug concentration in rapid (o) and slow (●) acetylators given a 20-mg slow intravenous infusion of hydralazine hydrochloride. Each point denotes the mean ± SE of five subjects. The inset shows a semilogarithmic plot of the mean data. Reproduced by permission from *J. Pharmacokin. Biopharm.*, 1980, *8*, 53.

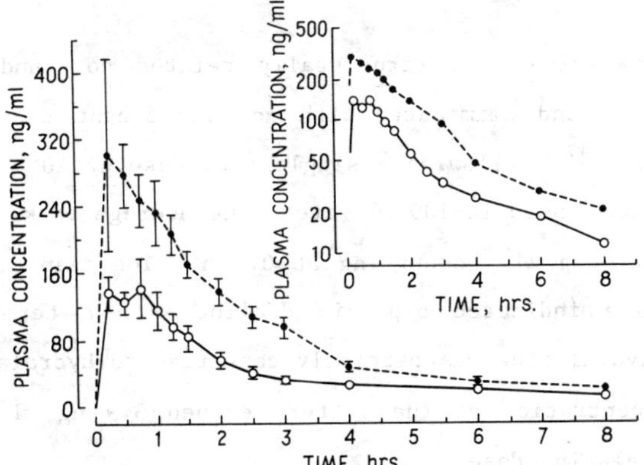

Figure 1.40 Time course of plasma drug concentration
in rapid (o) and slow (•) acetylators following ingestion of a 100 mg oral dose of hydralazine hydrochloride. Reproduced by permission from J. Pharmacokin.
Biopharm., 1980, 8, 53.

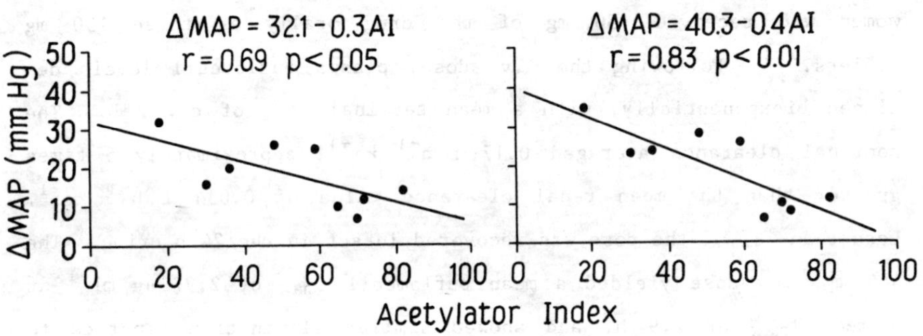

Figure 1.41 Relationships between peak reduction in
mean arterial pressure (ΔMAP) and acetylator index
(AI), following a single dose (left) and the fifth
dose (right) of hydralazine 1 mg kg^{-1} orally.
Reproduced by permission from Hypertension, 1981, 3,
580.

not generally regarded as being excreted unchanged via the kidneys,

reduced clearance in renal failure may be due either to impaired

metabolism or underestimates, by some investigators, of the amount of

unchanged drug cleared in urine.

Dihydralazine

Unlike hydralazine, the structurally related compound dihydralazine is absorbed and eliminated with no significant dependence on acetylator status.[747] Following a single p.o. dose of 20 mg dihydralazine sulphate suspended in 100 ml water, the average peak drug level in plasma was 47.6 ng ml^{-1} occurring at 0.9 h. The mean plasma concentration profile indicated biphasic decline with a terminal $t_{0.5}$ of _ca_. 5 h. Dihydralazine was partially converted to hydralazine; the mean plasma concentration of the latter reached 3.9 ng ml^{-1} at 1 h after the dihydralazine dose.

Buflomedil

The pharmacokinetics of buflomedil, a relatively new drug used for its peripheral vasodilator activity, was studied in 4 female patients who receive 100 mg buflomedil intravenously and 3 healthy women who received 450 mg of the drug orally as three 150 mg tablets.[748] Following the i.v. dose, plasma buflomedil levels declined biexponentially, with a mean terminal $t_{0.5}$ of _ca_. 2 h. The nonrenal clearance averaged 0.17 1 h^{-1} kg^{-1}, approximately 5 times greater than the mean renal clearance value of 0.034 1 h^{-1} kg^{-1}. Less than 18% of the dose was recovered intact in the 24 h urine. The 450 mg p.o. dose yielded a mean buflomedil C_{max} of 2.97 µg ml^{-1} at a mean t_{max} of 2.9 h, and showed similar elimination kinetics to that after i.v. administration.

Prazosin

The pharmacokinetics of the peripheral vasodilator prazosin have been reviewed.[749] In hypertensive patients who received a 2 mg i.v. dose, the drug had an overall distribution volume of 0.5 1 kg^{-1} and a terminal plasma $t_{0.5}$ of _ca_. 3 h.[750] Only 3.4% of the dose was recovered unchanged in 24 h urine. In the same patients, approximately 55% of a 2 mg p.o. dose was bioavailable, and was subsequently eliminated with the same $t_{0.5}$ as after i.v. administration. Virtually identical pharmacokinetic parameter values were observed by Grahnén et al.[751] in their patients who received single 0.5 mg p.o. and i.v. doses and increasing multiple p.o. doses up to 5 mg t.i.d. These investigators attributed the relatively low p.o. bioavailability of prazosin to incomplete absorption rather than first-pass metabolism, since the drug was cleared slowly from the body. Plasma clearances were 0.14 and 0.50 1 h^{-1} kg^{-1} for total and free prazosin, respectively. Prazosin was extensively bound to plasma albumin and α_1-acid glycoprotein, <u>ca</u>. 97% within the 1-30 ng ml^{-1} concentration range. Despite marked inter- and intra-patient variations in plasma prazosin levels, there appeared to be a linear correlation between prazosin dose and steady-state plasma concentration (r = 0.82, p < 0.001). After i.v. prazosin, the drug-induced hypotensive effect correlated with prazosin plasma concentration during the β-phase, as shown in Figure 1.42.[752] However, no such correlation was observed during maximal continuous therapy.

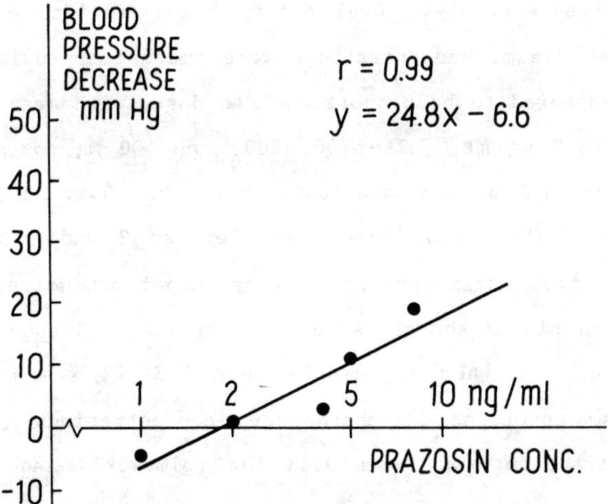

Figure 1.42 Correlation between plasma concentration of prazosin and decrease in systolic standing blood pressure after a single i.v. dose of 0.5 mg prazosin to one patient. Reproduced by permission from <u>Clin. Pharmacol. Ther.</u>, 1981, <u>30</u>, 447.

Prazosin elimination and plasma protein binding were similar between hypertensive patients with normal renal function and those with chronic renal failure.[753]   During a multiple dosing regimen of 3-8 mg d^{-1}, the two groups of patients also demonstrated similar antihypertensive responses to the drug. In a study comparing prazosin disposition in 7 young (22-32 yr) and 7 elderly (66-78 yr) healthy men,[754] it was shown that the mean bioavailability of prazosin from a 1 mg p.o. dose decreased with age from 68 to 48%.   This change was apparently due to decreased drug absorption in the elderly, since no significant effect of age was observed on prazosin clearance, approximately 4 ml min^{-1} kg^{-1} in both subject groups.

Tolmesoxide

The pharmacokinetics of the direct-acting vasodilator tolmesoxide have been studied in healthy subjects[755] and in hypertensive patients.[756] Following a 100 mg i.v. dose, plasma tolmesoxide levels declined biexponentially, with a mean terminal $t_{0.5}$ of 2.6 h.   The volume of distribution and total clearance averaged 0.71 l kg^{-1} and 242 ml min^{-1}, respectively.   Oral doses of tolmesoxide were rapidly absorbed. Peak plasma concentrations were reached approximately 1 h postdose and appeared to be proportional to dose, with mean values of 1.1, 3.8, and 6.2 µg ml^{-1} after 50, 200, and 400 mg doses, respectively. The overall p.o. bioavailability was <u>ca</u>. 85%. The elimination $t_{0.5}$ values after p.o. doses were between 2 and 3 h, similar to those after i.v. administration. A principal metabolite RX71112, that appeared in plasma shortly after p.o. or i.v. tolmesoxide, had a $t_{0.5}$ of 4-5 h.   Neither tolmesoxide nor RX71112 was extensively bound to plasma proteins at therapeutic concentrations (0.6-20 µg ml^{-1}). The fraction bound was 0.38 for tolmesoxide and 0.58 for RX71112.

Severe nausea and gastrointestinal side effects occurred at tolmesoxide doses of 600-900 mg daily.[756] These symptoms might be alleviated by administering the drug with food, which has been shown to delay the absorption of tolmesoxide and reduce its peak concentration in plasma, without significantly changing the overall bioavailability or pharmacologic response.[757]

Clonidine

The pharmacokinetics and clinical pharmacology of the centrally acting α_2-adrenoceptor agonist clonidine have been reviewed.[758,759] In 18 healthy, normotensive subjects, single p.o. doses of clonidine tablets were absorbed following a lag time of 19-22 min, and yielded peak plasma concentrations at 2.4-2.9 h.[760] The bioavailability appeared to be proportional to doses of 75, 150, and 250 µg, with mean peak plasma levels of 0.29, 0.61, and 1.16 ng ml^{-1}, respectively, and mean AUC values of 3.4, 5.7, and 13.8 ng h ml^{-1}, respectively. Average elimination $t_{0.5}$ values were 9 to 15 h. In 14 hypertensive patients, chronic p.o. doses of 0.1-0.6 mg clonidine twice daily also yielded plasma AUC values that showed direct correlation with dose (Figure 1.43).[761] The fall in diastolic blood pressure

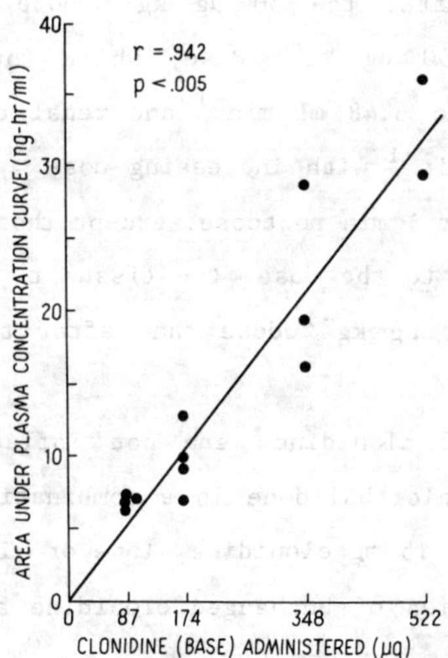

Figure 1.43   AUC as a function of clonidine dose. Reproduced by permission from <u>Clin. Pharmacol. Ther.</u>, 1981, <u>30</u>, 729.

in these patients also correlated well with plasma clonidine concentration. On the other hand, Frisk-Holmberg et al.[762] have suggested
dose-dependent pharmacokinetics during chronic therapy with clonidine.
In hypertensive patients who received single i.v. doses of 0.78-3.36
μg kg^{-1}, the mean elimination $t_{0.5}$ increased from 6.2 h to 12.8 h
with increasing doses, while the average plasma clearance decreased
from 9.94 to 2.61 ml min^{-1} kg^{-1}. The apparent volume of distribution, which averaged 3.45 1 kg^{-1}, did not change with dose.
Similarly, after multiple p.o. doses, 1.1 or 1.9 μg kg^{-1} twice
daily for 6-12 months, clonidine $t_{0.5}$ increased from a mean single
dose value of 8 h to 14.3 h. The p.o. bioavailability of clonidine
was reduced from a single dose value of 90% to <u>ca</u>. 65% after chronic
administration, probably due to decreased absorption secondary to
inhibition of GI motility and gastric emptying.

Additional data suggesting nonlinear kinetics of clonidine were
obtained from Sprague-Dawley rats who received rapid i.v. doses of 10,
50, or 250 μg kg^{-1}.[763] The drug showed rapid tissue distribution
after all doses, with an α-phase $t_{0.5}$ in plasma of less than 4 min.
The β-phase $t_{0.5}$ was 48 min after the 50 μg kg^{-1} dose but increased to 90 min after the 250 μg kg^{-1} dose, while total body
clearance decreased from 11.83 to 6.48 ml min^{-1} and renal clearance
decreased from 3.78 to 2.07 ml min^{-1} with increasing dose. Although
tissue clonidine concentrations at 1 min postdose, except those in the
heart, appeared linearly related to the dose, the tissue $t_{0.5}$ values
were always longer after the 250 μg kg^{-1} dose than after the lower
doses.

The disposition kinetics of clonidine were not influenced by
simultaneous administration of chlorthalidone in a combination product.[764] After 7 daily doses of 0.15 mg clonidine alone or with 15 mg
chlorthalidone, the renal excretion of unchanged clonidine accounted
for 63% of total clonidine dose.

Guanfacine

The pharmacokinetics of guanfacine were studied in 3 groups of hypertensive patients with normal renal function (GFR > 90 ml min^{-1}), moderate renal impairment (GFR 10-30 ml min^{-1}), and uraemia (GFR < 10 ml min^{-1}).[765] After a single 3 mg i.v. dose, no significant differences in plasma guanfacine concentrations or hypotensive effects were observed among the three patient groups. The mean $t_{0.5}$ was <u>ca.</u> 14 h and the volume of distribution ranged from 417 to 445 l. Although the 0-48 h urinary excretion of guanfacine averaged 57%, 14%, and 7.5% of the dose in order of decreasing renal function, reduced renal clearance was largely compensated by an increase in metabolic clearance, as shown in Figure 1.44. Similar results were obtained following multiple p.o. doses of guanfacine, 1 mg t.i.d. for 5 days, with nonrenal elimination playing an important role in patients with impaired renal function. The mean bioavailability from p.o. doses was approximately 60-70%.

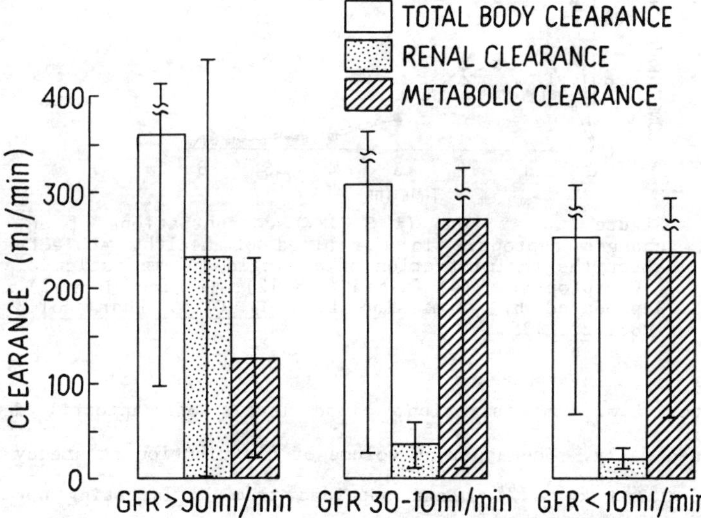

Figure 1.44 Mean total body clearance, renal clearance, and metabolic clearance of guanfacine in normal subjects, patients with moderately impaired renal function, and in uraemic patients. Reproduced by permission from <u>Clin. Pharmacokin.</u>, 1980, <u>5</u>, 476.

Captopril

The angiotensin-converting enzyme inhibitor, captopril, is efficiently absorbed after p.o. administration. Peak captopril concentrations in blood were 69.2, 364, and 800 ng ml^{-1} after doses of 10,
50, and 100 mg, all were reached within 1 h of dosing.[766-768]

The bioavailability of unchanged drug was 62% while the overall
absorption of radioactivity was <u>ca.</u> 70% of a ^{35}S or ^{14}C labeled dose
and appeared to be independent of dose size. Food given immediately
before the administration of ^{14}C-captopril reduced absorption by
35-40%, as indicated by blood levels of captopril (Figure 1.45), and
also cumulative excretion of radioactivity in urine.[769]

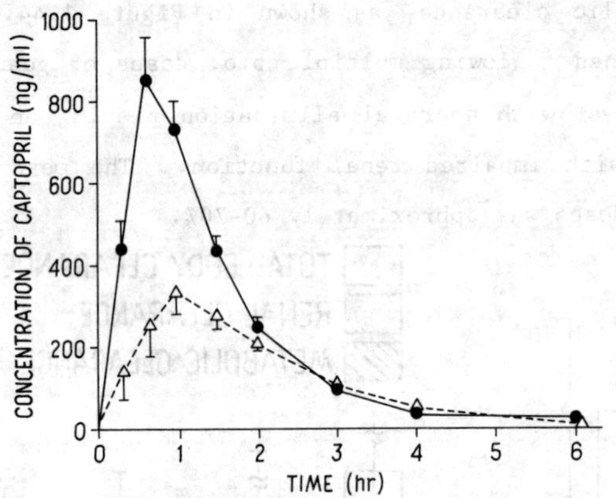

Figure 1.45   Mean (± S.E.M.) concentrations of unchanged captopril in the blood of healthy subjects
after the administration of a single 100 mg tablet of
^{14}C-captopril: (●) fasted (N = 12); (Δ) fed (N = 12).
Reproduced by permission from <u>J. Clin. Pharmacol.</u>,
1982, <u>22</u>, 135.

After i.v. administration, blood levels of captopril decayed
triexponentially. The apparent volume of distribution at steady-state
averaged 0.7 1 kg^{-1}.[766] Data obtained from 12 lactating normotensive women who received captopril tablets, 100 mg t.i.d. for 2 days,
showed negligible passage of drug into breast milk.[770] The mean
C_{max} in milk was 4.7 ng ml^{-1} at 3.8 h while that in blood was 713
ng ml^{-1} at 1.1 h postdose.

The mean terminal $t_{0.5}$ of captopril in blood was 1.9 h while the total body clearance averaged 0.76 l kg^{-1} h^{-1}.[766] Approximately 38% of the dose was excreted as unchanged drug in 24 h urine, which also contained small quantities (<u>ca</u>. 1.5% of dose) of captopril disulfide dimer, an autoxidation product.[766,768] Since the renal clearance of unchanged captopril exceeds inulin clearance, it appears that active tubular secretion is involved in the excretion of this compound. Concomitant administration of probenecid with intravenous ^{14}C-captopril in 4 healthy subjects reduced the mean total body clearance and renal clearance to 631 and 217 ml kg^{-1} h^{-1}, respectively, compared with 775 and 388 mg kg^{-1} h^{-1} when captopril was given alone.[771] The 24 h cumulative renal excretion of unchanged captopril decreased from 45.8 to 28.9% of dose, while that of metabolites increased from 32.1 to 55.2% of dose, in the presence of probenecid. The authors suggest that increased biotransformation of captopril in the presence of probenecid is probably due to increased residence time of captopril and not to any direct effect of probenecid on captopril metabolism. In patients with chronic renal failure, the mean $t_{0.5}$ of captopril following a 50 mg single p.o. dose was approximately double that observed in normal subjects.[767] The excretion of parent drug and major metabolites in 6 h urine of these patients was 1/5 to 1/4 of normal values.

In beagle dogs and rhesus monkeys with bile duct cannulation who received i.v. doses of ^{14}C-captopril as a constant infusion over 6 h, the mean terminal $t_{0.5}$ values in blood were 2.8 and 2.2 h, respectively.[772] The apparent distribution volumes averaged 2.5 l kg^{-1} in the dog and 3.6 l kg^{-1} in the monkey, suggesting extensive tissue distribution. Approximately 90-95% of the administered radioactivity was recovered in urine, while negligible quantities were found in the bile of both species. As in man, the majority of radioactivity in urine consisted of unchanged captopril, which amounted to 52.9 and 81.0% of dose in the dog and monkey, respectively.

Nicardipine

The pharmacokinetics of nicardipine have been studied after single[773] and repeated[774] doses in rats, dogs, monkeys, and humans. Despite its efficient absorption from the GI tract, the systemic bioavailability of nicardipine is relatively low, and increases with elevating doses, indicating a marked, but saturable, first-pass effect. In man, the mean absolute bioavailability of nicardipine increased from 6.5% of a 10 mg p.o. dose to 30.3% of a 40 mg dose. Nicardipine was extensively metabolized in the rat, dog, monkey, and man, with no unchanged drug detected in the urine. Following i.v. administration, the disappearance of nicardipine from plasma was rapid in all species tested. The longest terminal $t_{0.5}$, _ca_. 1 h, was observed in man.

Nifedipine, Verapamil, Diltiazem

Very limited pharmacokinetic data are available on the calcium ion antagonists nifedipine, verapamil, and diltiazem, as indicated in two recent reviews.[775,776]

Nifedipine

A single 5 mg p.o. dose of nifedipine in patients with essential hypertension induced a significant fall in blood pressure and rise in heart rate which paralleled the plasma concentration profile of nifedipine.[777] After chronic treatment, plasma nifedipine levels were significantly correlated with reduction in systolic and diastolic blood pressures.

Verapamil

Verapamil is cleared from the body predominantly by hepatic metabolism and, of the various metabolites, only norverapamil has pharmacologic activity.[778,779] Unchanged drug has an apparent distribution volume of 5 1 kg^{-1}, a plasma clearance of 0.8 1 h^{-1} kg^{-1}, and an elimination t$_{0.5}$ of <u>ca</u>. 5 h.[780] Due to extensive hepatic metabolism, verapamil is extensively cleared in the first pass after p.o. doses yielding a systemic availability of only 20%. Verapamil is 95% bound to plasma proteins[781] but can be displaced by other agents[782] with possible therapeutic consequences. Pharmacologic effects of verapamil are related to plasma levels, but effects are lower for a given plasma level after p.o. doses than after i.v. doses, possibly because of stereoselective elimination of the more active <u>l</u>-isomer by the liver after p.o. dosing.[783]

Diltiazem

Some pharmacokinetic data are available for diltiazem subsequent to development of a specific assay in plasma.[784] Peak plasma diltiazem levels are proportional to p.o. doses ranging from 60 to 120 mg, peak levels are achieved at 4 h, and the elimination t$_{0.5}$ is <u>ca</u>. 5 h.[785] Although side-effects were coincident with peak plasma levels in one study,[784] other studies have obtained poor correlations between cardiac or clinical effects and diltiazem levels in animals[786] or patients.[787]

Anticoagulants

The coumarins are currently the principal p.o. anticoagulants and attention here will be focused primarily on warfarin and other coumarin anticoagulents.

Warfarin

A bioavailability monograph has been presented for warfarin.[788] Studies in man based on relative areas under drug plasma-level curves indicate that warfarin is between 75 and 100% bioavailable after p.o. doses.[789] In these studies, plasma-level data were discussed in terms of a two-compartment model with elimination occurring from either the central or the peripheral compartment. Previous studies had shown that the two-compartment model with elimination occurring from the central compartment adequately describes warfarin blood levels after both p.o.[790] and i.v.[791] doses. Very similar pharmacokinetic constant values were obtained in all these studies, including a relatively small central compartment representing blood volume. Another study has utilized an additional compartment during the absorption processes representing warfarin in the gastric mucosa.[792] In this study, warfarin was efficiently absorbed from the human stomach and small intestine, when in the dissociated form. Inconsistencies between some previous reports on warfarin pharmacokinetics and metabolism are discussed by Benya and Wagner[793] in terms of drug instability to light and also during chromatography. A gas-chromatographic method, specific for unchanged warfarin, showed that metabolites of warfarin cannot be detected in plasma after single doses,[794] and have thus confirmed the validity of the results obtained in earlier studies on warfarin bioavailability and pharmacokinetics following p.o. doses to man.[795]

Active interest continues to center around the pharmacokinetics of warfarin and its enantiomers and their influence on observed pharmacologic effects. Studies in rats have demonstrated positive relationships between warfarin tissue distribution and its elimination rate constant, and also between the plasma concentration of warfarin that is required to inhibit prothrombin complex synthesis and its biological $t_{0.5}$.[796] Warfarin distribution volume and plasma clearance are also positively correlated with levels of circulating unbound drug.[797,798] However, poor correlations were obtained between liver:plasma concentration ratios and plasma free fraction values. This was attributed to similar warfarin binding characteristics to plasma and liver tissue.

Although warfarin is approximately 99% bound in rat plasma, the drug rapidly penetrates extravascular tissues.[799] Interpretation in terms of the two-compartment model indicated that liver, lung, heart, spleen, and brain tissue behave as part of the central compartment while the peripheral compartment is probably composed of lymph fluid into which free drug from plasma slowly equilibrates. Correlations between circulating warfarin levels and lowering of prothrombin activity,[800] and also direct inhibition of clotting factor synthesis,[801] were markedly improved when calculations were based on unbound rather than total drug levels.

The binding of warfarin to plasma proteins and to other tissues in disease states has received considerable interest.[802] In human studies, the protein binding of warfarin in the serum of patients with cardiovascular disease ranged from 98.1 to 99.6%, and there was no apparent relationship between binding and the concentration of total serum protein or albumin.[803] Although drug clearance correlated well with the free fraction of drug in serum, no such correlation was observed between the free fraction and prothrombin time. The serum protein binding of warfarin in normal adults is log-normally distributed[804] and the free fraction is significantly greater in women than in men.[805] Protein binding of warfarin may remain constant during prolonged periods in patients receiving fixed dosages of warfarin and other drugs,[806] and is not altered as a result of mild or moderate hepatic changes.[807] In renal impairment, however, the binding of warfarin to protein may be reduced, and linear correlations are reported between the free fraction and plasma creatinine and blood urea nitrogen.[808] The first of these is illustrated in Figure 1.46. Decreased protein binding is associated with a shorter mean warfarin elimination $t_{0.5}$ of 30 h in uraemia compared with 45 h in controls, although the pharmacological response to warfarin was similar in normal and ureamic subjects.

Other studies in rats have shown strong correlations between the warfarin elimination rate constant, and also the distribution volume V_d(area), and the free warfarin fraction,[810] and also that serum binding and the total clearance of warfarin may decrease after re-

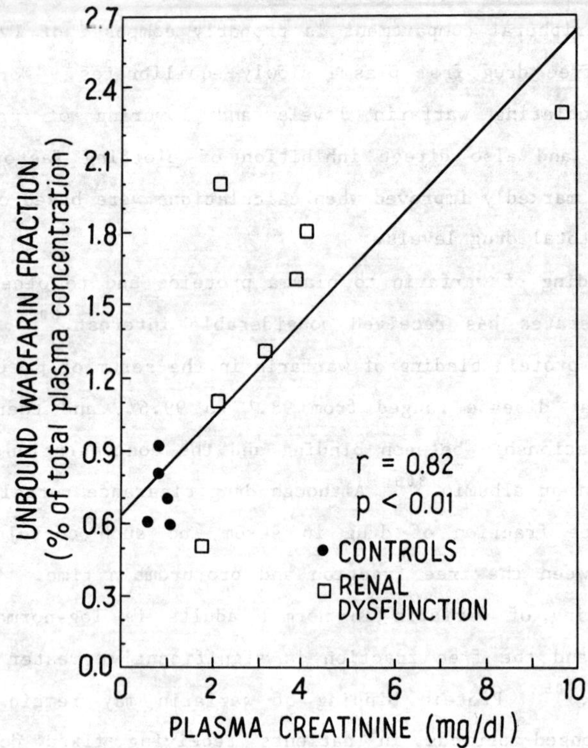

Figure 1.46   Relationship between binding of warfarin
to plasma proteins and plasma creatinine.   Reproduced
by permission from J. Clin. Pharmacol., 1976, 16, 468.

peated doses.[811] Although the latter effects might give rise to higher warfarin levels, they are compensated for by a requirement of higher drug levels to produce the same degree of anticoagulation.   Previously observed genetically-based differences in warfarin elimination
kinetics may be a consequence of differences in serum protein binding.
The degree of binding of racemic warfarin is trimodal with free fraction values of 0.0040, 0.0112, and 0.0166,[812] and the trimodal distribution reflects a similar distribution in warfarin clearance values.

     The anticoagulant activity of warfarin is a function of stereo-
chemical configuration of the unchanged drug,[813-816] but not of the

warfarin alcohol metabolites.[816] Although (+)-warfarin is cleared from plasma about twice as fast as (-)-warfarin in the rat,[817] in man (-)-warfarin is cleared from plasma _ca._ 40% faster than (+)-warfarin.[818] The relative distribution volumes for the enantiomorphs were not significantly different.[815] Plasma clearance of the four possible alcohols arising from metabolic reduction of the warfarin enantiomorphs was rapid (4.1-6.3% h^{-1}) with the exception of the (±)-alcohol which has a clearance of 1.7-2.4% h^{-1}, slower than that of the parent drug.[816] Radioactivity appearing in 96 h bile of rats amounted to 39.4% of a p.o. dose and 47.5% of an i.v. dose of ^{14}C-warfarin, and consisted of both unchanged drug and metabolites.[819] In contrast, radioactivity appearing in 96 h urine amounted to only 18.9 and 21.3%, respectively, of p.o. and i.v. doses. The rate of biliary excretion of radioactivity is increased by i.v. dosed oxyphenbutazone, owing to increased bile flow rate and possible redistribution of warfarin from tissue-binding sites.[820]

In one human study, five healthy subjects received, at one-month intervals, single p.o. doses of 0.75 mg kg^{-1} of S(-)-warfarin, R(+)-warfarin, and 1.5 mg kg^{-1} of racemate with one of the enantiomers labeled with a stable isotope (warfarin-d_5).[821] Analysis of plasma samples by gas chromatography-mass spectrometry showed that the mean $t_{0.5}$ values of S(-)- and R(+)-warfarin after separate administration were 1.2 and 2.3 d, respectively, while administration of the racemate did not alter the $t_{0.5}$ of either enantiomer. The apparent volume of distribution averaged 9-10 l in all cases.

Both enantiomers of warfarin have similar distribution characteristics in the rat and man, but the (S)-(-)-enantiomer has the greater pharmacological activity in both species. Differences in elimination kinetics of the enantiomers in rats have been used to predict changes in the rate of synthesis of prothrombin complex activity after single doses of the racemate.[822]

As an approach to a better understanding of plasma protein and tissue binding and their relative influence in dose-response relationships, Gibaldi and McNamara[823] used equation 1.22 to relate the

$$f_T = \frac{V_T \, (f_p)}{V_{d\beta} - V_p} \tag{1.22}$$

fraction of unbound drug in tissue, f_T, to the distribution volumes of plasma water, V_p, total body water minus plasma volume, V_T, the apparent drug volume at steady-state, $V_{d\beta}$, and the fraction of unbound drug in plasma, f_p. Application of their method to literature data prompted the conclusion that differences in plasma protein binding of warfarin in rats are associated with similar changes in tissue binding. This conclusion is consistent with previously observed high correlations between unbound drug in rat-liver homogenates and the unbound fraction in serum.

Many drug-drug interactions have been reported with warfarin. Although these are due primarily to displacement from protein binding sites, this is not the only mechanism. Potentiation of the hypoprothrombinaemic effect of warfarin in man by disulfiram[824] is due to inhibition of hepatic drug-metabolizing enzymes,[825] whereas the potentiation due to phenylbutazone and the recently introduced hypnotic triclofos is due to competitive displacement of warfarin from plasma albumin.[826,827] However phenylbutazone also causes inhibition of 7-hydroxylation of the potent (S)-(-)-enantiomer of warfarin.[828,829] Potentiation of warfarin effects by dextrothyroxine is due primarily to accelerated decline in the activities of clotting factors II and X rather than displacement of warfarin from protein-binding sites.[830,831] Co-administration of the benzodiazepines, nitrazepam, chlordiazepoxide, and diazepam, had no effect on plasma $t_{0.5}$ values or steady-state concentrations of warfarin in man,[832] and meprobamate caused only small changes in warfarin-controlled prothrombin times.[832]

Inhibition of warfarin anticoagulant activity by rifampicin in man is due to enhanced warfarin metabolism rather than impaired absorption.[834] This effect, clearly indicated in Figure 1.47, appears to result from induction of warfarin metabolizing enzymes in the smooth endoplasmic reticulum. Other studies have shown that warfarin metabolism may be induced by prolonged exposure to anaesthetic gases,[835] and have also confirmed that secobarbital and glutethimide reduce warfarin activity, presumably owing to enzyme induction, while chloral hydrate and methaqualone have little or no effect on warfarin activity.[836]

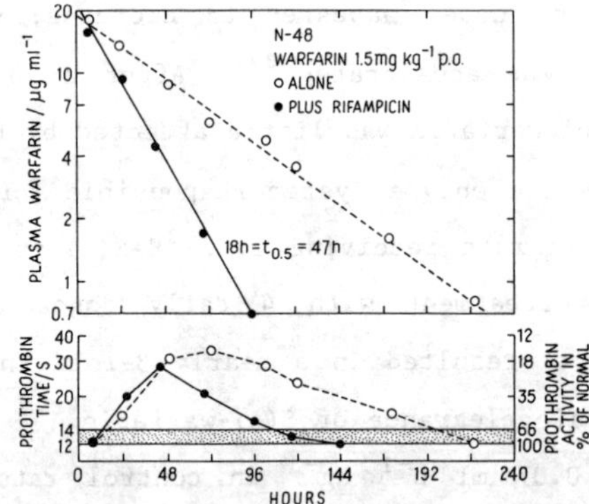

Figure 1.47 Plasma drug concentrations and one-stage prothrombin times after single doses of sodium warfarin with and without daily doses of rifampicin. Rifampicin, 600 mg daily p.o., was administered for three days before p.o. administration of sodium warfarin and during periods of hypoprothrombinaemia. Reproduced by permission from <u>Ann. Int. Med.</u>, 1974, <u>81</u>, 337.

The binding of warfarin to serum proteins is decreased in the presence of naproxen.[837] Previously reported similar interactions with clofibrate are now considered to be associated with the S-enantiomer of warfarin rather than with the less active R-enantiomer. Thus, clinical interactions between clofibrate and warfarin may be pharmacodynamic rather than pharmacokinetic in nature.[838] The R:S free fraction ratio is 1:3 in man and 1:6 in rats, and the ratios are independent of the free fraction. Similarity of this ratio in the rat and man rules out a species difference in binding as a contributory factor in the different rate of elimination of the R- and S-enantiomers in these two species.

Administration of ibuprofen to rats receiving warfarin caused a decrease in the biological $t_{0.5}$ and an increase in total clearance of warfarin, and these appear to be associated with displacement of bound warfarin in plasma.[839] Pretreatment with phenobarbital, however, had no effect on serum protein binding of either warfarin or dicumarol.[840] When rats were deprived of food, plasma protein binding of warfarin following 3 mg doses appeared to decrease, while the clearance of unbound drug was accelerated.[841] After a 10 mg dose, however, the disposition of warfarin was little affected by fasting.

Phenobarbital induces the enzyme system responsible for warfarin metabolism. Experiments in rats receiving i.v. ^{3}H-S(-)warfarin, 0.6 mg kg^{-1}, showed that pretreatment with 4 daily doses of phenobarbital (75 mg kg^{-1}, i.p.) resulted in a nearly 3-fold increase in both the total and intrinsic clearance of S(-)-warfarin.[842] The mean intrinsic clearance was 0.07 ml h^{-1} kg^{-1} in control rats and 0.2 ml h^{-1} kg^{-1} in rats pretreated with phenobarbital. Parallel decreases in warfarin $t_{0.5}$ and duration of anticoagulant effect were observed also in phenobarbital pretreated rats, while no statistically significant changes were noted in the apparent volume of distribution or the extent of warfarin binding to serum proteins. The plasma protein binding of ^{14}C-warfarin was also unaltered by the presence of pirprofen, a nonsteroidal antiinflammatory agent.[843]

Other Coumarin Anticoagulants

There have been several reports on the bioavailability of dicumarol, and particularly on the influence of formulation and particle size. Studies in dogs have demonstrated variable absorption from commercial tablets[844] and also capsules.[845] The bioavailability of dicumarol from p.o. doses is increased by magnesium oxide or hydroxide, but is significantly reduced by talc, colloidal magnesium aluminium silicate, aluminium hydroxide, and starch.[846] Increased absorption may be due to increased pH in the GI tract or formation of a readily absorbed magnesium-dicumarol chelate.

Striking similarities have been demonstrated between the pharmacokinetics of dicumarol and warfarin in the rat.[847] Although warfarin is about 30 times more potent that dicumarol based on effective total blood concentrations, their potencies are almost equivalent based on circulating free-drug levels. As the rate of dicumarol elimination in rats, and also the intensity of pharmacological effect, are both functions of the quantity of drug reaching the liver (liver:plasma ratio),[848] a positive relationship is obtained between drug $t_{0.5}$ and the plasma level required to produce a given intensity of pharmacological effect. Although the potentiating effect by phenylbutazone on warfarin activity is associated, at least in part, with protein-binding displacement, this could not be demonstrated for dicumarol using rat-liver homogenates.[849] Phenylbutazone also had little effect on dicumarol plasma:liver distribution ratios, and the exact mechanism of dicumarol potentiation by this agent has yet to be determined.

Plasma levels of dicumarol declined in triexponential fashion following i.v. doses to rats. Although all other kinetic parameters were largely independent of free fractions of this highly bound drug, a significant correlation was obtained between the free fraction and the terminal elimination rate constant.[850] Good correlations between total dicumarol clearance and the free drug fraction in serum appear to be a property shared by warfarin and other extensively bound compounds, whereas a high correlation between dicumarol clearance and the drug fraction resident in liver appears to be more specific for dicumarol and is of limited application.[851] Furthermore, the rate of dicumarol elimination in rats was significantly increased by phenobarbital pretreatment, while the serum:liver and serum:kidney drug concentration ratios were unchanged.[852] Thus, although linear relationships were observed between the fraction of drug in liver and elimination rate in both induced and control animals, the slopes of the regression lines were different.

Elimination of dicumarol followed first-order kinetics in two volunteers but was concentration-dependent in two other volunteers receiving 600 mg p.o. dicumarol.[853] Pretreatment with tolbutamide markedly increased the elimination rate of dicumarol in the first two subjects, but had no effect in the other two. The plasma level-response curve of dicumarol was unchanged by tolbutamide, but there was a small decrease in the area under the anticoagulant response versus time curve. Extensive first-pass metabolism is thought to be responsible for the systemic availability of less than 4% of p.o. dosed coumarin in man.[854]

Acenocoumarol is rapidly absorbed from p.o. doses, is avidly bound (98.7%) to plasma proteins, as are all other coumarin anticoagulants, and is extensively metabolized to compounds that show anticoagulant activity in mice.[855]

After single p.o. and i.v. doses of R(+)-, S(-)-, and R,S(±)-acenocoumarol in healthy subjects, the plasma concentrations of the R(+)-enantiomer were consistently higher than the S(-)-enantiomer.[856] Following 25 mg i.v. dose, the plasma clearance of S(-)-acenocoumarol was 14-15 l h^{-1}, approximately 10 times that of the R(+)-enantiomer, 1-1.5 l h^{-1}, while the plasma clearance of the racemate was approximately 2 l h^{-1}. The $t_{0.5}$ of S(-)-acenocoumarol was 2-4 h, compared with <u>ca</u>. 10 h for the R(+)-enantiomer, and the racemate. However, no differences between the two enantiomers and the racemate were observed in their extent of serum protein binding, approximately 98% at a concentration of 10 µg ml^{-1}. It appears that reported greater anticoagulant potency of R(+)- than S(-)-acenocoumarol is due to stereoselective differences in the clearance of the two enantiomers.

Orally administered coumarin is almost completely absorbed, although only <u>ca</u>. 1% of the dose is available to the systemic circulation as intact drug due to an extensive first-pass.[857] The bioavailability of coumarin from prolonged release tablets (4 x 15 mg) was 35% of that from a p.o. solution, indicating that the first-pass effect was enhanced in cases of sustained absorption. A much higher p.o. bioavailability of coumarin, <u>ca</u>. 45%, has been reported in the dog compared to man.[858]

Although elimination of the enantiomers of warfarin and other coumarins is stereospecific, no distinct differences were observed in the elimination rates of the S- and R- enantiomers of phenprocoumon in man, although the distribution volume and plasma clearance of S(-)-phenprocoumon were less than those for R(+)-phenprocoumon.[859] In terms of total anticoagulant effect, the S- enantiomer is 1.6-2.6 times more potent than the R- enantiomer, although the S- enantiomer is also more highly bound to plasma proteins. Unlike warfarin, differences in pharmacokinetic parameters between the enantiomers of phenprocoumon appear to be related to distribution rather than to stereospecific metabolism.

In rats, the antagonism of the hypoprothrombinaemic action of bishydroxycoumarin (BHC) by salicylate is due to displacement from plasma proteins, with consequent increases in liver uptake and biliary excretion.[860,861] Urinary excretion is unaffected. Plasma BHC levels in rats were significantly reduced by pentobarbital pretreatment, and to a lesser extent by glutethimide, owing to nonspecific microsomal enzyme induction.[862]

Heparin

Little information is available on the metabolism and pharmacokinetics of heparin. Anticoagulant effect is linearly related to the concentration of heparin in plasma,[863] as shown in a plot of the natural logarithm of activated partial thromboplastin time (APTT) versus heparin concentration (Figure 1.48).   The slope of the line ranged from 1.8 to 4.3 among 31 patients.   This indicates a smaller interpatient variability than that reported earlier by Cipolle et al.[864] who observed a nearly 600% variation in pretreatment heparin sensitivity.

Studies in man, using blood-clotting times to estimate heparin levels, have suggested that the rate of heparin elimination is decreased at high dose levels and also in renal impairment.[865]   However other studies based on bioassayed coagulation tests failed to demonstrate dose-dependent heparin elimination kinetics.[866]

Dose-dependent elimination was demonstrated in a subsequent study in which the heparin elimination $t_{0.5}$ increased from 40-50 min after a 50-100 U kg^{-1} dose to _ca_. 150 min following a 400 U kg^{-1} dose.[867]   Following a bolus i.v. dose of _ca_. 70 U kg^{-1} of beef lung

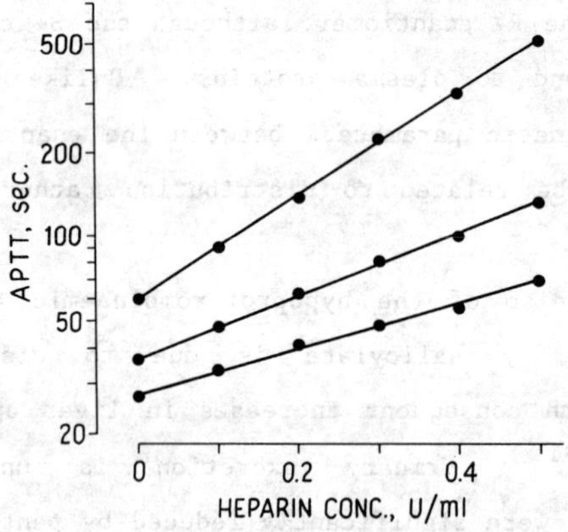

Figure 1.48   Relationship between activated partial thromboplastin time (APTT) and concentration of added heparin in plasma of three patients.   Reproduced by permission from _Clin. Pharmacol. Ther._, 1982, _32_, 503.

heparin, the mean $t_{0.5}$ of the drug was shorter in smokers (0.62 h) than in nonsmokers (0.97 h), and the clearance was more rapid in men (3.36 1 h^{-1}) than in women (1.83 1 h^{-1}).[866]

Dipyridamole

Oral doses of the antiplatelet agent dipyridamole were absorbed at a moderate rate in 6 normal young subjects after an initial lag time of 34-75 min.[868] The average systemic bioavailability was 43% of a 50 mg dose given after overnight fast. Dipyridamole was $>$ 99% bound to plasma proteins. The mean apparent distribution volume of dipyridamole after a 20 mg i.v. dose was 141 l. The terminal $t_{0.5}$ of dipyridamole was approximately 11.5 h after p.o. or i.v. administration, while the plasma clearance was 138 ml min^{-1}.

Tranexamic Acid

Tranexamic acid is used in the treatment of various fibrinolytic disorders. In 10 healthy subjects who received 2 g p.o. doses of tranexamic acid, fasted and with a standard meal in a crossover design, peak plasma concentrations averaged 14-15 µg ml^{-1} and occurred at a mean t_{max} of 2.8-2.9 h after both treatments.[869] The absolute bioavailability of p.o. tranexamic acid was approximately 34% compared to an i.v. dose, and was unaffected by food. The drug was excreted primarily via the kidneys, and greater than 95% of a 1 g i.v. dose was recovered intact in 72 h urine. The terminal $t_{0.5}$ in plasma was _ca_. 2 h, and the plasma clearance was 110-116 ml min^{-1}.

References

1. D.H. Huffman and D.L. Azarnoff, *J. Amer. Med. Assoc.*, 1972, *222*, 957.

2. B.F. Johnson, A.S.E. Fowle, S. Lader, J. Fox, and A.D. Munro-Faure, *Brit. Med. J.*, 1973, *iv*, 323.

3. J. Lindenbaum, *Pharmacol. Rev.*, 1973, *25*, 229.

4. D.J. Greenblatt, D.W. Duhme, J. Koch-Weser, and T.W. Smith, *New Engl. J. Med.*, 1973, *289*, 651.

5. J.C. Panisset, P. Biron, G. Tremblay, R. Nadeau, and A. Proulx, *Canad. Med. Assoc. J.*, 1973, *109*, 700.

6. N.A.J. Hamer and D.A. Chamberlain, *Brit. Med. J.*, 1973, *ii*, 177.

7. Editorial, *Lancet*, 1972, *ii*, 311.

8. B.F. Johnson, H. Greer, J. McCrerie, C. Bye, and A. Fowle, *Lancet*, 1973, *i*, 1473.

9. E. Steiness, V. Christensen, and H. Johansen, *Clin. Pharmacol. Ther.*, 1973, *14*, 949.

10. J. Lindenbaum, V.P. Butler, J.E. Murphy, and R.M. Cresswell, *Lancet*, 1973, *i*, 1215.

11. E.J. Fraser, R.H. Leach, and J.W. Poston, *Lancet*, 1972, *ii*, 541.

12. P.F. Binnion, M. McDermott, and D. Le Sher, *Lancet*, 1973, *i*, 1118.

13. J.G. Wagner, M. Christensen, E. Sakmar, D. Blair, J.D. Yates, P.W. Willis, A.J. Sedman, and R.G. Stoll, *J. Amer. Med. Assoc.*, 1973, *224*, 199.

14. E.J. Fraser, R.H. Leach, J.W. Poston, A.M. Bold, L.S. Culank, and A.B. Lipede, *J. Pharm. Pharmacol.*, 1973, *25*, 968.

15. V. Manninen, J. Melin, and P. Reissel, *Lancet*, 1972, *i*, 490.

16. T.R.D. Shaw, J.E. Carless, M.R. Howard, and K. Raymond, *Lancet*, 1973, *ii*, 209.

17. A.J. Jounela and A. Sothmann, *Lancet*, 1973, *i*, 202.

18. J. Lindenbaum, *Clin. Pharmacol. Ther.*, 1975, *17*, 296.

19. P.F. Binnion and M. Aristarco, *Clin. Pharmacol. Ther.*, 1974, *16*, 807.

20. A.G. Hibble, P. Isaac, and D.G. Grahame-Smith, *Lancet*, 1972, *ii*, 90.

21. L. Fleckenstein, B. Kroening, and M. Weintraub, *Clin. Pharmacol. Ther.*, 1974, *16*, 435.

22. B.F. Johnson and S. Lader, *Brit. J. Clin. Pharmacol.*, 1974, *1*, 329.

23. L. Nyberg, K.-E. Andersson, and A. Bertler, *Acta Pharm. Suecica*, 1974, *11*, 471.

24. D.H. Huffman, C.V. Manion, and D.L. Azarnoff, Clin. Pharmacol. Ther., 1974, 16, 310.

25. B.F. Johnson and C. Bye, Brit. Heart J., 1975, 37, 203.

26. W.J. Jusko, D.R. Conti, A. Molson, P. Kuritzky, J. Giller, and R. Schultz, J. Amer. Med. Assoc., 1974, 230, 1554.

27. F. Keller and N. Rietbrock, Int. J. Clin. Pharmacol., 1977, 15, 549.

28. D.J. Greenblatt, D.W. Duhme, J. Koch-Weser, and T.W. Smith, J. Amer. Med. Assoc., 1974, 229, 1774.

29. D.J. Greenblatt, D.W. Duhme, J. Koch-Weser, and T.W. Smith, Clin. Pharmacol. Ther., 1974, 16, 444.

30. J. Lindenbaum, M.H. Mellow, M.O. Blackstone, and V.P. Butler, New Engl. J. Med., 1971, 285, 1344.

31. J.P. Skelly and G. Knapp, J. Amer. Med. Assoc., 1973, 224, 243.

32. T.G. Vitti, D. Banes, and T.E. Byers, New Engl. J. Med., 1971, 285, 1433.

33. N. Sanchez, L.B. Sheiner, H. Halkin, and K.L. Melmon, Brit. Med. J., 1973, iv, 132.

34. P.F. Binnion, J. Clin. Pharmacol., 1976, 16, 461.

35. F.I. Marcus, J. Dickerson, S. Pippin, M. Stafford, and R. Bressler, Clin. Pharmacol. Ther., 1976, 20, 253.

36. P. Ghirardi, G. Catenazzo, O. Mantero, G.C. Merotti, and A. Marzo, J. Pharm. Sci., 1977, 66, 267.

37. J. Lindenbaum, Clin. Pharmacol. Ther., 1977, 21, 278.

38. F. Bochner, D.H. Huffman, D.D. Shen, and D.L. Azarnoff, J. Pharm. Sci., 1977, 66, 644.

39. R.P. Juhl, R.W. Summers, J.K. Guillory, S.M. Blaug, F.H. Cheng, and D.D. Brown, Clin. Pharmacol. Ther., 1976, 20, 387.

40. R. Brachtel and H.J. Gilfrich, Klin. Wschr., 1977, 55, 439.

41. M.C.B. van Oudtshoorn, Lancet, 1972, ii, 1153.

42. A.J. Jounela, P.J. Pentikäinen, and A. Sothmann, Eur. J. Clin. Pharmacol., 1975, 8, 365.

43. P.F. Binnion, Irish J. Med. Sci., 1974, 148, 346.

44. P.F. Binnion, M. McDermott, S.M. Kalman, J.E. Doherty, J.K. Bissett, and T.E. Ratts, Lancet, 1972, ii, 592.

45. S.A.H. Khalil, J. Pharm. Sci., 1974, 63, 1641.

46. S.A.H. Khalil, J. Pharm. Pharmacol., 1974, 26, 961.

47. J.C.K. Loo, M. Rowe, and I.J. McGilveray, J. Pharm. Sci., 1975, 64, 1727.

48. V. Manninen, A. Apajalahti, H. Simonen, and P. Reissel, Lancet, 1973, i, 1118.

49. V. Manninen, A. Apajalahti, J. Melin, and M. Karesoja, <u>Lancet</u>, 1973, <u>i</u>, 398.

50. S. Medin and L. Nyberg, Lancet, 1973, <u>i</u>, 1393.

51. W.H. Hall and J.E. Doherty, <u>Digestive Dis.</u>, 1971, <u>16</u>, 903.

52. K.S. Albert, J.W. Ayres, A.R. DiSanto, D.J. Weidler, E. Sakmar, M.R. Hallmark, R.G. Stoll, K.A. DeSante, and J.G. Wagner, <u>J. Pharm. Sci.</u>, 1978, <u>67</u>, 1582.

53. M.M. Applefeld, J. Adir, W.G. Crouthamel, and D.S. Roffman, <u>J. Clin. Pharmacol.</u>, 1981, <u>21</u>, 114.

54. K.-O. Haustein, <u>Eur. J. Clin. Pharmacol.</u>, 1981, <u>19</u>, 45.

55. H. Gault, J. Kalra, M. Ahmed, D. Kepkay, and J. Barrowman, <u>Clin. Pharmacol. Ther.</u>, 1980, <u>27</u>, 16.

56. H. Gault, J. Kalra, M. Ahmed, D. Kepkay, L. Longerich, and J. Barrowman, <u>Clin. Pharmacol. Ther.</u>, 1981, <u>29</u>, 181.

57. T. Hess, A. Krähenbühl, J. Luisier, and M. Weiss, <u>Schweiz. Med. Wschr.</u>, 1981, <u>111</u>, 1434.

58. T.R.D. Shaw and M.R. Howard, <u>Lancet</u>, 1972, <u>ii</u>, 493.

59. B. Beermann, <u>Lancet</u>, 1973, <u>i</u>, 375.

60. B. Beermann, <u>Eur. J. Clin. Pharmacol.</u>, 1972, <u>5</u>, 11.

61. H.J. Dengler, G. Bodem, and K. Wirth, Proc. 5th Int. Congr. Pharmacol., San Francisco, 1972, Karger, Basel, 1973, <u>Vol. 3</u>, p. 112.

62. R. Thomas and S. Aldous, <u>Lancet</u>, 1973, <u>ii</u>, 1267.

63. B. Beermann, K. Hellström, A. Rosen, and B. Werner, <u>Eur. J. Clin. Pharmacol.</u>, 1972, <u>5</u>, 19.

64. H.J. Dengler, G. Bodem, and K. Wirth, <u>Arzneim.-Forsch.</u>, 1973, <u>23</u>, 64.

65. R.H. Reuning, R.A. Sams, and R.E. Notari, <u>J. Clin. Pharmacol.</u>, 1973, <u>13</u>, 127.

66. K.H. Damm, W. Braun, and H. Heckert, <u>Arch. Pharmakol.</u>, 1973, <u>277</u>. 267.

67. E.E. Ohnhaus, P. Spring, and L. Dettli, <u>Eur. J. Clin. Pharmacol.</u>, 1972, <u>5</u>, 34.

68. N.D. Kim, L.E. Bailey, and P.E. Dresel, <u>J. Pharmacol. Exp. Ther.</u>, 1972, <u>181</u>, 377.

69. J. Morrison and T. Killip, <u>Clin. Res.</u>, 1970, <u>18</u>, 668.

70. W. Shapiro, K. Narahara, and K. Neblett, <u>Circulation</u>, 1970, <u>42, suppl. 3</u>, 110.

71. C.A. Bush, J.H. Caldwell, R.P. Lewis, N.J. Greenberger, and A.M. Weissler, <u>Circulation</u>, 1970, <u>42, suppl. 3</u>, 111.

72. Å. Bertler and A. Redfors, <u>Acta Pharmacol. Toxicol.</u>, 1971, <u>29, suppl. 3</u>, 281.

73. R.J. Hoeschen and V. Proveda, Canad. Med. Assoc. J., 1971, 105, 170.

74. G.A. Beller, T.W. Smith, W.H. Abelmann, E. Haber, and W.B. Hood, Jr., New Engl. J. Med., 1971, 284, 989.

75. S.W. Rabkin and G. Grupp, Pharmacologist, 1971, 13, 198.

76. R.D. Schoenwald, J. Pharm. Sci., 1974, 63, 411.

77. W.G. Kramer, R.P. Lewis, T.C. Cobb, W.F. Forester, Jr., J.A. Visconti, L.A. Wanke, H.G. Boxenbaum, and R.H. Reuning, J. Pharmacokin. Biopharm., 1974, 2, 299.

78. J.G. Wagner, J. Clin. Pharmacol., 1974, 14, 329.

79. J.R. Koup, D.J. Greenblatt, W.J. Jusko, T.W. Smith, and J. Koch-Weser, J. Pharmacokin. Biopharm., 1975, 3, 181.

80. L. Nyberg, K.-E. Andersson, and Å. Bertler, Acta Pharm. Suecia, 1974, 11, 459.

81. L.I. Harrison and M. Gibaldi, J. Pharm. Sci., 1977, 66, 1679.

82. G. Hartel, K. Kyllonen, E. Merikallio, K. Ojala, V. Manninen, and P. Reissell, Clin. Pharmacol. Ther., 1976, 19, 153.

83. H. Allonen, K.E. Andersson, E. Lisalo, J. Kanto, L.G. Stromblad, and G. Wettrell, Acta Pharmacol. Toxicol., 1977, 41, 193.

84. J.K. Aronson, D.G. Grahame-Smith, K.F. Hallis, A. Hibble, and F. Wigley, Brit. J. Clin. Pharmacol., 1977, 4, 213.

85. J.K. Aronson and D.G. Grahame-Smith, Brit. J. Clin. Pharmacol., 1977, 4, 223.

86. D.J. Chapple, R. Hughes, and B.F. Johnson, Brit. J. Pharmacol., 1976, 57, 23.

87. W.D. Hager, P. Fenster, M. Mayersohn, D. Perrier, P. Graves, F.I. Marcus, and S. Goldman, New Engl. J. Med., 1979, 300, 1238.

88. B. Moezzi, V. Fatourechi, R. Khozain, and B. Eslami, Jpn. Heart J., 1978, 19, 366.

89. J.M. Gayes, D.J. Greenblatt, B.L. Lloyd, J.S. Harmatz, and T.W. Smith, J. Clin. Pharmacol., 1978, 18, 16.

90. R. Krakauer and E. Steiness, Clin. Pharmacol. Ther., 1978, 24, 454.

91. W.G. Kramer, A.J. Kolibash, R.P. Lewis, M.S. Bathala, J.A. Visconti, and R.H. Reuning, J. Pharmacokin. Biopharm., 1979, 7, 47.

92. H. Smulyan and R.H. Eich, Amer. J. Cardiol., 1976, 37, 716.

93. T. Jogestrand and K. Sundqvist, Eur. J. Clin. Pharmacol., 1981, 19, 89.

94. T. Jogestrand, F. Ericsson, and K. Sundqvist, Eur. J. Clin. Pharmacol., 1981, 19, 97.

95. J. Bonelli, H. Rameis, and H. Waginger, Int. J. Clin. Pharmacol. Ther. Toxicol., 1981, 19, 93.

96. J.R. Koup, <u>Int. J. Clin. Pharmacol. Ther. Toxicol.</u>, 1980, <u>18</u>, 236.

97. R. Krasula, R. Yanagi, A.R. Hastreiter, S. Levisky, and L.F. Soyka, <u>J. Pediatr.</u>, 1974, <u>84</u>, 265.

98. G. Wettrell and K.-E. Andersson, <u>Eur. J. Clin. Pharmacol.</u>, 1975, <u>9</u>, 49.

99. R. Gorodischer, J. Krasner, and S.J. Yaffe, <u>Res. Comm. Chem. Path. Pharmacol.</u>, 1974, <u>9</u>, 387.

100. E. Iisalo and M. Dahl, <u>Acta Paediat. Scand.</u>, 1974, <u>63</u>, 699.

101. G. Wettrell, K.-E. Andersson, Å. Bertler, and N.R. Lundström, <u>Acta Paediat. Scand.</u>, 1974, <u>63</u>, 705.

102. A.C.V. Giardina, K.H. Ehlers, J.B. Morrison, and M.A. Engle, <u>Circulation</u>, 1975, <u>51</u>, 713.

103. J.M. Neutze, J.D. Rutherford, and P.J. Hurley, <u>NZ Med. J.</u>, 1977, <u>86</u>, 7.

104. R. Gorodischer, W.J. Jusko, and S.J. Yaffe, <u>Res. Comm. Chem. Path. Pharmacol.</u>, 1977, <u>16</u>, 363.

105. G. Wettrell, <u>Eur. J. Clin. Pharmacol.</u>, 1977, <u>11</u>, 329.

106. H. Halkin, M. Radomsky, P. Millman, S. Almog, L. Blieden, and H. Boichis, <u>Eur. J. Clin. Pharmacol.</u>, 1978, <u>13</u>, 113.

107. L. Nyberg and G. Wettrell, <u>Clin. Pharmacokin.</u>, 1978, <u>3</u>, 453.

108. P.K. Ng, J. Cote, D. Schiff, and R.L. Collins-Nakai, <u>Res. Comm. Chem. Path. Pharmacol.</u>, 1981, <u>34</u>, 207.

109. W. Berman, Jr., J. Musselman, and R. Shortencarrier, <u>J. Pharmacokin. Biopharm.</u>, 1982, <u>10</u>, 173.

110. D.J. Weidler, N.S. Jallad, H.S. Movahhed, E. Sakmar, and J.G. Wagner, <u>Res. Commun. Chem. Path. Pharmacol.</u>, 1978, <u>19</u>, 57.

111. E. Tsutsumi, H. Fujiki, H. Takeda, and H. Fukushima, <u>J. Clin. Pharmacol.</u>, 1979, <u>19</u>, 200.

112. D.D. Brown, J.C. Dormois, G.N. Abraham, K. Lewis, and K. Dixon, <u>Clin. Pharmacol. Ther.</u>, 1976, <u>20</u>, 395.

113. A.D. Malcolm, F.Y. Leung, J.C.A. Fuchs, and J.E. Duarte, <u>Clin. Pharmacol. Ther.</u>, 1977, <u>21</u>, 567.

114. R.G. McAllister, Jr., S.M. Howell, M.S. Gomer, and J.B. Selby, <u>J. Clin. Pharmacol.</u>, 1976, <u>16</u>, 110.

115. J. Bonelli, H. Haydl, K. Hruby, and G. Kaik, <u>Int. J. Clin. Pharmacol.</u>, 1978, <u>16</u>, 302.

116. B. Cusack, J. Kelly, K. O'Malley, J. Noel, J. Lavan, and J. Horgan, <u>Clin. Pharmacol. Ther.</u>, 1979, <u>25</u>, 772.

117. H.R. Ochs, G. Bodem, and D.J. Greenblatt, <u>J. Clin. Pharmacol.</u>, 1981, <u>21</u>, 396.

118. E.B. Leahey, Jr., J.T. Bigger, Jr., V.P. Butler, Jr., J.A. Reiffel, G.C. O'Connell, L.E. Scaffidi, and J.N. Rottman, <u>Amer. J. Cardiol.</u>, 1981, <u>48</u>, 1141.

119. E. Steiness, S. Waldorff, P.B. Hansen, H. Kjaergård, J. Buch, and H. Egeblad, Clin. Pharmacol. Ther., 1980, 27, 791.

120. R. Dahlqvist, G. Ejvinsson, and K. Schenck-Gustafsson, Brit. J. Clin. Pharmacol., 1980, 9, 413.

121. S. Waldorff, P.B. Hansen, H. Kjaergard, J. Buch, H. Egeblad, and E. Steiness, Clin. Pharmacol. Ther., 1981, 30, 1972.

122. M. Wandell, J.R. Powell, W.D. Hager, P.E. Fenster, P.E. Graves, K.A. Conrad, and S. Goldman, Clin. Pharmacol. Ther., 1980, 28, 425.

123. K.E. Pedersen, A. Dorph-Pedersen, S. Hvidt, N.A. Klitgaard, and F. Nielsen-Kudsk, Clin. Pharmacol. Ther., 1981, 30, 311.

124. K.E. Pedersen, A. Dorph-Pedersen, S. Hvidt, N.A. Klitgaard, K. Kjaer, and F. Nielsen-Kudsk, Clin. Pharmacol. Ther., 1982, 32, 562.

125. P.E. Fenster, K.A. Comess, C.D. Hanson, and P.R. Finley, Clin. Pharmacol. Ther., 1982, 32, 428.

126. J.G. Wagner, K.D. Popat, S.K. Das, E. Sakmar, and H. Movahhed, J. Pharmacokin. Biopharm., 1981, 9, 147.

127. H.R. Ochs, D.J. Greenblatt, and G. Bodem, Clin. Pharmacol. Ther., 1980, 28, 340.

128. J.E. Doherty, J.K. Bissett, J.J. Kane, N. DeSoyza, M.L. Murphy, W.J. Flanigan, and G.V. Dalrymple, Int. J. Clin. Pharmacol. Biopharm., 1975, 12, 89.

129. J.G. Wagner, J.D. Yates, P.W. Willis, E. Sakmar, and R.G. Stoll, Clin. Pharmacol. Ther., 1974, 15, 291.

130. H. Halkin, L.B. Sheiner, C.C. Peck, and K.L. Melmon, Clin. Pharmacol. Ther., 1975, 17, 385.

131. J.R. Koup, W.J. Jusko, C.M. Elwood, and R.K. Kohli, Clin. Pharmacol. Ther., 1975, 18, 9.

132. W.J. Jusko, S.J. Szefler, and A.L. Goldfarb, J. Clin. Pharmacol., 1974, 14, 525.

133. W.J. Jusko and M. Weintraub, Clin. Pharmacol. Ther., 1974, 16, 449.

134. J.K. Aronson and D.G. Grahame-Smith, Brit. J. Clin. Pharmacol., 1976, 3, 1045.

135. W.J.F. van der Vijgh and P.L. Oe, Int. J. Clin. Pharmacol., 1977, 15, 249.

136. W.J.F. van der Vijgh and P.L. Oe, Int. J. Clin. Pharmacol., 1977, 15, 225.

137. D.J. Sumner, A.J. Russell, and B. Whiting, Brit. J. Clin. Pharmacol., 1976, 3, 221.

138. M.F. Paulson and P.G. Welling, J. Clin. Pharmacol., 1976, 16, 660.

139. J.H. Caldwell and C.T. Cline, Clin. Pharmacol. Ther., 1976, 19, 410.

140. G. Tsujimoto, T. Sasaki, T. Ishizaki, T. Suganuma, and H. Hirayama, Brit. J. Clin. Pharmacol., 1982, 13, 493.

141. M.H. Gault, D. Sugden, C. Maloney, M. Ahmed, and M. Tweeddale, Clin. Pharmacol. Ther., 1979, 25, 499.

142. E. Steiness, Clin. Pharmacol. Ther., 1978, 23, 511.

143. R.D. Okada, W.D. Hager, P.E. Graves, M. Mayersohn, D.G. Perrier, and F.I. Marcus, Circulation, 1978, 58, 1196.

144. W.J.F. van der Vijgh and P.L. Oe, Int. J. Clin. Pharmacol., 1978, 16, 540.

145. J.T. Slattery and J.R. Koup, Clin. Pharmacokin., 1979, 4, 395.

146. T.P. Gibson and H.A. Nelson, Clin. Pharmacol. Ther., 1980, 27, 219.

147. L.F. Soyka, Ped. Clin. N. Amer., 1972, 19, 241.

148. R.W. Jelliffe, J. Buell, and R. Kalaba, Ann. Int. Med., 1972, 77, 891.

149. C.C. Peck, L.B. Sheiner, C.M. Martin, D.T. Combs, and K.L. Melmon, New Engl. J. Med., 1973, 289, 441.

150. N.J.B. Christiansen, K. Kølendorf, K. Siersbaek-Nielsen, and J.M. Hansen, Acta Med. Scand., 1973, 194, 257.

151. A. Redfors, Brit. Heart J., 1972, 34, 383.

152. M.J. Stewart and W. Simpson, Lancet, 1972, ii, 493.

153. J.E. Doherty, New Engl. J. Med., 1971, 285, 1540.

154. N.A. Cohen, Lancet, 1972, i, 535.

155. J.D. Hobson and A. Zettner, J. Amer. Med. Assoc., 1973, 223, 147.

156. D. Citrin, I.H. Stevenson, and K. O'Malley, Scottish Med. J., 1972, 17, 275.

157. W. Shapiro, K. Taubert, and K. Narahara, Arch. Int. Med., 1972, 130, 31.

158. J. Morrison and T. Killip, Circulation, 1973, 47, 341.

159. D.D. Brown and G.N. Abraham, J. Lab. Clin. Med., 1973, 82, 201.

160. R.W. Jelliffe and G. Brooker, Amer. J. Med., 1974, 57, 63.

161. F.I. Marcus, Amer. J. Med., 1975, 58, 452.

162. J.G. Wagner, J. Clin. Pharmacol., 1974, 14, 379.

163. W.L. Chiou, J. Clin. Pharmacol., 1975, 15, 272.

164. N.J. Greenberger and F.B. Thomas, J. Lab. Clin. Med., 1973, 81, 241.

165. J.Q. Russell and C.D. Klaassen, J. Pharmacol. Exp. Ther., 1973, 186, 455.

166. J.Q. Russell and C.D. Klaassen, J. Pharmacol. Exp. Ther., 1972, 183, 513.

167. C.D. Klaassen, J. Pharmacol. Exp. Ther., 1972, 183, 520.

168. W. Schaumann, F. Zielske, K. Kohler, and K. Koch, Arch. Pharmakol., 1972, 272, 32.

169. N. Rietbrock, U. Abshagen, K. von Bergmann, and H. Kewitz, Arch. Pharmakol., 1972, 274, 171.

170. G. Härtel, V. Manninen, J. Melin, and A. Apajalahti, Ann. Clin. Res., 1973, 5, 87.

171. B. Beermann, Eur. J. Clin. Pharmacol., 1972, 5, 28.

172. W. Doering, E. König, D. Kronski, and D. Hall, Deut. Med. Woch., 1973, 98, 2274.

173. M.C. Castle and G.L. Lage, Biochem. Pharmacol., 1972, 21, 1449.

174. U. Abshagen, Arch. Pharmakol., 1973, 278, 91.

175. N. Rietbrock, U. Abshagen, K. von Bergmann, and H. Kewitz, Arch. Pharmakol., 1972, 274, 171.

176. M.C. Castle and G.L. Lage, Res. Comm. Chem. Path. Pharmacol., 1973, 5, 99.

177. M.C. Castle and G.L. Lage, Drug Metab. Dispos., 1973, 1, 590.

178. P.H. Hinderling, E.R. Garrett, and R.C. Wester, J. Pharm. Sci., 1977, 66, 242.

179. P.H. Hinderling, E.R. Garrett, and R.C. Wester, J. Pharm. Sci., 1977, 66, 314.

180. P.H. Hinderling and E.R. Garrett, J. Pharm. Sci., 1977, 66, 326.

181. F. Keller H.P. Blumenthal K. Maertin, and N. Reitbrock, Eur. J. Clin. Pharmacol., 1977, 12, 387.

182. N. Rietbrock, J. Guggenmos, J. Kuhlmann, and U. Hess, Eur. J. Clin. Pharmacol., 1976, 9, 373.

183. J. Marinow, A. Olcay, W. Schaumann, and W. Weiss, Eur. J. Clin. Pharmacol., 1977, 11, 213.

184. J.H. Wood, J. Amer. Pharm. Assoc., 1976, NS.16, 467.

185. L. Storstein, Clin. Pharmacol. Ther., 1976, 20, 6.

186. L. Storstein and H. Janssen, Clin. Pharmacol. Ther., 1976, 20, 15.

187. L. Storstein, Clin. Pharmacol. Ther., 1976, 20, 158.

188. H.F. Vöhringer, N. Rietbrock, P. Spurny, J. Kuhlmann, H. Hampl, and R. Baethke, Clin. Pharmacol. Ther., 1976, 19, 387.

189. L. Storstein, Clin. Pharmacol. Ther., 1976, 21, 536.

190. H.F. Vöhringer and N. Rietbrock, Clin. Pharmacol. Ther., 1974, 16, 796.

191.   J.-O. Branstad, U. Meresaar, and A. Agren, <u>Acta Pharm. Suecica</u>, 1972, <u>9</u>, 129.

192.   L. Storstein, <u>Clin. Pharmacol. Ther.</u>, 1975, <u>17</u>, 313.

193.   U. Peters, T.-U. Hausamen, and F. Grosse-Brockhoff, <u>Deut. Med. Woch.</u>, 1974, <u>99</u>, 2381.

194.   H.-F. Vöhringer, L. Weller, and N. Rietbrock, <u>Arch. Pharmacol.</u>, 1975, <u>287</u>, 129.

195.   M.A. Donovan, C.M. Castleden, J.E.F. Pohl, and C.A. Kraft, <u>Brit. J. Clin. Pharmacol.</u>, 1981, <u>11</u>, 401.

196.   T.W. Smith, R. Selden, and W. Findley, <u>Clin. Res.</u>, 1971, <u>19</u>, 356.

197.   J.R. Benotti, L.J. Lesko, and J.E. McCue, <u>J. Clin. Pharmacol.</u>, 1982, <u>22</u>, 425.

198.   F. Chanoine, M.S. Benedetti, J.-F. Ancher, and P. Dostert, <u>Arzneim.-Forsch.</u>, 1981, <u>31</u>, 1430.

199.   B.I. Sasyniuk and R.I. Ogilvie, <u>Ann. Rev. Pharmacol.</u>, 1975, <u>15</u>, 131.

200.   J. Koch-Weser, <u>Clin. Pharmacokin.</u>, 1977, <u>2</u>, 389.

201.   C. Graffner, G. Johnsson, and J. Sjogren, <u>Clin. Pharmacol. Ther.</u>, 1975, <u>17</u>, 414.

202.   E. Karlsson, <u>Eur. J. Clin. Pharmacol.</u>, 1973, <u>6</u>, 245.

203.   D. Fremstad, S. Dahl, S. Jacobsen, P.K.M. Lunde, K.J. Nadland, A.A. Marthinsen, T. Waaler, and K.H. Landmark, <u>Eur. J. Clin. Pharmacol.</u>, 1973, <u>6</u>, 251.

204.   J. Birkhead, T. Evans, P. Mumford, E. Martinez, and D. Jewitt, <u>Brit. Heart J.</u>, 1976, <u>38</u>, 77.

205.   T. Cunningham, G. Sloman, and G. Nyberg, <u>Med. J. Austral.</u>, 1977, <u>1</u>, 370.

206.   W. Campbell, W. J. Tilstone, D.H. Lawson, I. Hutton, and T.D.V. Lawrie, <u>Brit. J. Clin. Pharmacol.</u>, 1976, <u>3</u>, 1023.

207.   T.C. Smith and A.W. Kinkel, <u>Curr. Ther. Res.</u>, 1980, <u>27</u>, 217.

208.   J. Dreyfuss, J.T. Bigger, A.I. Cohen, and E.C. Schreiber, <u>Clin. Pharmacol. Ther.</u>, 1972, <u>13</u>, 366.

209.   A. Hunter and C.D. Klaassen, <u>Proc. Soc. Exp. Biol. Med.</u>, 1972, <u>139</u>, 1445.

210.   B.L. Kamath, C.-M. Lai, S.D. Gupta, M.J. Durrani, and A. Yacobi, <u>J. Pharm. Sci.</u>, 1981, <u>70</u>, 299.

211.   P.G. Basseches and G.J. DiGregorio, <u>J. Pharm. Sci.</u>, 1982, <u>71</u>, 1256.

212.   H. Weily and E. Genton, <u>Clin. Res.</u>, 1971, <u>19</u>, 169.

213.   E.G.V. Giardina, J.T. Biggar, Jr., R.H. Heissenbuttel, and E. Yu, <u>Clin. Res.</u>, 1971, <u>19</u>, 349.

214.   H.S. Weily and E. Genton, <u>Arch. Int. Med.</u>, 1972, <u>130</u>, 366.

215. C.V. Manion, D. Lalka, D.T. Baer, and M.B. Meyer, J. Pharm. Sci., 1977, 66, 983.

216. J.S. Dutcher, J.M. Strong, S.V. Lucas, W. Lee, and A.J. Atkinson, Clin. Pharmacol. Ther., 1977, 22, 447.

217. D.E. Drayer, D.T. Lowenthal, R.L. Woosley, A.S. Nies, A. Schwartz, and M.M. Reidenberg, Clin. Pharmacol. Ther., 1977, 22, 63.

218. A.J. Atkinson, Jr., F.A. Krumlovsky, C.M. Huang, and F. del Greco, Clin. Pharmacol. Ther., 1976, 20, 585.

219. E.V. Giardina, J. Dreyfus, J.T. Bigger, Jr., J.M. Shaw, and E.C. Schreiber., Clin. Pharmacol. Ther., 1976, 19, 339.

220. P. du Souich and S. Erill, Eur. J. Clin. Pharmacol., 1978, 14, 21.

221. P. du Souich and S. Erill, Clin. Pharmacol. Ther., 1977, 22, 588.

222. R.L. Galeazzi, L.Z. Benet, and L.B. Sheiner, Clin. Pharmacol. Ther., 1976, 20, 278.

223. R.L. Galeazzi, C. Omar-Amberg, and G. Karlaganis, Clin. Pharmacol. Ther., 1981, 29, 440.

224. E. Karlsson, L. Molin, B. Norlander, and F. Sjoqvist, Brit. J. Clin. Pharmacol., 1974, 1, 467.

225. T.P. Gibson, J. Matusik, E. Matusik, H.A. Nelson, J. Wilkinson, and W.A. Briggs, Clin. Pharmacol. Ther., 1975, 17, 395.

226. M.M. Reidenberg, D.E. Drayer, M. Levy, and H. Warner, Clin. Pharmacol. Ther., 1975, 17, 722.

227. C. Graffner, J. Pharmacokin. Biopharm., 1975, 3, 69.

228. J. Elson, J.M. Strong, W.-K. Lee, and A.J. Atkinson, Jr., Clin. Pharmacol. Ther., 1975, 17, 134.

229. J.M. Strong, J.S. Dutcher, W.-K. Lee, and A.J. Atkinson, Jr., J. Pharmacokin. Biopharm., 1975, 3, 223.

230. J. Dreyfuss, J.T. Bigger, Jr., A.I. Cohn, and E.C. Schreiber, Clin. Pharmacol. Ther., 1972, 13, 366.

231. J.M. Strong, J.S. Dutcher, W.-K. Lee, and A.J. Atkinson, Jr., Clin. Pharmacol. Ther., 1975, 18, 613.

232. D. Lalka, M.G. Wyman, B.N. Goldreyer, T.M. Ludden, and D.S. Cannom, J. Clin. Pharmacol., 1978, 18, 397.

233. J.J. Lima, D.R. Conti, A.L. Goldfarb, L.H. Golden, and W.J. Jusko, Eur. J. Clin. Pharmacol., 1978, 13, 303.

234. E. Karlsson, Clin. Pharmacokin., 1978, 3, 97.

235. P. Schröder, N.A. Klitgaard, and E. Simonsen, Eur. J. Clin. Pharmacol., 1979, 15, 63.

236. T.P. Gibson, A.J. Atkinson, E. Matusik, L.D. Nelson, and W.A. Briggs, Kidney Int., 1977, 12, 422.

237. G.P. Stec, A.J. Atkinson, M.J. Nevin, J.-P. Thenot, T.I. Ruo, T.P. Gibson, P. Ivanovich, and F. del Greco, *Clin. Pharmacol. Ther.*, 1979, 26, 618.

238. M.M. Reidenberg, M. Camacho, J. Kluger, and D.E. Drayer, *Clin. Pharmacol. Ther.*, 1980, 28, 732.

239. M.G. Wyman, B.N. Goldreyer, D.S. Cannom, T.M. Ludden, and D. Lalka, *J. Clin. Pharmacol.*, 1981, 21, 20.

240. S. Singh, H. Gelband, A.V. Mehta , K. Kessler, A. Casta, and A.S. Pickoff, *Clin. Pharmacol. Ther.*, 1982, 32, 607.

241. T.M. Ludden and M.H. Crawford, *Clin. Pharmacol. Ther.*, 1982, 31, 343.

242. R.E. Kates, P. Jaillon, D.S. Rubenson, and R.A. Winkle, *Clin. Pharmacol. Ther.*, 1980, 28, 52.

243. J.E. Brown and D.G. Shand, *Clin. Pharmacokin.*, 1982, 7, 125.

244. S.J. Connolly and R.E. Kates, *Clin. Pharmacokin.*, 1982, 7, 206.

245. W.D. Mason, J.O. Covinsky, J.L. Valentine K.L. Kelly, O.H. Weddle, and B.L. Martz, *J. Pharm. Sci.*, 1976, 65, 1325.

246. D.J. Greenblatt, H.J. Pfeifer, H.R. Ochs, K. Franke, D.S. MacLaughlin, T.W. Smith, and J. Koch-Weser, *J. Pharmacol. Exp. Ther.*, 1977, 202, 365.

247. T.W. Guentert, R.A. Upton, N.H.G. Holford, A. Bostrom, and S. Riegelman, *J. Pharmacokin. Biopharm.*, 1980, 8, 243.

248. I.J. McGilveray, K.K. Midha, M. Rowe, N. Beaudoin, and C. Charette, *J. Pharm. Sci.*, 1981, 70, 524.

249. T. Huynh-Ngoc, M. Chabot, and G. Sirois, *J. Pharm. Sci.*, 1978, 67, 1456.

250. J.D. Strum, J.W. Ebersole, J.M. Jaffe, J.L. Colazzi, and R.I. Poust, *J. Pharm. Sci.*, 1978, 67, 568.

251. C.T. Ueda, B.J. Williamson, and B.S. Dzindzio, *Clin. Pharmacol. Ther.*, 1976, 20, 260.

252. R. Henning and G. Nyberg, *Eur. J. Clin. Pharmacol.*, 1973, 6, 239.

253. W.A. Mahon, M. Mayersohn, and T. Inaba, *Clin. Pharmacol. Ther.*, 1976, 19, 566.

254. K.A. Conrad, B.L. Molk, and C.A. Chidsey, *Circulation*, 1977, 55, 1.

255. G. Gaul and E. Aldor, *Arzneim.-Forsch.*, 1981, 31, 1486.

256. C.G. Regardh, G. Johnsson, P. Lundborg, and B.A. Persson, *Arzneim.-Forsch.*, 1977, 27, 1716.

257. G.M. Frigo, E. Perucca, M. Teggia-Droghi, G. Gatti, A. Mussini, and J. Salerno, *Brit. J. Clin. Pharmacol.*, 1977, 4, 449.

258. C.T. Ueda and B.S. Dzindzio, *Brit. J. Clin. Pharmacol.*, 1981, 11, 571.

259. J. Spénard, G. Sirois, and M.A. Gagnon, Brit. J. Clin. Pharmacol., 1982, 13, 752.

260. U. Otto and L. Paalzow, Acta Pharmacol. Toxicol., 1975, 36, 415.

261. T.W. Guentert, N.H.G. Holford, P.E. Coates, R.A. Upton, and S. Riegelman, J. Pharmacokin. Biopharm, 1979, 7, 315.

262. T.W. Guentert, R.A. Upton, N.H.G. Holford, and S. Riegelman, J. Pharmacokin. Biopharm., 1979, 7, 303.

263. W.D. Wosilait, Life Sci., 1974, 14, 2189.

264. W.D. Wosilait, Res. Comm. Chem. Path. Pharmacol., 1975, 12, 147.

265. V.E. Isaacs and R.D. Schoenwald, J. Pharm. Sci., 1974, 63, 1119.

266. K.M. Kessler, D.T. Lowenthal, H. Warner, T. Gibson, W. Briggs, and M.M. Reidenberg, New Engl. J. Med., 1974, 290, 706.

267. D. Fremstad, O.G. Nilsen, L. Storstein, J. Amlie, and S. Jacobsen, Eur. J. Clin. Pharmacol., 1979, 15, 187.

268. E. Woo and D.J. Greenblatt, J. Pharm. Sci., 1979, 68, 466.

269. R.E. Kates and M.F. Blanford, J. Clin. Pharmacol., 1979, 19, 378.

270. H.R. Ochs, D.J. Greenblatt, E. Woo, K. Franke, and T.W. Smith, Pharmacology, 1978, 17, 301.

271. C.T. Ueda and B.S. Dzindzio, Clin. Pharmacol. Ther., 1978, 23, 158.

272. C.T. Ueda and B.S. Dzindzio, Eur. J. Clin. Pharmacol., 1979, 16, 101.

273. D.E. Drayer, D.T. Lowenthal, K.M. Restivo, A. Schwartz, C.E. Cook, and M.M. Reidenberg, Clin. Pharmacol. Ther., 1978, 24, 31.

274. S. Yosselson-Superstine, Y. Yanuka, and S. Ishai, Int. J. Clin. Pharmacol. Ther. Toxicol., 1982, 20, 181.

275. K. M. Kessler and G.O. Perez, Clin. Pharmacol. Ther., 1981, 30, 121.

276. A.S. Pickoff, K.M. Kessler, S. Singh, G.S. Wolff, D.F. Tamer, O.L. Garcia, and H. Gelband, Dev. Pharmacol. Ther., 1981, 3, 108.

277. T.W. Guentert and S. Øie, J. Pharm. Sci., 1982, 71, 325.

278. J. Russo, Jr., M.E. Russo, R.A. Smith, and L.K. Pershing, J. Clin. Pharmacol., 1982, 22, 264.

279. D.E. Drayer, M. Hughes, B. Lorenzo, and M.M. Reidenberg, Clin. Pharmacol. Ther., 1980, 27, 72.

280. P. Jaillon and R.E. Kates, J. Pharmacol. Exp. Ther., 1980, 213, 33.

281. C.T. Ueda, D.S. Hirschfeld, M.M. Scheinman, M. Rowland, B.J. Williamson, and B.S. Dzindzio, Clin. Pharmacol. Ther., 1976, 19, 30.

282. C.T. Ueda, B.E. Ballard, and M. Rowland, J. Pharmacol. Exp. Ther., 1977, 200, 459.

283. C.A. Neff, L.D. Davis, and J.D. Baggot, Amer. J. Vet. Res., 1972, 33, 1521.

284. D.J. Greenblatt, V. Bolognini, J. Koch-Weser, J.S. Harmatz, J. Amer. Med. Assoc., 1976, 236, 273.

285. N.I. Benowitz and W. Meister, Clin. Pharmacokin., 1978, 3, 177.

286. E. Perucca and A. Richens, Brit. J. Clin. Pharmacol., 1979, 8, 21.

287. G.G. deBoer, D.D. Breimer, H. Mattie, J. Pronk, and J.M. Gubbens-Stibbe, Clin. Pharmacol. Ther., 1979, 26, 701.

288. K.K. Adjepon-Yamoah, D.B. Scott, and L.F. Prescott, Brit. J. Anaesthesia, 1973, 45, 143.

289. A.G. deBoer, D.D. Breimer, J. Pronk, and J.M. Gubbens-Stibbe, J. Pharm. Sci., 1980, 69, 804.

290. T. Nishihata, J.H. Rytting, and T. Higuchi, J. Pharm. Sci., 1982, 71, 869.

291. K.K. Adjepon-Yamoah, D.B. Scott, and L.F. Prescott, Eur. J. Clin. Pharmacol., 1974, 7, 397.

292. E. Karlsson, P. Collste, and M.D. Rawlins, Eur. J. Clin. Pharmacol., 1974, 7, 455.

293. M.M. Bassan, S.R. Weinstein, and W.J. Mandel, Amer. Heart J., 1974, 87, 302.

294. D. Shen and M. Gibaldi, J. Clin. Pharmacol., 1974, 14, 339.

295. L. Ryden, H. Wasir, T.-B. Conradsson, and B. Olsson, Brit. Heart J., 1972, 34, 1012.

296. L.S. Cohen, J.E. Rosenthal, D.W. Horner, J.M. Atkins, O.A. Matthews, and S.J. Sarnoff, Amer. J. Cardiol., 1972, 28, 520.

297. K. Okumura, H. Sezaki, and K. Kakemi, Chem. Pharm. Bull. (Japan), 1972, 20, 1607.

298. D. Oltmanns, Ch. Lübben, R. Pentz, and C.-P. Siegers, Int. J. Clin. Pharmacol. Ther. Toxicol., 1982, 20, 582.

299. J.A.H. Forrest, N.D.C. Finlayson, K.K. Adjepon-Yamoah, and L.F. Prescott, Brit. Med. J., 1977, 1, 1384.

300. J. LeLorier, D. Grenon, Y. Latour, G. Caille, G. Dumont, A. Brosseau, and A. Solignac, Ann. Internal Med., 1977, 87, 700.

301. L.F. Prescott, K.K. Adjepon-Yamoah, and R.G. Talbot, Brit. Med. J., 1976, 1, 939.

302. K. Ahmad and F. Medzihradsky, Res. Comm. Chem. Path. Pharmacol., 1971, 2, 813.

303. J.B. Keenaghan and R.N. Boyes, J. Pharmacol. Exp. Ther., 1972, 180, 454.

304. N. Benowitz, R.P. Forsyth, K.L. Melmon, and M. Rowland, Clin. Pharmacol. Ther., 1974, 16, 87.

305. N. Benowitz, R.P. Forsyth, K.L. Melmon, and M. Rowland, <u>Clin. Pharmacol. Ther.</u>, 1974, <u>16</u>, 99.

306. K.A. Collinsworth, J.M. Strong, A.J. Atkinson, Jr., R.A. Winkle, F. Perlroth, and D.C. Harrison, <u>Clin. Pharmacol. Ther.</u>, 1975, <u>18</u>, 59.

307. H. Halkin, P. Meffin, K.L. Melmon, and M. Rowland, <u>Clin. Pharmacol. Ther.</u>, 1975, <u>17</u>, 669.

308. P.A. Routledge, D.G. Shand, A. Barchowsky, G. Wagner, and W.W. Stargel, <u>Clin. Pharmacol. Ther.</u>, 1981, <u>30</u>, 154.

309. A. Barchowsky, D.G. Shand, W.W. Stargel, G.S. Wagner, and P.A. Routledge, <u>Brit. J. Clin. Pharmacol.</u>, 1982, <u>13</u>, 411.

310. P.A. Routledge, A. Barchowsky, T.D. Bjornsson, B.B. Kitchell, and D.G. Shand, <u>Clin. Pharmacol. Ther.</u>, 1980, <u>27</u>, 347.

311. M. Finster, H.O. Morishima, R.N. Boyes, and B.G. Covino, <u>Anaesthesiology</u>, 1972, <u>36</u>, 159.

312. M. Esquivel, T.F. Blaschke, G.H. Snidow, and P.J. Meffin, <u>J. Pharm. Pharmacol.</u>, 1978, <u>30</u>, 804.

313. N. Vicuna, D. Lalka, S.R. Burrow, A.J. McLean, P. du Souich, and J.L. McNay, <u>Res. Commun. Chem. Path. Pharmacol.</u>, 1978, <u>22</u>, 485.

314. H.O. Morishima, M. Finster, H. Pedersen, A. Fukunaga, R.A. Ronfeld, H.G. Vassallo, and B.G. Covino, <u>Anaesthesiology</u>, 1979, <u>50</u>, 431.

315. W.L. Blankenbaker, C.A. DiFazio, and F.A. Berry, <u>Anaesthesiology</u>, 1975, <u>42</u>, 325.

316. L.A. Bauer, T. Brown, M. Gibaldi, L. Hudson, S. Nelson, V. Raisys, and J.P. Shea, <u>Clin. Pharmacol. Ther.</u>, 1982, <u>31</u>, 433.

317. R.A. Zito and P.R. Reid, <u>J. Clin. Pharmacol.</u>, 1981, <u>21</u>, 100.

318. A.T. Elvin, A.F.D. Cole, J.A. Pieper, S.H. Rolbin, and D. Lalka, <u>Clin. Pharmacol. Ther.</u>, 1981, <u>30</u>, 455.

319. T.L. Svendsen, M. Tangφ, S. Waldorff, E. Steiness, and J. Trap-Jensen, <u>Brit. J. Clin. Pharmacol.</u>, 1982, <u>13</u>, 223S.

320. C.A. DiFazio and R.E. Brown, <u>Anaesthesiology</u>, 1972, <u>36</u>, 238.

321. R.L. Williams, T.F. Blaschke, P.J. Meffin, K.L. Melmon, and M. Rowland, <u>Clin. Pharmacol. Ther.</u>, 1976, <u>20</u>, 290.

322. R.L. Nation, E.J. Triggs, and M. Selig, <u>Brit. J. Clin. Pharmacol.</u>, 1977, <u>4</u>, 439.

323. P.D. Thomson, K.L. Melmon, J.A. Richardson, K. Cohn, W. Steinbrunn, R. Cudihee, and M. Rowland, <u>Ann. Int. Med.</u>, 1973, <u>78</u>, 499.

324. D. Lalka, M.B. Meyer, B.R. Duce, and A.T. Elvin, <u>Clin. Pharmacol. Ther.</u>, 1976, <u>19</u>, 757.

325. R.A. Winkle, P.J. Meffin, J.W. Fitzgerald, and D.C. Harrison, <u>Circulation</u>, 1976, <u>54</u>, 884.

326. R.A. Ronfeld, E.M. Wolshin, and A.J. Block, <u>Clin. Pharmacol. Ther.</u>, 1982, <u>31</u>, 384.

327. U. Klotz and E. Golbs, Arzneim.-Forsch., 1980, 30, 619.

328. P.J. Meffin, E.W. Robert, R.A. Winkle, S. Harapat, F.A. Peters, and D.C. Harrison, J. Pharmacokin. Biopharm., 1979, 7, 29.

329. D.B. Haughey and J.J. Lima, Eur. J. Clin. Pharmacol., 1982, 22, 185.

330. J.L. Cunningham, D.D. Shen, I. Shudo, and D.L. Azarnoff, Brit. J. Clin. Pharmacol., 1978, 5, 343.

331. D.K. Dubetz, N.N. Brown, W.D. Hooper, M.J. Eadie, and J.H. Tyrer, Brit. J. Clin. Pharmacol., 1978, 6, 279.

332. G. Forssell, C. Graffner, R. Nordlander, and O. Nyquist, Eur. J. Clin. Pharmacol., 1980, 17, 209.

333. K.M. Giacomini, S.E. Swezey, K. Turner-Tamiyasu, and T.F. Blaschke, J. Pharmacokin. Biopharm., 1982, 10, 1.

334. S.M. Bryson, J.R. Lawrence, W.H. Steele B.C. Campbell, H.L. Elliott, and D.J. Sumner, Eur. J. Clin. Pharmacol., 1982, 23, 453.

335. J.R. Lawrence, S.M. Bryson, D.J. Sumner, B.C. Campbell, and B. Whiting, Biopharm. Drug Dispos., 1979, 1, 51.

336. D.D. Shen, J.L. Cunningham, I. Shudo, and D.L. Azarnoff, Biopharm. Drug Dispos., 1980, 1, 133.

337. A. Johnston, J.A. Henry, S.J. Warrington, and N.A.J. Hamer, Brit. J. Clin. Pharmacol., 1980, 10, 245.

338. A.J. Jounela, P.J. Pentikäinen, and K. Oksanen, Int. J. Clin. Pharmacol. Ther. Toxicol., 1982, 20, 276.

339. S.M. Bryson, C.J. Cairns, and B. Whiting, Brit. J. Clin. Pharmacol., 1982, 13, 417.

340. K. Landmark, J.E. Bredesen, E. Thaulow, S. Simonsen, and J.P. Amlie, Eur. J. Clin. Pharmacol., 1981, 19, 187.

341. K.F. Ilett, B.W. Madsen, and J.D. Woods, Clin. Pharmacol. Ther., 1979, 26, 1.

342. A. Karim, C. Kook, R.L. Novotney, J. Zagarella, and J. Campion, Drug Metab. Dispos., 1978, 6, 338.

343. P.H. Hinderling and E.R. Garrett, J. Pharmacokin. Biopharm., 1976, 4, 199.

344. P.H. Hinderling and E.R. Garrett, J. Pharmacokin. Biopharm., 1976, 4, 231.

345. I. Hirshleifer, Curr. Ther. Res., 1973, 15, 616.

346. S.G. Hastings, Arch. Int. Pharmacodyn., 1973, 203, 117.

347. H. Maier-Lenz, L. Ringwelski, and A. Windorfer, Arzneim.-Forsch., 1980, 30, 320.

348. S. Sved, W.M. McLean, and I.J. McGilveray, J. Pharm. Sci., 1981, 70, 1368.

349. P.K. Noonan and R.C. Wester, J. Pharm. Sci., 1980, 69, 365.

350. P.R. Imhof, A. Sieber, J. Hodler, P. Müller, B. Ott, P. Fankhauser, L.-C. Chu, and A. Gérardin, Eur. J. Clin. Pharmacol., 1982, 23, 99.

351. E.F. McNiff, A. Yacobi, F.M. Young-Chang, L.H. Golden, A. Goldfarb, and H.-L. Fung, J. Pharm. Sci., 1981, 70, 1054.

352. E.M. Johnson, A.B. Harkey, D.J. Blehm, and P. Needleman, J. Pharmacol. Exp. Ther., 1972, 182, 56.

353. D.F. Assinder, L.F. Chasseaud, J.O. Hunter, R.J. Jung, and T. Taylor, Arzneim.-Forsch., 1977, 27, 156.

354. T. Taylor, L.F. Chasseaud, and E. Doyle, Biopharm. Drug Dispos., 1980, 1, 149.

355. R.A. Morrison, H.-L. Fung, D. Höhmann, T. Meinertz, and E. Jähnchen, J. Pharm. Sci., 1982, 71, 721.

356. P.A. Cossum and M.S. Roberts, Eur. J. Clin. Pharmacol., 1981, 19. 181.

357. T. Taylor, D.A. O'Kelly, R.M. Major, A. Darragh, and L.F. Chasseaud, Arzneim.-Forsch., 1978, 28, 1426.

358. D.F. Assinder, L.F. Chasseaud, and T. Taylor, J. Pharm. Sci., 1977, 66, 775.

359. V. Gladigau, G. Neurath, M. Dünger, K. Schnelle, and K.I. Johnson, Arzneim.-Forsch., 1981, 31, 835.

360. K.I. Johnson, V. Gladigau, and K. Schnelle, Arzneim.-Forsch., 1981, 31, 1026.

361. L.F. Chasseaud, E. Doyle, and T. Taylor, Biopharm. Drug Dispos., 1981, 2, 273.

362. S.J. Shane, J.J. Iazzetta, A.W. Chisholm, J.F. Berka, and D. Leung, Brit. J. Clin. Pharmacol., 1978, 6, 37.

363. D. Mansel-Jones, T. Taylor, E. Doyle, L.F. Chasseaud, A. Darragh, D.A. O'Kelly, and H. Over, J. Clin. Pharmacol., 1978, 18, 544.

364. H.-L. Fung, E.F. McNiff, D. Ruggirello, A. Darke, U. Thadani, and J.O. Parker, Brit. J. Clin. Pharmacol., 1981, 11, 579.

365. E. Doyle and L.F. Chasseaud, J. Pharm. Sci., 1981, 70, 1270.

366. T. Taylor, L.F. Chasseaud, R. Major, and E. Doyle, Biopharm. Drug Dispos., 1981, 2, 255.

367. U. Abshagen, G. Betzien, R. Endele, and B. Kaufmann, Eur. J. Clin. Pharmacol., 1981, 20, 269.

368. S. Spörl-Radun, G. Betzien, B. Kaufmann, V. Liede, and U. Abshagen, Eur. J. Clin. Pharmacol., 1980, 18, 237.

369. M.G. Bogaert, M.T. Rosseel, J. Boelaert, and R. Daneels, Eur. J. Clin. Pharmacol., 1981, 21, 73.

370. I.W.F. Davidson, H.S. Miller, Jr., and F.J. DiCarlo, J. Pharm. Sci., 1971, 60, 274.

371. I.W.F. Davidson, H.S. Miller, Jr., and F.J. DiCarlo, J. Pharmacol. Exp. Ther., 1970, 175, 42.

372. I.W.F. Davidson, F.O. Rollins, F.J. DiCarlo, and H.S. Miller, Jr., Clin. Pharmacol. Ther., 1971, 12, 972.

373. I.D. Bradbrook, P. Feldschreiber, P.J. Morrison, H.J. Rogers, and R.G. Spector, Eur. J. Clin. Pharmacol., 1981, 19, 301.

374. P.J. Pentikäinen, I.H. Koivula, and H.A. Hiltunen, Eur. J. Clin. Pharmacol., 1982, 23, 261.

375. M. Eichelbaum, A. Somogyi, G.E. von Unruh, and H.J. Dengler, Eur. J. Clin. Pharmacol., 1981, 19, 133.

376. A. Johnston, C.D. Burgess, and J. Hamer, Brit. J. Clin. Pharmacol., 1981, 12, 397.

377. D.L. Keefe, Y.-G. Yee, and R.E. Kates, Clin. Pharmacol. Ther., 1981, 29, 21.

378. J.G. Wagner, A.P. Rocchini, and J. Vasiliades, Clin. Pharmacol. Ther., 1982, 32, 172.

379. P. Anderson, U. Bondesson, and C. Sylvén, Eur. J. Clin. Pharmacol., 1982, 23, 49.

380. B.G. Woodcock, W. Schulz, G. Kober, and N. Rietbrock, Clin. Pharmacol. Ther., 1981, 30, 52.

381. R.E. Kates, D.L.D. Keefe, J. Schwartz, S. Harapat, E.B. Kirsten, and D.C. Harrison, Clin. Pharmacol. Ther., 1981, 30, 44.

382. B.G. Woodcock, I. Rietbrock, H.F. Vöhringer, and N. Rietbrock, Clin. Pharmacol. Ther., 1981, 29, 27.

383. A. Somogyi, M. Albrecht, G. Kliems, K. Schäfer, and M. Eichelbaum, Brit. J. Clin. Pharmacol., 1981, 12, 51.

384. B.G. Woodcock and N. Rietbrock, Brit. J. Clin. Pharmacol., 1982, 13, 240.

385. E.L. Kinney, R.M. Moskowitz, and R. Zelis, J. Clin. Pharmacol., 1981, 21, 337.

386. M. Anastasiou-Nana, G.M. Levis, and S. Moulopoulos, Int. J. Clin. Pharmacol. Ther. Toxicol., 1982, 20, 524.

387. F. Andreasen, H. Agerbaek, P. Bjerregaard, and H. Gøtzsche, Eur. J. Clin. Pharmacol., 1981, 19, 293.

388. R. Kannan, K. Nademanee, J.A. Hendrickson, H.J. Rostami, and B.N. Singh, Clin. Pharmacol. Ther., 1982, 31, 438.

389. E.R. Garrett, J.R. Green, Jr., and M. Bialer, Biopharm. Drug Dispos., 1982, 3, 129.

390. P.G. Welling, J.H. Thomsen, A.L. Shug, and F.L.S. Tse, Int. J. Clin. Pharmacol. Biopharm., 1979, 17, 56.

391. R.J. Wills, J.H. Thomsen, and P.G. Welling, Drugs Exp. Clin. Res., 1979, 5, 19.

392. A. Bizzi, M. Cini, S. Garattini, G. Mingardi, L. Licini, and G. Mecca, Lancet, 1979, 1, 882.

393. G. Johnsson and C.G. Regårdh, Clin. Pharmacokin., 1976, 1, 233.

394. D.G. Shand, Postgrad. Med. J., 1976, 52 (suppl. 4), 22.

395. J. Meier, Cardiology, 1979, 64 (suppl. 1), 1.

396. D.G. Shand, Drugs, 1974, 7, 39.

397. T. Suzuki, S. Isozaki, R. Ishida, Y. Saitoh, and F. Nakagawa, Chem. Pharm. Bull. (Japan), 1974, 22, 1639.

398. C.A. Chidsey, P. Morselli, G. Bianchetti, A. Morganti, G. Leonetti, and A. Zanchetti, Circulation, 1975, 52, 313.

399. P.J. Meffin, R.A. Winkle, F.A. Peters, and D.C. Harrison, Clin. Pharmacol. Ther., 1977, 22, 557.

400. A.A. Gulaid, I.M. James, C.M. Kaye, O.R.W. Lewellen, E. Roberts, M. Sankey, J. Smith, R. Templeton, and R.J. Thomas, Biopharm. Drug Dispos., 1981, 2, 103.

401. A. Roux, B. Flouvat, N.P. Chau, B. Letac, and M. Lucsko, Brit. J. Clin. Pharmacol., 1980, 9, 215.

402. C.M. Kaye and A.D. Long, Brit. J. Clin. Pharmacol., 1976, 3, 196.

403. P.J. Meffin, S.R. Harapat, and D.C. Harrison, Res. Comm. Chem. Path. Pharmacol., 1976, 15, 31.

404. M.A. Martin, F.C. Phillips, G.T. Tucker, and A.J. Smith, Eur. J. Clin. Pharmacol., 1978, 14, 383.

405. P.J. Meffin, R.A. Winkle, F.A. Peters, and D.C. Harrison, Clin. Pharmacol. Ther., 1978, 24, 542.

406. T.J. Coombs, C.J. Coulson, and V.J. Smith, Brit. J. Clin. Pharmacol., 1980, 9, 395.

407. R. Zaman, D.B. Jack, and M.J. Kendall, Brit. J. Clin. Pharmacol., 1981, 12, 427.

408. A. Roux, P. Aubert, J. Guedon, and B. Flouvat, Eur. J. Clin. Pharmacol., 1980, 17, 339.

409. K. Ohashi, S.J. Warrington, C.M. Kaye, G.W. Houghton, M. Dennis, R. Templeton, and P. Turner, Brit. J. Clin. Pharmacol., 1981, 12, 561.

410. B. Flouvat, A. Roux, B. Delhotal, D. Lemaigre, M. Leroy, and F. Liot, Int. J. Clin. Pharmacol. Ther. Toxicol., 1982, 20, 358.

411. C.-G. Regårdh, Acta Pharmacol. Toxicol., 1975, 37, 2.

412. N.-O. Bodin, K.O. Borg, R. Johansson, H. Obainwu, and R. Svensson, Acta Pharmacol. Toxicol., 1974, 35, 261.

413. M.D. Rawlins, P. Collste, M. Frisk-Holmberg, M. Lind, J. Östman, and F. Sjoqvist, J. Clin. Pharmacol., 1974, 7, 353.

414. G. Alvan, M. Lind, B. Mellstrom, and C. von Bahr, J. Pharmacokin. Biopharm., 1977, 5, 193.

415. G. Alvan, K. Piafsky, M. Lind, and C. von Bahr, Clin. Pharmacol. Ther., 1977, 22, 316.

416. P. Collste, P. Seideman, K.-O. Borg, K. Haglund, and C. von Bahr, Clin. Pharmacol. Ther., 1979, 25, 423.

417. G. Alvan, M. Lind, B. Mellstrom, and C. von Bahr, J. Pharmacokin. Biopharm., 1977, 5, 193.

418. K.M. Piafsky and O. Borga, Clin. Pharmacol. Ther., 1977, 22, 545.

419. B. Åblad, M. Ervik, J. Hallgren, G. Johnsson, and L. Solvell, Eur. J. Clin. Pharmacol., 1972, 5, 44.

420. P. Collste K. Haglund, M. Frisk-Holmberg, and M.D. Rawlins, Eur. J. Clin. Pharmacol., 1976, 10, 85.

421. P. Collste, K. Haglund, M. Frisk-Holmberg, M.L.E. Orme, M.D. Rawlins, and J. Ostman, Eur. J. Clin. Pharmacol., 1976, 10, 89.

422. C. Bengtsson, G. Johnsson, and C.-G. Regårdh, Clin. Pharmacol. Ther., 1975, 17, 400.

423. K.O. Borg, E. Carlsson, L. Ek, and R. Johansson, Acta Pharmacol. Toxicol., 1975, 36, 24.

424. J.D. Fitzgerald, R. Ruffin, K.E. Smedstad, R. Roberts, and J. McAinsh, Eur. J. Clin. Pharmacol., 1978, 13, 81.

425. W.D. Mason, N. Winter, G. Kochad, I. Cohen, and R. Bell, Clin. Pharmacol. Ther., 1979, 25, 408.

426. F.J. Conway, J.D. Fitzgerald, J. McAinsh, D.J. Rowlands, and W.T. Simpson, Brit. J. Clin. Pharmacol., 1976, 3, 267.

427. J. McAinsh, W.T. Simpson, B.F. Holmes, J. Young, and S.H. Ellis, Biopharm. Drug Dispos., 1980, 1, 323.

428. J. McAinsh, W. Bastain, J. Young, and J.D. Harry, Biopharm. Drug Dispos., 1981, 2, 147.

429. E. Riva, P.L. Farina, R. Sega, G. Tognoni, W. Bastain, and J. McAinsh, Eur. J. Clin. Pharmacol., 1980, 17, 333.

430. C.G. Regårdh, P. Lundborg, and B.A. Persson, Biopharm. Drug Dispos., 1981, 2, 79.

431. F.E. Ros, H.C. Innemee, and P.A. Van Zwieten, Docum. Ophthal., 1979, 48, 291.

432. A. Melander, B. Niklasson, I. Ingemarsson, H. Liedholm, B. Schersten, and N.-O. Sjoberg, Eur. J. Clin. Pharmacol., 1978, 14, 93.

433. W.J.F. van der Vijgh, P.A. Majid, P.J. de Feyter, R. Wardeh, and E.E. van der Wall, Int. J. Clin. Pharmacol. Ther. Toxicol., 1980, 18, 375.

434. B. Hallengren, O.R. Nilsson, B.E. Karlberg, A. Melander, L. Tegler, and E. Wahlin-Boll, Eur. J. Clin. Pharmacol., 1982, 21, 379.

435. W.D. Mason, G. Kochak, N. Winer, and I. Cohen, J. Pharm. Sci., 1980, 69, 344.

436. J. Sassard, N. Pozet, J. McAinsh, J. Legheand, and P. Zech, Eur. J. Clin. Pharmacol., 1977, 12, 175.

437. S.H. Wan, R.T. Koda, and R.F. Maronde, Brit. J. Clin. Pharmacol., 1979, 7, 569.

438. J. McAinsh, B.F. Holmes, S. Smith, D. Hood, and D. Warren, Clin. Pharmacol. Ther., 1980, 28, 302.

439. B. Flouvat, S. Decourt, P. Aubert, L. Potaux, M. Domart, A. Goupil, and A. Baglin, Brit. J. Clin. Pharmacol., 1980, 9, 379.

440. W. Kirch, H. Kohler, E. Mutshler, and M. Schafer, Eur. J. Clin. Pharmacol., 1981, 19, 65.

441. P.C. Rubin, P.J.W. Scott, K. McLean, A. Pearson, D. Ross, and J.L. Reid, Brit. J. Clin. Pharmacol., 1982, 13, 235.

442. A. Amery, J. DePlaen, P. Lijnen, J. McAinsh, and T. Reybrouck, Clin. Pharmacol. Ther., 1977, 22, 691.

443. Internal document, Warner-Lambert/Parke-Davis Research Division, 1984.

444. L. Balant, R.J. Francis, T.N. Tozer, A. Marmy, J.-M. Tschopp, and J. Fabre, J. Pharmacokin. Biopharm., 1980, 8, 421.

445. W.J. Louis, N. Christophidis, M. Brignell, V. Vijayasekaran, J. McNeil, and F.J.E. Vajda, Aust. N.Z. J. Med., 1978, 8, 602.

446. D.A. Richards, J.G. Maconochie, R.E. Bland, R. Hopkins, E.P. Woodings, and L.E. Martin, Eur. J. Clin. Pharmacol., 1977, 11, 85.

447. G.L. Sanders, D.M. Davies, and M.D. Rawlins, Brit. J. Clin. Pharmacol., 1980, 10, 121.

448. R. Mäntylä, H. Allonen, J. Kanto, T. Kleimola, and R. Sellman, Brit. J. Clin. Pharmacol., 1980, 9, 435.

449. J. Kanto, H. Allonen, T. Kleimola, and R. Mantyla, Int. J. Clin. Pharmacol. Ther. Toxicol., 1981, 19, 41.

450. A.J. Wood, D.G. Ferry, and R.R. Bailey, Brit. J. Clin. Pharmacol., 1982, 13, 81S.

451. J. Bonelli, G. Hitzenberger, W. Krause, H. Wendt, and U. Speck, Int. J. Clin. Pharmacol. Ther. Toxicol., 1980, 18, 169.

452. U. Abshagen, G. Betzien, B. Kaufmann, and G. Endele, Eur. J. Clin. Pharmacol., 1982, 21, 293.

453. C.-G. Regårdh and G. Johnsson, Clin. Pharmacokin., 1980, 5, 557.

454. C.-G. Regårdh, G. Johnsson, L. Jordö, and L. Sölvell, Acta Pharmacol. Toxicol., 1975, 36, 45.

455. C.-G. Regårdh, K.O. Borg, R. Johansson, G. Johnsson, and L. Palmer, J. Pharmacokin. Biopharm., 1974, 2, 347.

456. M.J. Kendall, D. Brown, A. Grieve, and V.A. John, Eur. J. Drug Metab. Pharmacokin., 1977, 4, 73.

457. G. Johnsson, G.C. Regårdh, and L. Somell, Acta Pharmacol. Toxicol., 1975, 36 (suppl. 5), 31.

458. K.O. Borg, E. Fellenius, R. Johansson, and M. Wallborg, Acta Pharmacol. Toxicol., 1975, 36, 104.

459. R.C. Browning, V.A. John, R.J.L. Till, and W. Theobald, Brit. J. Clin. Pharmacol., 1981, 12, 600.

460. G. Johnsson, L. Jordö, P. Lundborg, C.-G. Regårdh, and O. Ronn, Int. J. Clin. Pharmacol. Ther. Toxicol., 1980, 18, 292.

461. A.J. Uusitalo and O. Keyriläinen, Ann. Clin. Res., 1979, 11, 199.

462. M.B. Comerford and E.M.M. Besterman, Ann. Clin. Res., 1982, 14, 27.

463. C.P. Quarterman, M.J. Kendall, and P.G. Welling, Eur. J. Clin. Pharmacol., 1979, 15, 97.

464. M.J. Kendall, V.A. John, C.P. Quarterman, and P.G. Welling, Eur. J. Clin. Pharmacol., 1980, 17, 87.

465. P. Collste, K. Haglund, and C. Von Bahr, Clin. Pharmacol. Ther., 1980, 27, 441.

466. M.G. Myers and J.J. Thiessen, Clin. Pharmacol. Ther., 1980, 27, 756.

467. D.B. Jack, M.J. Kendall, S. Dean, S.J. Laugher, and R. Zaman, Biopharm. Drug Dispos., 1982, 3, 47.

468. D.B. Jack, C.P. Quarterman, R. Zaman, and M.J. Kendall, Eur. J. Clin. Pharmacol., 1982, 23, 37.

469. K. Haglund, P. Seideman, P. Collste, L.-O. Borg, and C. von Bahr, Clin. Pharmacol. Ther., 1979, 26, 326.

470. A.J. Wood, Brit. J. Clin. Pharmacol., 1977, 4, 240.

471. C.P. Dawes, M.J. Kendall, and V.A. John, Brit. J. Clin. Pharmacol., 1978, 5, 217.

472. C.P. Quarterman, M.J. Kendall, and D.B. Jack, Brit. J. Clin. Pharmacol., 1981, 11, 287.

473. L. Jordo, P.O. Attman, M. Aurell, L. Johansson, J. Johnsson, and C.-G. Regårdh, Clin. Pharmacokin., 1980, 5, 169.

474. K.-J. Hoffmann, C.-G. Regardh, M. Aurell, M. Ervik, and L. Jordö, Clin. Pharmacokin., 1980, 5, 181.

475. K.-U. Seiler, K.J. Schuster, G.-J. Meyer, W. Niedermayer, and O. Wassermann, Clin. Pharmacokin., 1980, 5, 192.

476. C.-G. Regårdh, L. Jordö, M. Ervik, P. Lundborg, R. Olsson, and O. Ronn, Clin. Pharmacokin., 1981, 6, 375.

477. J. Dreyfuss, J.M. Shaw, and J.J. Ross, Xenobiotica, 1978, 8, 503.

478. R.G. Devlin, K.L. Duchin, and P.M. Fleiss, Brit. J. Clin. Pharmacol., 1981, 12, 393.

479. L. Brunner, P. Imhof, and D. Jack, Eur. J. Clin. Pharmacol., 1975, 8, 3.

480. B. Åblad, M. Ervik, J. Hallgren, G. Johnsson, and L. Solvell, Eur. J. Clin. Pharmacol., 1972, 5, 44.

481. G.H. Evans and D.G. Shand, Clin. Pharmacol. Ther., 1973, 14, 487.

482. A. Bobik, G.L. Jennings, P.I. Korner, P. Ashley, and G. Jackman, Brit. J. Clin. Pharmacol., 1979, 7, 545.

483. C.P. Dawes, M.J. Kendall, and P.G. Welling, Brit. J. Clin. Pharmacol., 1979, 7, 299.

484. J.J. Vallner, H.W. Jun, T.E. Needham, J.T. Stewart, W. Brown, H. Frazer, and I.L. Honigberg, J. Clin. Pharmacol., 1977, 17, 231.

485. H.W. Jun, S.L. Hayes, J.J. Vallner, I.L. Honigberg, A.E. Rojos, and J.T. Stewart, J. Clin. Pharmacol., 1979, 13, 415.

486. J.F. Giudicelli, C. Richer, M. Chauvin, N. Idrissi, and A. Berdeaux, Brit. J. Clin. Pharmacol., 1977, 4, 135.

487. S.D. Sharma, A.D. Mehra, and B.J. Vakil, Curr. Ther. Res., 1980, 27, 576.

488. R. Gugler, W. Herold, and J.L. Dengler, Eur. J. Clin. Pharmacol., 1974, 7, 17.

489. J. Meier, Acta Med. Scand., 1977, 606 (suppl.), 65.

490. G.L. Jennings, A. Bobik, E.T. Fagan, and P.I. Korner, Brit. J. Clin. Pharmacol., 1979, 7, 245.

491. R. Gugler and G. Bodem, Eur. J. Clin. Pharmacol., 1978, 13, 13.

492. L.A. Salako, A.O. Falase, A. Rogon, and R.A. Adio, Eur. J. Clin. Pharmacol., 1979, 15, 299.

493. J.L. Kiger, D. Lavene, M.F. Guillaume, M. Guerrett, and J. Longchampt, Int. J. Clin. Pharmacol., 1976, 13, 228.

494. D. Lavene, Y.A. Weiss, M.E. Safar, Y. Loria, N. Agorus, D. Georges, and P.L. Milliez, J. Clin. Pharmacol., 1977, 17, 501.

495. N.P. Chau, Y.A. Weiss, M.E. Safar, D.E. Lavene, D.R. Georges, and P.L. Milliez, Clin. Pharmacol. Ther., 1977, 22, 505.

496. E.E. Ohnhaus, E. Nüesch, J. Meier, and F. Kalberer, Eur. J. Clin. Pharmacol., 1974, 7, 25.

497. E.E. Ohnhaus, U. Munch, and J. Meier, Eur. J. Clin. Pharmacol., 1982, 22, 247.

498. E.E. Ohnhaus, H. Heidemann, J. Meier, and G. Maurer, Eur. J. Clin. Pharmacol., 1982, 22, 423.

499. R. Gugler, W. Hobel, G. Bodem, and H.J. Dengler, Clin. Pharmacol. Ther., 1975, 17, 127.

500. S.R. Johansson, M. McCall, C. Wilhelmsson, and J.A. Vedin, Clin. Pharmacol. Ther., 1980, 27, 593.

501. C. Heierli, H. Thoelen, P. Radielovic, Int. J. Clin. Pharmacol., 1977, 15, 65.

502. D.G. Shand, Drugs, 1974, 7, 39.

503. S.G. Carruthers, J.G. Kelly, D.G. McDevitt, R.G. Shanks, and M.J. Walsh, Brit. Med. J., 1973, ii, 177.

504. S.G. Carruthers, J.G. Kelly, D.G. McDevitt, and R.G. Shanks, Clin. Pharmacol. Ther., 1974, 15, 497.

505.   C.M. Kaye and C.R. Kumana, Brit. J. Clin. Pharmacol., 1974, 1, 169.

506.   H.E. Barber and G.R. Bourne, Brit. J. Pharmacol., 1971, 41, 513.

507.   B. Scales and M.B. Cosgrove, J. Pharmacol. Exp. Ther., 1970, 175, 338.

508.   W.H. Aellig, B.N.C. Prichard, and B. Scales, Brit. J. Pharmacol., 1970, 40, 573P.

509.   C.M. Kaye, D.G. Robinson, and P. Turner, Brit. J. Pharmacol., 1973, 49, 115P.

510.   D.G. Shand, R.E. Rangno, and G.H. Evans, Pharmacology, 1972, 8, 344.

511.   C.R. Cleaveland and D.G. Shand, Clin. Pharmacol. Ther., 1972, 13, 181.

512.   G.H. Evans and D.G. Shand, Clin. Pharmacol. Ther., 1973, 14, 487.

513.   D.J. Coltart and D.G. Shand, Brit. Med. J., 1970, iii, 731.

514.   C.R. Cleaveland and D.G. Shand, Clin. Res., 1971, 19, 348.

515.   C.T. Dollery, D.S. Davies, and M.E. Conolly, Arch. Int. Pharmacodyn., 1971, 192, suppl., 214.

516.   C.E. McLean and B.C. Deane, Angiology, 1970, 21, 536.

517.   J.W. Paterson, M.E. Conolly, C.T. Dollery, A. Hayes, and R.G. Cooper, Pharmacologia Clinica, 1970, 2, 127.

518.   A. Hayes and R.G. Cooper, J. Pharmacol. Exp. Ther., 1971, 176, 302.

519.   D.G. Shand, E.M. Nuckolls, and J.A. Oates, Clin. Pharmacol. Ther., 1970, 11, 112.

520.   J.J. MacKichan, D.R. Pyszezynski, and W.J. Jusko, Biopharm. Drug Dispos., 1980, 1, 159.

521.   R. Gomeni, G. Bianchetti, R. Sega, and P.L. Morselli, J. Pharmacokin. Biopharm., 1977, 5, 183.

522.   J.J. MacKichan, D.R. Pyszczynski, and W.J. Jusko, Res. Commun. Chem. Path. Pharmacol., 1978, 20, 531.

523.   L. Borgström, C.-G. Johansson, H. Larsson, and R. Lenander, J. Pharmacokin. Biopharm., 1981, 9, 419.

524.   G.P. Mould, J. Clough, B.A. Morris, G. Stout, and V. Marks, Biopharm. Drug Dispos., 1981, 2, 49.

525.   R.T. Krediet, A.J. Dunning, and L. Offerhaus, Eur. J. Clin. Pharmacol., 1980, 18, 391.

526.   H.R. Ochs, E. Grube, D.J. Greenblatt, M. Knuchel, and G. Bodem, Klin. Wschr., 1982, 60, 521.

527.   R. Roscoe, J. Cooper, T.W. Wilson, N.N. Joshi, and K.K. Midha, Biopharm. Drug Dispos., 1982, 3, 105.

528. C.M. Castleden, C.F. George, and M.D. Short, <u>Brit. J. Clin. Pharmacol.</u>, 1978, <u>5</u>, 121.

529. J. McAinsh, N.S. Baber, R. Smith, and J. Young, <u>Brit. J. Clin. Pharmacol.</u>, 1978, <u>6</u>, 115.

530. Y. Garceau, I. Davis, and J. Hasegawa, <u>J. Pharm. Sci.</u>, 1978, <u>67</u>, 1360.

531. R.E. Vestal, D.M. Kornhauser, J.W. Hollifield, and D.G. Shand, <u>Clin. Pharmacol. Ther.</u>, 1979, <u>25</u>, 19.

532. M. Chiariello, M. Volpe, F. Rengo, B. Trimarco, R. Violini, B. Ricciardelli, and M. Condorelli, <u>Clin. Pharmacol. Ther.</u>, 1979, <u>26</u>, 433.

533. R.U. Grundy, J. McAinsh, and D.C. Taylor, <u>J. Pharm. Pharmacol.</u>, 1974, <u>26</u>, 65P.

534. H.G. Dobbs, V.A. Skoutakis, S.R. Acchiardo, and B.R. Dobbs, <u>Curr. Ther. Res.</u>, 1977, <u>21</u>, 887.

535. A. Melander, K. Danielson, B. Schersten, and E. Wahlin, <u>Clin. Pharmacol. Ther.</u>, 1977, <u>22</u>, 108.

536. A.J. McLean, C. Isbister, A. Bobik, and F.J. Dudley, <u>Clin. Pharmacol. Ther.</u>, 1981, <u>30</u>, 31.

537. T. Walle, T.C. Fagan U.K. Walle, M.-J. Oexmann, E.C. Conradi, and T.E. Gaffney, <u>Clin. Pharmacol. Ther.</u>, 1981, <u>30</u>, 790.

538. A.J. McLean, H. Skews, A. Bobik, and F.J. Dudley, <u>Clin. Pharmacol. Ther.</u>, 1980, <u>27</u>, 726.

539. J. McAinsh, B.F. Holmes, N.S. Baber, and J. Young, <u>Biopharm. Drug Dispos.</u>, 1981, <u>2</u>, 167.

540. P. Fenster, D. Perrier, M. Mayersohn, and F.I. Marcus, <u>Clin. Pharmacol. Ther.</u>, 1980, <u>27</u>, 450.

541. B.S. Grabowski, W.J. Cady, W.W. Young, and J.F. Emery, <u>Int. J. Clin. Pharmacol. Ther. Toxicol.</u>, 1980, <u>18</u>, 317.

542. D.C. Taylor and R. Grundy, <u>J. Pharm. Pharmacol.</u>, 1980, <u>32</u>, 499.

543. J. McAinsh, N.S. Baber, B.F. Holmes, J. Young, and S.H. Ellis, <u>Biopharm. Drug Dispos.</u>, 1981, <u>2</u>, 39.

544. W.J. Leahey J.D. Neill, M.P.S. Varma, and R.G. Shanks, <u>Brit. J. Clin. Pharmacol.</u>, 1980, <u>9</u>, 33.

545. R.E. Schneider, J. Babb, H. Bishop, M. Mitchard, A.M. Hoare, and C.F. Hawkins, <u>Brit. Med. J.</u>, 1976, <u>2</u>, 794.

546. B.T. Cooper, W.T. Cooke, M.L. Lucas, and J.A. Blair, <u>Brit. Med. J.</u>, 1976, <u>2</u>, 1135.

547. B.T. Cooper, W.T. Cooke, M.L. Lucas, and J.A. Blair, <u>Brit. Med. J.</u>, 1977, <u>1</u>, 445.

548. K.M. Piafsky, O. Borga, I. Odar-Cederlöf, C. Johansson, and F. Sjöqvist, <u>New Engl. J. Med.</u>, 1978, <u>299</u>, 1435.

549. H. Bishop, R.E. Schneider, and P.G. Welling, <u>Biopharm. Drug Dispos.</u>, 1981, <u>2</u>, 291.

550. R.E. Schneider and H. Bishop, <u>Clin. Pharmacokin.</u>, 1982, <u>7</u>, 281.

551. P.A. Routledge, W.W. Stargel, G.S. Wagner, and D.G. Shand, <u>Brit. J. Clin. Pharmacol.</u>, 1980, <u>9</u>, 438.

552. T.K. Daneshmend and C.J.C. Roberts, <u>Brit. J. Clin. Pharmacol.</u>, 1982, <u>13</u>, 817.

553. A.J.J. Wood, K. Carr, R.E. Vestal, S. Belcher, G.R. Wilkinson, and D.G. Shand, <u>Brit. J. Clin. Pharmacol.</u>, 1978, <u>6</u>, 345.

554. T. Walle, E.C. Conradi, U.K. Walle, T.C. Fagan, and T.E. Gaffney, <u>Clin. Pharmacol. Ther.</u>, 1978, <u>24</u>, 668.

555. D.M. Kornhauser, A.J.J. Wood, R.E. Vestal, G.R. Wilkinson, R.A. Branch, and D.G. Shand, <u>Clin. Pharmacol. Ther.</u>, 1978, <u>23</u>, 165.

556. E.A. Taylor, D. Jefferson, J.D. Carroll, and P. Turner, <u>Brit. J. Clin. Pharmacol.</u>, 1981, <u>12</u>, 549.

557. J.R. Plachetka, N.W. Salomon, and J.G. Copeland, <u>Clin. Pharmacol. Ther.</u>, 1981, <u>30</u>, 745.

558. M. Wood, D.G. Shand, and A.J.J. Wood, <u>Anesthesiology</u>, 1979, <u>51</u>, 512.

559. B. Silber, M. Lo, and S. Riegelman, <u>Res. Comm. Chem. Path. Pharmacol.</u>, 1980, <u>27</u>, 419.

560. S.K. Gardner, W.J. Cady, and Y.S. Ong, <u>Int. J. Clin. Pharmacol. Ther. Toxicol.</u>, 1980, <u>18</u>, 421.

561. T. Walle, E.C. Conradi, U.K. Walle, T.C. Fagan, and T.E. Gaffney, <u>Clin. Pharmacol. Ther.</u>, 1980, <u>27</u>, 22.

562. D.W. Schneck, J.F. Pritchard, T.P. Gibson, J.E. Vary, and A.H. Hayes, Jr., <u>Clin. Pharmacol. Ther.</u>, 1980, <u>27</u>, 744.

563. G.H. Evans, A.S. Nies, and D.G. Shand, <u>J. Pharmacol. Exp. Ther.</u>, 1973, <u>186</u>, 114.

564. G.H. Evans and D.G. Shand, <u>Clin. Pharmacol. Ther.</u>, 1973, <u>14</u>, 494.

565. G.H. Evans, G.R. Wilkinson, and D.G. Shand, <u>J. Pharmacol. Exp. Ther.</u>, 1973, <u>186</u>, 447.

566. D.G. Shand, R.A. Branch, G.H. Evans, A.S. Nies, and G.R. Wilkinson, <u>Drug Metab. Dispos.</u>, 1973, <u>1</u>, 679.

567. R.A. Branch, A.S. Nies, and D.G. Shand, <u>Drug Metab. Dispos.</u>, 1973, <u>1</u>, 687.

568. A. Breckenridge, P. Buranapong, C.T. Dollery, C.F. George, D. Macerlean, and M. L'E Orme, <u>Brit. J. Pharmacol.</u>, 1973, <u>48</u>, 336P.

569. T. Suzuki, Y. Saitoh, S. Isozaki, and R. Ishida, <u>J. Pharm. Sci.</u>, 1973, <u>62</u>, 345.

570. T. Suzuki, Y. Saitoh, S. Isozaki, and R. Ishida, <u>Chem. Pharm. Bull. (Japan)</u>, 1972, <u>20</u>, 2731.

571. D.G. Shand, G.H. Evans, and A.S. Nies, <u>Life Sci.</u>, 1971, <u>10</u>, 1417.

572. H.I. Pirttiaho, E.A. Sotaniemi, R.O. Pelkonen, U. Pitkanen, M. Anttila, and H. Sundqvist, Brit. J. Clin. Pharmacol., 1980, 9, 399.

573. K. Tawara, K. Kawashima, H. Ishikawa, K. Yamamoto, K. Saito, A. Ebihara, and S. Yoshida, Eur. J. Clin. Pharmacol., 1981, 19, 197.

574. J. Feely, A. Forrest, A. Gunn, W. Hamilton, I. Stevenson, and J. Crooks, Clin. Pharmacol. Ther., 1980, 28, 759.

575. R.J. Sawchuk, J. Robayo, and K.W. Miller, Brit. J. Clin. Pharmacol., 1974, 1, 440.

576. R.H. Cotham and D. Shand, Clin. Pharmacol. Ther., 1975, 18, 535.

577. F.M. Williams, B.N. Singh, P.K. Ambler, and R. Dorrington, Clin. Exp. Pharmacol. Physiol., 1976, 3, 473.

578. J.D. Rutherford, B.N. Singh, P.K. Ambler, and R.M. Norris, Clin. Exp. Pharmacol. Physiol., 1976, 3, 297.

579. A. Lehtonen, J. Kanto, and T. Kleimola, Eur. J. Clin. Pharmacol., 1977, 11, 155.

580. E. Vervloet, B.F.M. Pluym, J. Cilissen, K. Kohlen, and W.H.M. Merkus, Clin. Pharmacol. Ther., 1977, 22, 853.

581. D.G. McDevitt, M. Frisk-Holmberg, J.W. Hollifield, and D.G. Shand, Clin. Pharmacol. Ther., 1976, 20, 152.

582. M. Esler, A. Zweifler, O. Randall, and V. DeQuattro, Clin. Pharmacol. Ther., 1977, 22, 299.

583. D. Perrier and M. Gibaldi, J. Clin. Pharmacol., 1974, 14, 415.

584. M. Gibaldi and D. Perrier, J. Pharm. Sci., 1972, 61, 952.

585. R. Zacest and J. Koch-Weser, Pharmacology, 1972, 7, 178.

586. C.R. Cleaveland and D.G. Shand, Clin. Pharmacol. Ther., 1972, 13, 191.

587. H. Imura, Y. Kato, M. Ikeda, M. Morimoto, M. Yawata, and M. Fukase, J. Clin. Endocrinol., 1968, 28, 1079.

588. J. Wilson, Biochem. Pharmacol., 1969, 18, 2029.

589. C.F. George, M. L'E. Orme, P. Buranapong, D. Macerlean, A.M. Breckenridge, and C.T. Dollery, J. Pharmacokin. Biopharm., 1976, 4, 17.

590. D.T. Lowenthal, W.A. Briggs, T.P. Gibson, H. Nelson, and W.J. Cirksena, Clin. Pharmacol. Ther., 1974, 16, 761.

591. R.A. Branch, J. James, and A.E. Read, Gut, 1974, 15, 837.

592. C.M. Castleden, C.M. Kaye, and R.L. Parsons, Brit. J. Clin. Pharmacol., 1975, 2, 303.

593. R.A. Branch and D.G. Shand, Clin. Pharmacokin., 1976, 1, 264.

594. G. Bianchetti, G. Graziani, D. Brancaccio, A. Morganti, G. Leonetti, M. Manfrin, R. Sega, R. Gomeni, C. Ponticelli, and P.L. Morselli, Clin. Pharmacokin., 1976, 1, 373.

595. R.E. Vestal, A.J.J. Wood, R.A. Branch, D.G. Shand, and G.R. Wilkinson, Clin. Pharmacol. Ther., 1979, 26, 8.

596. R.G. McAllister, D.W. Bourne, T.G. Tan, J.L. Erickson, C.C. Wachtel, and E.P. Todd, Clin. Pharmacol. Ther., 1979, 25, 1.

597. A.J.J. Wood, D.M. Kornhauser, G.R. Wilkinson, D.G. Shand, and R.A. Branch, Clin. Pharmacokin., 1978, 3, 478.

598. J.G. Kelly and D.G. McDevitt, Brit. J. Clin. Pharmacol., 1978, 6, 123.

599. W.J. Stone and T. Walle, Clin. Pharmacol. Ther., 1980, 28, 449.

600. C.F. George, T. Fenyvesi, M.E. Conolly, and C.T. Dollery, Eur. J. Clin. Pharmacol., 1972, 4, 74.

601. G. Karlberg, D. Lundberg, and H. Åberg, Acta Pharmacol. Toxicol., 1974, 34, 222.

602. C.M. Cottrill, R.G. McAllister, Jr., L. Gettes, and J.A. Noonan, J. Pediatr., 1977, 91, 812.

603. H. Sundquist, M. Anttilla, A. Simon, and J.W. Reich, J. Clin. Pharmacol., 1979, 79, 557.

604. P. Kahela, M. Anttila, R. Tikkanen, and H. Sundquist, Acta Pharmacol. Toxicol., 1979, 44, 7.

605. T. Ishizaki, H. Hirayama, K. Tawara, H. Nakaya, M. Sato, and K. Sato, J. Pharmacol. Exp. Ther., 1980, 212, 173.

606. T.B. Tjandramaga, J. Thomas, R. Verbeeck, R. Verbesselt, R. Verberckmoes, and P.J. DeSchepper, Brit. J. Pharmacol., 1976, 3, 259.

607. M. Anttila, M. Arstila, M. Pfeffer, R. Tikkanen, V. Vallinkoski, and H. Sundqvist, Acta Pharmacol. Toxicol., 1976, 32, 118.

608. H.C. Brown, S.C. Carruthers, J.G. Kelly, D.G. McDevitt, and R.G. Shanks, Eur. J. Clin. Pharmacol., 1976, 9, 367.

609. K. Schnelle, G. Klein, and A. Schinz, J. Clin. Pharmacol., 1979, 19, 516.

610. P.J. Neuvonen, E. Elonen, and L. Tarssanen, Acta Pharmacol. Toxicol., 1979, 45, 52.

611. G. Berglund, R. Descamps, and J.A. Thomis, Eur. J. Clin. Pharmacol., 1980, 18, 321.

612. G.B. Park, R.F. Koss, A.F. DeFelice, S.K. O'Neil, and J. Edelson, Arch. Int. Pharmacodyn. Ther., 1982, 259, 4.

613. A. Bobik, G.J. Jennings, P. Ashley, and P.I. Korner, Eur. J. Clin. Pharmacol., 1979, 16, 243.

614. O.F. Else, H. Sorenson, and I.R. Edwards, Eur. J. Clin. Pharmacol., 1978, 14, 431.

615. J.A. Vedin, J.K. Kristianson, and C.-E. Wilhelmsson, Eur. J. Clin. Pharmacol., 1982, 23, 43.

616. J.B. Fourtillan, P. Courtois, M.A. Lefebvre, and J. Girault, Eur. J. Clin. Pharmacol., 1981, 19, 193.

617. G. Alvan, B. Calissendorff, P. Seideman, K. Widmark, and G. Widmark, <u>Clin. Pharmacokin.</u>, 1980, <u>5</u>, 95.

618. R. El-Rashidy, <u>Biopharm. Drug Dispos.</u>, 1981, <u>2</u>, 197.

619. B.N. Singh, F.M. Williams, R.M.L. Whitlock, J. Collett, and C. Chew, <u>Clin. Pharmacol. Ther.</u>, 1980, <u>28</u>, 159.

620. T. Ishizaki and K. Tawara, <u>Cardiology</u>, 1979, <u>64 (suppl. 1)</u>, 25.

621. D.T. Lowenthal, J.M. Pitone, M.B. Affrime, J. Shirk, P. Busby, K.E. Kim, J. Nacarrow, C.D. Swartz, and G. Onesti, <u>Clin. Pharmacol. Ther.</u>, 1978, <u>23</u>, 606.

622. D.E. Resetarits and T.R. Bates, <u>J. Pharm. Sci.</u>, 1979, <u>68</u>, 126.

623. V.P. Shah, V.K. Prasad, B.E. Cabana, and P. Sojka, <u>Curr. Ther. Res.</u>, 1978, <u>24</u>, 366.

624. J.P. Hunt, V.P. Shah, V.K. Prasad, and B.E. Cabana, <u>Acad. Pharm. Sci.</u>, 1978, <u>8</u>, 195.

625. A.B. Straughn, A.P. Melikian, and M.C. Meyer, <u>J. Pharm. Sci.</u>, 1979, <u>68</u>, 1099.

626. R.H. Barbhaiya, T.A. Phillips, and P.G. Welling, <u>J. Pharm. Sci.</u>, 1981, <u>70</u>, 291.

627. M.A. Osman, R.B. Patel, D.S. Irwin, W.A. Craig, and P.G. Welling, <u>Biopharm. Drug Dispos.</u>, 1982, <u>3</u>, 89.

628. V.P. Shah, J.P. Hunt, V.K. Prasad, and B.E. Cabana, <u>J. Pharm. Sci.</u>, 1981, <u>70</u>, 833.

629. P.G. Welling, R.H. Barbhaiya, R.B. Patel, T.S. Foster, V.P. Shah, J.P. Hunt, and V.K. Prasad, <u>Curr. Ther. Res.</u>, 1982, <u>31</u>, 379.

630. V.P. Shah, J. Lee, J.P. Hunt, V.K. Prasad, B.E. Cabana, and T. Foster, <u>Curr. Ther. Res.</u>, 1981, <u>29</u>, 823.

631. P.G. Welling, D.M. Walter, R.B. Patel, R.H. Barbhaiya, W.A. Porter, G.L. Amidon, T.S. Foster, V.P. Shah, J.P. Hunt, and V.K. Prasad, <u>Curr. Ther. Res.</u>, 1981, <u>29</u>, 815.

632. V.P. Shah, P. Knight, V.K. Prasad, and B.E. Cabana, <u>J. Pharm. Sci.</u>, 1982, <u>71</u>, 822.

633. P.G. Welling and R.H. Barbhaiya, <u>J. Pharm. Sci.</u>, 1982, <u>71</u>, 32.

634. P.G. Welling and V.P. Shah, <u>Am. J. Hosp. Pharm.</u>, 1984, <u>41</u>, 450.

635. W.F. Ebling, A.F. Murro, F.J. Voelker, D.E. Resetarits, and T.R. Bates, <u>J. Pharm. Sci.</u>, 1981, <u>70</u>, 224.

636. J.H. Gustafson and L.Z. Benet, <u>J. Pharmacokin. Biopharm.</u>, 1981, <u>9</u>, 461.

637. R.H. Barbhaiya, W.A. Craig, H.P. Corrick-West, and P.G. Welling, <u>J. Pharm. Sci.</u>, 1982, <u>71</u>, 245.

638. B. Beermann and M. Groschinsky-Grind, <u>Eur. J. Clin. Pharmacol.</u>, 1978, <u>13</u>, 125.

639. B. Beermann and M. Groschinsky-Grind, <u>Eur. J. Clin. Pharmacol.</u>, 1977, <u>12</u>, 297.

640. I.J. McGilveray, R.D. Hossie, and G.L. Mattok, <u>Canad. J. Pharm.</u>
      <u>Sci.</u>, 1973, <u>8</u>, 13.

641. R.H. Barbhaiya, R.B. Patel, H.P. Corrick-West, R.S. Joslin, and
      P.G. Welling, <u>Biopharm. Drug Dispos.</u>, 1982, <u>3</u>, 329.

642. R.L. Williams, R.O. Davies, R.S. Berman, G.I. Holmes, P. Huber,
      W.L. Gee, E.T. Lin, and L.Z. Benet, <u>J. Clin. Pharmacol.</u>, 1982,
      <u>22</u>, 32.

643. B. Beermann and M. Groschinsky-Grind, <u>Eur. J. Clin. Pharmacol.</u>,
      1978, <u>13</u>, 385.

644. L. Jordö, G. Johnsson, P. Lundborg, B.A. Persson, C.-G. Regårdh,
      and O. Ronn, <u>Brit. J. Clin. Pharmacol.</u>, 1979, <u>7</u>, 563.

645. L. Backman, B. Beermann, M. Groschinsky-Grind, and D. Hallberg,
      <u>Clin. Pharmacokin.</u>, 1979, <u>4</u>, 63.

646. B. Beermann, M. Groshinsky-Grind, and A. Rosen, <u>Clin.</u>
      <u>Pharmacol. Ther.</u>, 1976, <u>19</u>, 531.

647. G.J. Yakatan, R.B. Smith, E.L. Frome, and J.T. Doluisio, <u>J.</u>
      <u>Clin. Pharmacol.</u>, 1977, <u>17</u>, 37.

648. O. Brφrs, S. Jacobsen, and E. Arnesen, <u>Eur. J. Clin. Pharmacol.</u>,
      1978, <u>14</u>, 29.

649. O. Brφrs and S. Jacobsen, <u>Eur. J. Clin. Pharmacol.</u>, 1979, <u>15</u>,
      281.

650. P.J. McNamara, W.A. Colburn, and M. Gibaldi, <u>J. Clin.</u>
      <u>Pharmacol.</u>, 1978, <u>18</u>, 190.

651. O. Brφrs and S. Jacobsen, <u>Eur. J. Clin. Pharmacol.</u>, 1979, <u>16</u>,
      125.

652. O. Brφrs, J.F.W. Haffner, and S. Jacobsen, <u>Eur. J. Clin.</u>
      <u>Pharmacol.</u>, 1979, <u>15</u>, 287.

653. L. Borgström, C.-G. Johansson, H. Larsson, and R. Lenander, <u>J.</u>
      <u>Pharmacokin. Biopharm.</u>, 1981, <u>9</u>, 431.

654. M. Schäfer-Korting and E. Mutschler, <u>Eur. J. Clin. Pharmacol.</u>,
      1982, <u>21</u>, 315.

655. B. Beermann, M. Groschinsky-Grind, and B. Lindström, <u>Clin.</u>
      <u>Pharmacol. Ther.</u>, 1977, <u>22</u>, 385.

656. B. Beermann, M. Groschinsky-Grind, B. Lindström, and B. Wikland,
      <u>Eur. J. Clin. Pharmacol.</u>, 1978, <u>13</u>, 119.

657. C.C. Hobbs and T.M. Twomey, <u>Clin. Pharmacol. Ther.</u>, 1978, <u>23</u>,
      241.

658. R.E. Cutler and A.D. Blair, <u>Clin. Pharmacokin.</u>, 1979, <u>4</u>, 279.

659. L.Z. Benet, <u>J. Pharmacokin. Biopharm.</u>, 1979, <u>7</u>, 1.

660. B. Beermann and M. Groschinsky-Grind, <u>Clin. Pharmacokin.</u>, 1980,
      <u>5</u>, 221.

661. M.R. Kelly, R.E. Cutler, A.W. Forrey, and B.M. Kimpel, <u>Clin.</u>
      <u>Pharmacol. Ther.</u>, 1974, <u>15</u>, 178.

662. E.S. Waller, S.F. Hamilton, J.W. Massarella, M.A. Sharanevych, R.V. Smith, G.J. Yakatan, and J.T. Doluisio, J. Pharm. Sci., 1982, 71, 1105.

663. E. Dalén and B. Lindström, Brit. J. Clin. Pharmacol., 1978, 6, 537.

664. M.H. Rubinstein and J.M. Rughani, Drug Devel. Indust. Pharm., 1978, 4, 541.

665. B. Beermann, Clin. Pharmacol. Ther., 1982, 32, 584.

666. F. Andreasen, C.K. Christensen, F.K. Jacobsen, J. Jansen, C.E. Mogensen, and O.L. Pedersen, Eur. J. Clin. Invest., 1982, 12, 247.

667. F. Andreasen, O. Lederball Pedersen, and E. Mikkelsen, Eur. J. Clin. Pharmacol., 1978, 14, 237.

668. D.E. Smith, D.C. Brater, E.T. Lin, and L.Z. Benet, J. Pharmacokin. Biopharm., 1979, 7, 265.

669. M. Homeida, C. Roberts, and R.A. Branch, Clin. Pharmacol. Ther., 1977, 22, 402.

670. J. Honari, A.D. Blair, and R.D. Cutler, Clin. Pharmacol. Ther., 1977, 22, 395.

671. D.C. Brater, Clin. Pharmacol. Ther., 1978, 24, 548.

672. M. Homeida, C. Roberts, and R.A. Branch, Clin. Pharmacol. Ther., 1977, 22, 402.

673. D.E. Smith, W.L. Gee, D.C. Brater, E.T. Lin, and L.Z. Benet, J. Pharm. Sci., 1980, 69, 571.

674. H.J. Rogers, P. Morrison, F.R. House, and I.D. Bradbrook, Int. J. Clin. Pharmacol. Ther. Toxicol., 1982, 20, 8.

675. E. Riva, P. Farina, G. Tognoni, S. Bottino, C. Orrico, and G. Pardi, Eur. J. Clin. Pharmacol., 1978, 14, 560.

676. B. Beermann, M. Groschinsky-Grind, L. Fahraeus, and B. Lindstrom, Clin. Pharmacol. Ther., 1978, 24, 560.

677. P. Vert, M. Broquaire, M. Legagneur, and P.L. Morselli, Eur. J. Clin. Pharmacol., 1982, 22, 39.

678. E. Riva, E. Fossali, and A. Bettinelli, Eur. J. Clin. Pharmacol., 1982, 21, 303.

679. E. Keller, G. Hoppe-Seyler, and P. Schollmeyer, Clin. Pharmacol. Ther., 1982, 32, 442.

680. D.E. Smith, J.G. Gambertoglio, F. Vincenti, and L.Z. Benet, Clin. Pharmacol. Ther., 1981, 30, 105.

681. R.K. Verbeeck, R.V. Patwardhan, J.-P. Villeneuve, G.R. Wilkinson, and R.A. Branch, Clin. Pharmacol. Ther., 1982, 31, 719.

682. R. Fuller, C. Hoppel, and S.T. Ingalls, Clin. Pharmacol. Ther., 1981, 30, 461.

683. C. Allgulander, B. Beermann, and A. Sjögren, Clin. Pharmacokin., 1980, 5, 570.

684. G. Gonzàlez, A. Arancibia, M.I. Rivas, P. Caro, and C. Antezana, Eur. J. Clin. Pharmacol., 1982, 22, 315.

685. M.M. Hammarlund and L.K. Paalzow, Biopharm. Drug Dispos., 1982, 3, 345.

686. R.K. Verbeeck, J.F. Gerkens, G.R. Wilkinson, and R.A. Branch, J. Pharmacol. Exp. Ther., 1981, 216, 479.

687. G.J. Yakatan, D.D. Maness, J. Scholler, W.M.J. Novick, Jr., and J.T. Doluisio, J. Pharm. Sci., 1976, 65, 1456.

688. A. Nomura, H. Yasuda, K. Katoh, T. Akimoto, K. Miyazaki, and T. Arita, Clin. Pharmacol. Ther., 1982, 32, 303.

689. R.E. Cutler, A.W. Forrey, G. Christopher, and B.M. Kimpel, Clin. Pharmacol. Ther., 1974, 15, 588.

690. C.M. Huang, A.J. Atkinson, M. Levin, N.W. Levin and A. Quintanilla, Clin. Pharmacol. Ther., 1974, 16, 659.

691. F. Andreasen, H.E. Hansen, and E. Mikkelsen, Eur. J. Clin. Pharmacol., 1978, 13, 41.

692. W.J. Tilstone and A. Fine, Clin. Pharmacol. Ther., 1978, 23, 644.

693. A. Rane, J.P. Villeneuve, W.H. Stone, A.S. Nies, G.R. Wilkinson, and R.A. Branch, Clin. Pharmacol. Ther., 1978, 24, 199.

694. M. Nakano, K. Fujii, and S. Goto, Chem. Pharm. Bull., 1979, 27, 101.

695. H.J. Rose, K. O'Malley, and A.W. Pruitt, Clin. Pharmacol. Ther., 1977, 21, 141.

696. B. Beermann, E. Dalen, and B. Lindstrom, Clin. Pharmacol. Ther., 1977, 22, 70.

697. P. Chennavasin, R.A. Johnson, and D.C. Brater, J. Pharmacokin. Biopharm., 1981, 9, 623.

698. M.G. Lee, M.-L. Chen, and W.L. Chiou, Res. Comm. Chem. Path. Pharmacol., 1981, 34, 17.

699. W. Sadee, S. Riegelman, and S.C. Jones, J. Pharm. Sci., 1972, 61, 1129.

700. W. Sadee, S. Riegelman, and S.C. Jones, J. Pharm. Sci., 1972, 61, 1132.

701. A. Karim, R.E. Ranney, and H.I. Maibach, J. Pharm. Sci., 1971, 60, 708.

702. W. Sadee, M. Dagcioglu, and R. Schröder, J. Pharmacol. Exp. Ther., 1973, 185, 686.

703. A. Karim, J. Zagarella, T.C. Hutsell, A. Chao, and B.J. Baltes, Clin. Pharmacol. Ther., 1976, 19, 170.

704. M.J. Tidd, L.E. Ramsay, J.R. Shelton, and R.F. Palmer, Int. J. Clin. Pharmacol., 1977, 15, 205.

705. J.M. Clarke, L.E. Ramsay, J.R. Shelton, M.J. Tidd, S. Murray, and R.F. Palmer, J. Pharm. Sci., 1977, 66, 1429.

706. G.T. McInnes, M.J. Asbury, L.E. Ramsay, J.R. Shelton, and I.R. Harrison, J. Clin. Pharmacol., 1982, 22, 410.

707. H. Rameis, G. Hitzenberger, and H. Horwatitsch, Int. J. Clin. Pharmacol. Ther. Toxicol., 1982, 20, 327.

708. A.Y. Chao, D.R. Sanvordeker, J. Zagarella, K. Mattes, B. Nicholova, and A. Karim, J. Pharm. Sci., 1976, 65, 1630.

709. A. Melander, K. Danielson, B. Schersten, T. Thulin, and E. Wahlin, Clin. Pharmacol. Ther., 1977, 22, 100.

710. A. Karim, J. Zagarella, J. Hribar, and M. Dooley, Clin. Pharmacol. Ther., 1976, 19, 158.

711. A. Karim, J. Zagarella, T.C. Hutsell, and M. Dooley, Clin. Pharmacol. Ther., 1976, 19, 177.

712. U. Abshagen, H. Rennekamp, and G. Luszpinski, Eur. J. Clin. Pharmacol., 1977, 11, 169.

713. G.M. Bell, L. Fananapazir, and J.L. Anderton, Brit. J. Clin. Pharmacol., 1981, 12, 585.

714. L.E. Ramsay, I.R. Harrison, J.R. Shelton, and C.W. Vose, Eur. J. Clin. Pharmacol., 1976, 10, 43.

715. L.M. Hofmann, M.I. Krupnick, and H.A. Garcia, J. Pharmacol. Exp. Ther., 1972, 180, 1.

716. P. Collste, M. Garle, M.D. Rawlins, and F. Sjoqvist, Eur. J. Clin. Pharmacol., 1976, 9, 319.

717. W. Riess, U.C. Dubach, D. Burckhardt, W. Theobald, P. Vuillard, and M. Zimmerli, Eur. J. Clin. Pharmacol., 1977, 12, 375.

718. H.L.J. Fleuren and J.M. van Rossum, J. Pharmacokin. Biopharm., 1977, 5, 359.

719. R.L. Williams, C.D. Blume, E.T. Lin, N.H.G. Holford, and L.Z. Benet, J. Pharm. Sci., 1982, 71, 533.

720. D.L. Davies, A.F. Lant, N.R. Millard, A.J. Smith, J.W. Ward, and G.M. Wilson, Clin. Pharmacol. Ther., 1974, 15, 141.

721. P.J. Pentikäinen, P.J. Neuvonen, M. Kekki, and A. Penttila, J. Pharmacokin. Biopharm., 1980, 8, 219.

722. H.L. Elliott, A.F. Ansari, B.C. Campbell, and J.R. Lawrence, Eur. J. Clin. Pharmacol., 1982, 21, 311.

723. R.R. Brodie, L.F. Chasseaud, A. Darragh, T. Taylor, and L.M. Walmsley, Biopharm. Drug Dispos., 1982, 3, 361.

724. H.L.J. Fleuren, C.P.W. Verwey-van Wissen, and J.M. van Rossum, Eur. J. Clin. Pharmacol., 1980, 17, 59.

725. P.E. Grebow and J.A. Treitman, J. Pharm. Sci., 1981, 70, 1310.

726. P.E. Grebow, J.A. Treitman, E.P. Barry, D.J. Blasucci, S.T. Portelli, N.C. Tantillo, R.A. Vukovich, and E.S. Neiss, Eur. J. Clin. Pharmacol., 1982, 22, 295.

727. A.J. Smith and R.N. Smith, Brit. J. Pharmacol., 1973, 48, 646.

728. M.F. Grayson, A.J. Smith, and R.N. Smith, Brit. J. Pharmacol.,
      1971, 43, 473P.

729. J.H. Nodine, K.N. Modi, M. Rhodes, V. Paz-Martinez, L. Ibarra,
      and R.J. Santos, Clin. Pharmacol. Ther., 1973, 14, 196.

730. E.J. Belair, A.I. Cohen, and J. Yelnosky, Brit. J. Pharmacol.,
      1972, 45, 476.

731. A.I. Cohen, A.D. Hartman, O.N. Hinsvark, P.F. Kraus, and W.
      Zazulak, J. Pharm. Sci., 1973, 62, 931.

732. T.M. Ludden, J.L. McNay, Jr., A.M.M. Shepherd, and M.S. Lin,
      Clin. Pharmacokin., 1982, 7, 185.

733. T.M. Ludden, A.M.M. Shepherd, J.L. McNay, and M.-S. Lin, Clin.
      Pharmacol. Ther., 1980, 28, 736.

734. A.M.M. Shepherd, T.M. Ludden, J.L. McNay, and M.-S. Lin, Clin.
      Pharmacol. Ther., 1980, 28, 804.

735. T.M. Ludden, J.L. McNay, Jr., A.M.M. Shepherd, and M.S. Lin,
      Arthritis Rheumatism, 1981, 24, 987.

736. M.M. Reidenberg, D. Drayer, A.L. DeMarco, and C.T. Bello, Clin.
      Pharmacol. Ther., 1973, 14, 970.

737. R. Zacest and J. Koch-Weser, Clin. Pharmacol. Ther., 1972, 13,
      420.

738. J.A. Timbrell, S.J. Harland, and V. Facchini, Clin. Pharmacol.
      Ther., 1980, 28, 350.

739. J.A. Timbrell, S.J. Harland, and V. Facchini, Clin. Pharmacol.
      Ther., 1981, 29, 337.

740. R.J. Walden, R. Hernandez, D. Witts, B.R. Graham, and B.N.C.
      Prichard, Eur. J. Clin. Pharmacol., 1981, 20, 53.

741. A. Melander, K. Danielson, A. Hanson, B. Rudell, B. Schersten,
      T. Thulin, and E. Wahlin, Clin. Pharmacol. Ther., 1977, 22, 104.

742. T. Talseth, Clin. Pharmacol. Ther., 1977, 21, 715.

743. D.D. Shen, J.P. Hosler, R.L. Schroder, and D.L. Azarnoff, J.
      Pharmacokin. Biopharm., 1980, 8, 53.

744. P.A. Reece, I. Cozamanis, and R. Zacest, Clin. Pharmacol. Ther.,
      1980, 28, 769.

745. A.M.M. Shepherd, J.L. McNay, T.M. Ludden, M.-S. Lin, and G.E.
      Musgrave, Hypertension, 1981, 3, 580.

746. T. Talseth, Eur. J. Clin. Pharmacol., 1976, 10, 311.

747. A.R. Waller, L.F. Chasseaud, T. Taylor, A. Darragh, and D.A.
      O'Kelly, Biopharm. Drug Dispos., 1979, 1, 59.

748. E. Rey, G. Barrier, Ph. d'Athis, D. de Lauture, M.O. Richard,
      J.P. Lirzin, C. Sureau, and G. Olive, Int. J. Clin. Pharmacol.
      Ther. Toxicol., 1980, 18, 437.

749. P. Jaillon, Clin. Pharmacokin., 1980, 5, 365.

750. N. Ph. Chau, B.L. Flouvat, E. Le Roux, and M.E. Safar, Clin.
      Pharmacol. Ther., 1980, 28, 6.

751. A. Grahnén, P. Seideman, B. Lindström, K. Haglund, and C. von Bahr, Clin. Pharmacol. Ther., 1981, 30, 439.

752. P. Seideman, A. Grahnén, K. Haglund, B. Lindstrom, and C. von Bahr, Clin. Pharmacol. Ther., 1981, 30, 447.

753. D.T. Lowenthal, D. Hobbs, M.B. Affrine, T.M. Twomey, E.W. Martinez, and G. Onesti, Clin. Pharmacol. Ther., 1980, 27, 779.

754. P.C. Rubin, P.J.W. Scott, and J.L. Reid, Brit. J. Clin. Pharmacol., 1981, 12, 401.

755. J.G. Lloyd-Jones, R. Henson, J.D. Nichols, D. Greenslade, and J.M. Clifford, Eur. J. Clin. Pharmacol., 1981, 19, 119.

756. J.H. Silas, F.C. Phillips, S. Freestone, G.T. Tucker, and L.E. Ramsay, Eur. J. Clin. Pharmacol., 1981, 19, 113.

757. H.L. Elliott, P.A. Meredith, K. McLean, M.A. Hughes, and J.L. Reid, Eur. J. Clin. Pharmacol., 1982, 21, 287.

758. D.T. Lowenthal, J. Cardiovasc. Pharmacol., 1980, 2, S29.

759. J.L. Reid, Brit. J. Clin. Pharmacol., 1981, 12, 295.

760. S.N. Anavekar, B. Jarrott, M. Toscano, and W.J. Louis, Eur. J. Clin. Pharmacol., 1982, 23, 1.

761. M.J. Hogan, J.D. Wallin, and L.-C. Chu, Clin. Pharmacol. Ther., 1981, 30, 729.

762. M. Frisk-Holmberg, L. Paalzow, and P.O. Edlund, Brit. J. Clin. Pharmacol., 1981, 12, 653.

763. E.L. Conway and B. Jarrott, J. Pharmacokin. Biopharm., 1982, 10, 187.

764. D. Arndts, J. Doevendans, G. Arendt, and G. Rippen, Arzneim.-Forsch., 1981, 31, 1954.

765. W. Kirch, H. Köhler, W. Braun, and Ch.v. Gizycki, Clin. Pharmacokin., 1980, 5, 476.

766. K.L. Duchin, S.M. Singhvi, D.A. Willard, B.H. Migdalof, and D.N. McKinstry, Clin. Pharmacol. Ther., 1982, 31, 452.

767. K. Onoyama, H. Hirakata, K. Iseki, S. Fujimi, T. Omae, M. Kobayashi, and Y. Kawahara, Hypertension, 1981, 3, 456.

768. K.J. Kripalani, D.N. McKinstry, S.M. Singhvi, D.A. Willard, R.A. Vukovich, and B.H. Migdalof, Clin. Pharmacol. Ther., 1980, 27, 636.

769. S.M. Singhvi, D.N. McKinstry, J.M. Shaw, D.A. Willard, and B.H. Migdalof, J. Clin. Pharmacol., 1982, 22, 135.

770. R.G. Devlin and P.M. Fleiss, J. Clin. Pharmacol., 1981, 21, 110.

771. S.M. Singhvi, K.L. Duchin, D.A. Willard, D.N. McKinstry, and B.H. Migdalof, Clin. Pharmacol. Ther., 1982, 32, 182.

772. S.M. Singhvi, A.E. Peterson, J.J. Ross, Jr., J.M. Shaw, G.R. Keim, and B.H. Migdalof, J. Pharm. Sci., 1981, 70, 1108.

773. S. Higuchi and Y. Shiobara, Xenobiotica, 1980, 10, 447.

774. S. Higuchi, H. Sasaki, and T. Seki, Xenobiotica, 1980, 10, 897.

775. M. Eichelbaum, Clin. Invest. Med., 1980, 3, 13.

776. R.G. McAllister, Jr., J. Cardiovasc. Pharmacol., 1982, 4, S340.

777. K. Aoki, K. Sato, Y. Kawaguchi, and M. Yamamoto, Eur. J. Clin. Pharmacol., 1982, 23, 197.

778. G. Remberg, M. Ende, M. Eichelbaum, and M. Schomerus, Arzneim.-Forsch., 1980, 30, 398.

779. G. Neugebauer, Cardiovasc. Res., 1978, 12, 247.

780. R.G. McAllister and E.B. Kirsten, Clin. Pharmacol. Ther., 1982, 31, 418.

781. M. Schomerus, B. Spiegelhalder, B. Stieren, and M. Eichelbaum, Cardiovasc. Res., 1976, 10, 605.

782. C.L. Yong, R.L. Kunka, and T.R. Bates, Res. Comm. Chem. Path. Pharmacol., 1980, 30, 329.

783. K. Satoh, T. Yanagisawa, and N. Taira, Cardiovasc. Pharmacol., 1980, 2, 309.

784. V. Rovei, M. Mitchard, and P.L. Morselli, J. Chromatogr., 1977, 138, 391.

785. E.L. Kinney, R.M. Moskowitz, and R. Zelis, J. Clin. Pharmacol., 1981, 21, 337.

786. M. Lievre, J. Descotes, J.L. Brazier, Q.T. Chah, and G. Faucon, Arch. Int. Pharmacodyn. Ther., 1981, 252, 272.

787. S.J. Rosenthal, R. Ginsburg, I.H. Lamb, D.S. Baim, and J.S. Schroeder, Amer. J. Cardiol., 1980, 46, 1027.

788. T.J. Benya, J. Amer. Pharm. Assoc., 1976, NS16, 271.

789. A. Breckenridge and M. Orme, Clin. Pharmacol. Ther., 1973, 14, 955.

790. J.G. Wagner, P.G. Welling, K.P. Lee, and J.E. Walker, J. Pharm. Sci., 1971, 60, 666.

791. R.A. O'Reilly, P.G. Welling, and J.G. Wagner, Thrombos. Diathes. Haemorrh., 1971, 25, 178.

792. M. Siurala, O. Mustala, K. Pyörälä, M. Kekki, M. Aireksinen, J. Jussila, H. Salmi, and R. Julkunen, Acta Hepato-Gastro-enterologica, 1972, 19, 190.

793. T.J. Benya and J.G. Wagner, Canad. J. Pharm. Sci., 1976, 11, 70.

794. K.K. Midha, I.J. McGilveray, and J.K. Cooper, J. Pharm. Sci., 1974, 63, 1725.

795. P.G. Welling, K.P. Lee, U. Khanna, and J.G. Wagner, J. Pharm. Sci., 1970, 59, 1621.

796. A. Yacobi, L.B. Wingard, and G. Levy, J. Pharm. Sci., 1974, 63, 868.

797. A. Yacobi and G. Levy, J. Pharm. Sci., 1975, 64, 1660.

798. G. Levy and A. Yacobi, *J. Pharm. Sci.*, 1974, *63*, 805.

799. T.J. Benya and J.G. Wagner, *J. Pharmacokin. Biopharm.*, 1975, *3*, 237.

800. A. Yacobi and G. Levy, *Res. Comm. Chem. Path. Pharmacol.*, 1975, *12*, 405.

801. G. Levy, *J. Pharmacokin. Biopharm.*, 1973, *1*, 541.

802. K. Bachmann and R. Shapiro, *Clin. Pharmacokin.*, 1977, *2*, 110.

803. A. Yacobi, J.A. Udall, and G. Levy, *Clin. Pharmacol. Ther.*, 1976, *19*, 552.

804. A. Yacobi, T. Lampman, and G. Levy, *Clin. Pharmacol. Ther.*, 1977, *21*, 283.

805. A. Yacobi, R.G. Stoll, A.R. DiSanto, and G. Levy, *Res. Comm. Chem. Path. Pharmacol.*, 1976, *12*, 743.

806. A. Yacobi, J.A. Udall, and G. Levy, *Clin. Pharmacol. Ther.*, 1976, *20*, 300.

807. R.L. Williams, W.L. Schary, T.F. Blaschke, P.J. Meffin, K.L. Melmon, and M. Rowland, *Clin. Pharmacol. Ther.*, 1976, *20*, 90.

808. K. Bachmann, R. Shapiro, and J. Mackiewicz, *J. Clin. Pharmacol.*, 1976, *16*, 468.

809. K. Bachmann, R. Shapiro, and J. Mackiewicz, *J. Clin. Pharmacol.*, 1977, *17*, 292.

810. A. Yacobi and G. Levy, *J. Pharm. Sci.*, 1977, *66*, 567.

811. A. Yacobi and G. Levy, *J. Pharm. Sci.*, 1977, *66*, 1275.

812. J.T. Slattery, A. Yacobi, and G. Levy, *Life Sci.*, 1976, *19*, 447.

813. A. Breckenridge and M. L'E. Orme, *Life Sci.*, 1972, *11*, 337.

814. D.S. Hewick, *J. Pharm. Pharmacol.*, 1972, *24*, 661.

815. D.S. Hewick and J. McEwen, *J. Pharm. Pharmacol.*, 1973, *25*, 458.

816. R.J. Lewis, W.F. Trager, A.J. Robinson, and K.K. Chan, *J. Lab. Clin. Med.*, 1973, *81*, 925.

817. A. Yacobi and G. Levy, *J. Pharmacokin. Biopharm.*, 1974, *2*, 239.

818. A. Breckenridge, M. Orme, H. Wesseling, R.J. Lewis, and R. Gibbons, *Clin. Pharmacol. Ther.*, 1974, *15*, 424.

819. R. Losito and M.-A. Rousseau, *Thrombos. Diathes. Haemorrh.*, 1972, *27*, 300.

820. W.D. Wosilait and L.L. Eisenbrandt, *Res. Comm. Chem. Path. Pharmacol.*, 1972, *4*, 413.

821. C. Hignite, J. Uetrecht, C. Tschanz, and D. Azarnoff, *Clin. Pharmacol. Ther.*, 1980, *28*, 99.

822. G. Levy, R.A. O'Reilly, and L.B. Wingard, Jr., *Res. Comm. Chem. Path. Pharmacol.*, 1974, *7*, 359.

823. M. Gibaldi and P.J. McNamara, *J. Pharm Sci.*, 1977, *66*, 1211.

824.   E. Rothstein, J. Amer. Med. Assoc., 1972, 221, 1052.

825.   R.A. O'Reilly, Ann. Int. Med., 1973, 78, 73.

826.   E.M. Sellers, M. Lang, J. Koch-Weser, and R.W. Colman, Clin. Pharmacol. Ther., 1972, 13, 911.

827.   H.W. Jun, L.A. Luzzi, and P.L. Hsu, J. Pharm. Sci., 1972, 61, 1835.

828.   W.L. Schary, R.J. Lewis, and M. Rowland, Res. Comm. Chem. Path. Pharmacol., 1975, 10, 663.

829.   R.J. Lewis, W.F. Trager, K.K. Chan, A. Breckenridge, M. Orme, M. Rowland, and W. Schary, J. Clin. Invest., 1974, 53, 1607.

830.   R.A. O'Reilly, M.A. Sahud, and A.J. Robinson, Thrombos. Diathes. Haemorrh., 1972, 27, 309.

831.   M. Weintraub, R.T. Breckenridge, and P.F. Griner, J. Lab. Clin. Med., 1973, 81, 273.

832.   M.L'E. Orme, A. Breckenridge, and R.V. Brooks, Brit. Med. J., 1972, iii, 611.

833.   L. Gould, A. Michael, S. Fisch, and R.F. Comprecht, J. Amer. Med. Assoc., 1972, 220, 1460.

834.   R.A. O'Reilly, Ann. Int. Med., 1974, 81, 337.

835.   M.M. Ghoneim, M. Delle, W.R. Wilson, and J.J. Ambre, Anaesthesiology, 1975, 43, 333.

836.   J.A. Udall, Amer. J. Cardiol., 1975, 35, 67.

837.   A. Yacobi and G. Levy, Res. Comm. Chem. Path. Pharmacol., 1976, 15, 369.

838.   T.D. Bjornsson, P.J. Meffin, and T.F. Blaschke, J. Pharmacokin. Biopharm., 1977, 5, 495.

839.   J.T. Slattery, A. Yacobi, and G. Levy, J. Pharm. Sci., 1977, 66, 943.

840.   A. Yacobi, J.T. Slattery, and G. Levy, J. Pharm. Sci., 1977, 66, 941.

841.   R. Laliberte, S. Chakrabarti, and J. Brodeur, J. Pharmacol. Exp. Ther., 1977, 200, 44.

842.   A. Yacobi, J.T. Slattery, and G. Levy, J. Pharm. Sci., 1980, 69, 634.

843.   R.C. Luders and D. Chao, J. Pharm. Sci., 1981, 70, 1370.

844.   M.J. Akers, J.L. Lach, and L.J. Fischer, J. Pharm. Sci., 1973, 62, 1192.

845.   J.F. Nash, L.D. Bechtel, L.R. Lowary, B.E. Rodda, and H.A. Rose, Drug Development Comm., 1974-75, 1, 443.

846.   M.J. Akers, J.L. Lach, and L.J. Fischer, J. Pharm. Sci., 1973, 62, 391.

847.   A. Yacobi, C.-M. Lai, and G. Levy, J. Pharm. Sci., 1975, 64, 1995.

848. E. Jähnchen and G. Levy, J. Pharmacol. Exp. Ther., 1974, 188, 293.

849. E. Jähnchen, L.B. Wingard, and G. Levy, J. Pharmacol. Exp. Ther., 1973, 187, 176.

850. A. Yacobi, C. Lai, and G. Levy, J. Pharm. Sci., 1977, 66, 1741.

851. C. Lai and G. Levy, J. Pharm. Sci., 1977, 66, 1739.

852. C. Lai, A. Yacobi, and G. Levy, J. Pharmacol. Exp. Ther., 1976, 199, 74.

853. E. Jähnchen, T. Meinertz, H.J. Gilfrich, and U. Groth, Eur. J. Clin. Pharmacol., 1976, 10, 349.

854. W.A. Ritschel, M.E. Brady, H.S.I. Tan, K.A. Hoffmann, I.M. Yiu, and K.W. Grummich, Eur. J. Clin. Pharmacol., 1977, 12, 457.

855. W. Dieterle, J.W. Faigle, C. Montigel, M. Sulc, and W. Theobald, Eur. J. Clin. Pharmacol., 1977, 11, 367.

856. J. Godbillon, J. Richard, A. Gerardin, T. Meinertz, W. Kasper, and E. Jahnchen, Brit. J. Clin. Pharmacol., 1981, 12, 621.

857. W.A. Ritschel and K.A. Hoffmann, J. Clin. Pharmacol., 1981, 21, 294.

858. W.A. Ritschel and K.W. Grummich, Arzneim.-Forsch., 1981, 31, 643.

859. E. Jahnchen, T. Meinertz, H. Gilfrich, U. Groth, and A. Martini, Clin. Pharmacol. Ther., 1976, 20, 342.

860. H.S. Buttar, B.B. Coldwell, and G.H. Thomas, Brit. J. Pharmacol., 1973, 48, 278.

861. B.H. Thomas, B.B. Coldwell, H.S. Buttar, and W. Zeitz, Canad. J. Physiol. Pharmacol., 1973, 51, 205.

862. J. Zaroslinski, R. Browne, and L. Possley, Arch. Int. Pharmacodyn., 1972, 195, 185.

863. L.R. Whitfield, J.J. Schentag, and G. Levy, Clin. Pharmacol. Ther., 1982, 32, 503.

864. R.J. Cipolle, R.D. Seifert, B.A. Neilan, D.E. Zaske, and E. Haus, Clin. Pharmacol. Ther., 1981, 29, 387.

865. P.J. Perry, G.R. Herron, and J.C. King, Clin. Pharmacol. Ther., 1974, 16, 514.

866. J.W. Estes, Curr. Ther. Res., 1975, 18, 45.

867. T.D. Bjornsson, J. Pharm. Sci., 1982, 71, 1186.

868. C. Mahony, K.M. Wolfram, D.M. Cocchetto, and T.D. Bjornsson, Clin. Pharmacol. Ther., 1982, 31, 330.

869. A. Pilbrant, M. Schannong, and J. Vessman, Eur. J. Clin. Pharmacol., 1981, 20, 65.

2 Drugs Acting on the Central Nervous System

Introduction

Psychopharmacological agents, and in particular the tricyclic antidepressants, are often used in large quantities over prolonged periods. As the side effects of many of these agents are not immediately obvious, patients may often be exposed to excessive doses.[1] It is desirable, therefore, to understand their dose-response relationships and pharmacokinetics in order to optimize therapy. However, despite the increasing practice of monitoring circulating levels of psychotropic drugs in patients,[2,3] there is still little information regarding optimum dosage schedules or dose-response or drug level-response relationships.[4,5]

At a Ciba Foundation Symposium in July 1979 it was concluded that, while there is some evidence for a therapeutic range within which optimal response is obtained, the value of monitoring psychotropic drugs is doubtful.[6] Some of the problems associated with pharmacokinetic interactions are discussed by Kaumeier.[7] Four studies attempting to establish relationships between circulating tricyclic drug levels and clinical outcome produced four dissimilar sets of results.[8] The observed differences may have been due partly to the variability of plasma protein binding among the patients studied, and partly to the overall heterogeneity of the patient populations. Other studies in depressed patients failed to obtain meaningful correlations between circulating levels of nortriptyline and changes in the Hamilton, Chronholm-Ottoson, and Beck rating scales.[9,10]

In a subsequent review of the literature on therapeutic implications of tricyclic antidepressant levels, however, Luchins and

Ananth[11] concluded that, while present evidence precluded the possibility of defining generally therapeutic ranges of drug levels for depressed patients, routine plasma level determinations may be useful in cases of intractable depression. Another study reported good correlations between the incidence of adverse clinical findings in patients and total circulating tricyclic antidepressant levels.[12] Correlations obtained between 10 adverse effects and drug levels are shown in Figure 2.1. The results are expressed in terms of circulating drug levels less than or greater than 1 µg ml^{-1} and show very

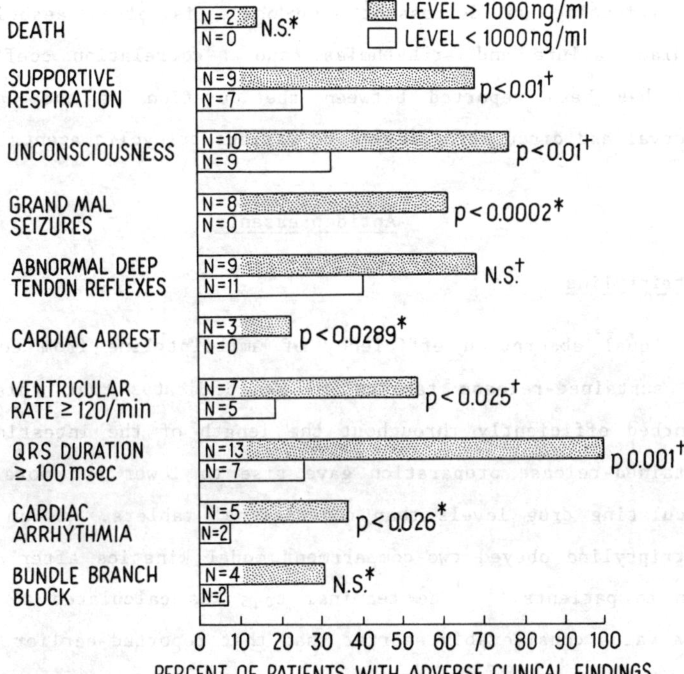

Figure 2.1 Forty patients grouped into those with maximum tricyclic levels above (N = 13) and below (N = 28) 1000 ng ml^{-1}. (*) Fisher exact probability; (†) test of the difference between two proportions. Reproduced by permission from <u>Clin. Pharmacol. Ther.</u>, 1977, <u>21</u>, 47.

high correlations. The exact compounds involved for each individual were not specified. The protein binding characteristics of a number of tricyclic agents were described by an expression of the form of equation 2.1,[13] where K is the affinity constant, k_c is related to

$$\log K = 2.3 \pm 0.05(SD)\log k_c - 0.17 \pm 0.01 R_m - 0.54 \qquad (2.1)$$

charge transfer, and R_m is a hydrophobicity parameter. The results were interpreted to indicate that the major factor in the binding is electronic in nature, with only a small contribution due to drug hydrophobicity.

Tricyclic antidepressant overdosage is often associated with cardiac failure and arrhythmias, and a correlation coefficient of +0.7 has been reported between the duration of the cardiac QRS interval and circulating levels of various tricyclic agents.[14]

Antidepressants

Amitriptyline

Equal absorption efficiency of amitriptyline from conventional and sustained-release tablets in man indicates that this drug is absorbed efficiently throughout the length of the intestine.[15] The sustained-release preparation gave rise to lower but more prolonged circulating drug levels than conventional tablets. Serum levels of amitriptyline obeyed two-compartment model kinetics after i.v. infusion to patients.[16] The terminal $t_{0.5}$ was calculated to be <u>ca</u>. 17 h, a value considerably shorter than that reported earlier for normal volunteers, but similar to $t_{0.5}$ values reported earlier for patients.

Varying estimates have been described of the $t_{0.5}$ of amitriptyline in plasma. A value of 13 h was obtained in one study,[17] but blood sampling was terminated at 30 h postdosing. In other studies, in which sampling was continued throughout 96 h, mean $t_{0.5}$ values of 36 and 22 h have been reported.[18,19] Plasma levels of amitriptyline obey two-compartment model kinetics after p.o. dosing, and the demethylated metabolite, nortriptyline, is eliminated at a similar rate to the parent drug. Steady-state levels of amitriptyline following repeated doses are accurately predicted from single-dose data. Mean plasma levels of these compounds following single doses to four volunteers are shown in Figure 2.2. Salivary levels of amitriptyline exceed those in plasma and the monitoring of drug levels in saliva may be useful in some patients.[20]

In 10 adult female patients who received 75 mg daily doses of amitriptyline as a single nightly dose or 3 x 25 mg divided doses, mean steady-state plasma levels of amitriptyline and the metabolite, nortriptyline, were similar during the two dosage regimens, though with considerable interpatient variation.[21] Amitriptyline concentrations were between 19 and 66 ng ml^{-1} from the single dose and between 21 and 70 ng ml^{-1} from the divided doses. Corresponding nortriptyline levels were 16-72 and 17-69 ng ml^{-1}.

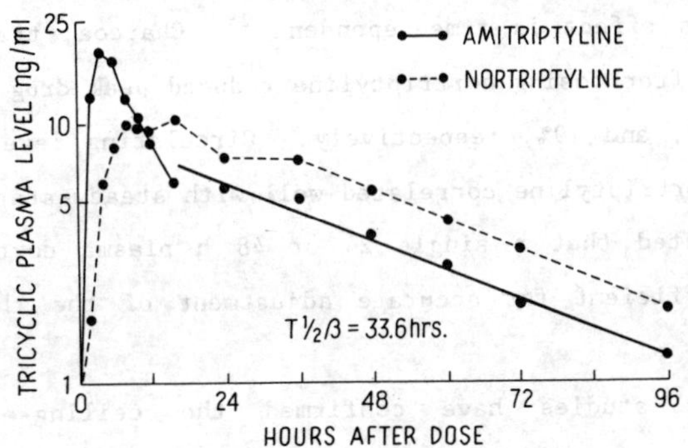

Figure 2.2 Semilogarithmic plot of the mean amitriptyline and nortriptyline plasma levels in four subjects after a single p.o. dose of 75 mg amitriptyline hydrochloride. Reproduced by permission from <u>J. Clin. Pharmacol.</u>, 1978, <u>18</u>, 462.

Nortriptyline

Area analysis showed that the bioavailability of nortriptyline following p.o. doses was <u>ca</u>. 66% of that following i.m. administration.[22] Higher metabolite levels following the p.o. dose and a similar overall drug $t_{0.5}$ after p.o. and i.m. doses suggested that differences in bioavailability from the two dosage routes were due to first-pass metabolism. The influence of hepatic clearance on the bioavailability of p.o. dosed nortriptyline may be calculated by means of equation 2.2[23] where f is the fraction of a p.o. dose that reaches

$$f = \frac{\text{flow rate}}{\text{flow rate} + \left[D/\int_o^\infty C_o \cdot dt\right]} \qquad (2.2)$$

the systemic circulation intact, flow rate is the rate of hepatic blood flow, D is the p.o. dose, and the integral represents the area under the plasma level curve. Predicted bioavailability values using equation 2.2 agreed closely with those observed by other investigators.[24,25]

Although nortriptyline is normally efficiently absorbed from the GI tract,[26,27] absorption is significantly reduced by activated charcoal.[28] This effect is time-dependent.[29] Charcoal treatment at 0.5, 2, and 4 h after dosing nortriptyline reduced peak drug levels in plasma by 77, 37, and 19%, respectively. Circulating levels from a single dose of nortriptyline correlated well with steady-state levels, and it is suggested that a single 24 or 48 h plasma nortriptyline level may be sufficient for accurate adjustment of the therapeutic dose.[30]

Two further studies have confirmed the ceiling-effect of nortriptyline plasma levels and therapeutic efficacy. Kragh-Sörensen et al.[31] recommended a plasma level of 50-150 ng ml^{-1} for optimal antidepressive effect, while Ziegler et al.[32] obtained a significantly better response on the Hamilton Depression Scale in patients with nortriptyline levels between 50 and 140 ng ml^{-1} than in those with levels between 140 and 260 ng ml^{-1}. Åsberg[33] suggested a curvilinear relationship with a reduction in effect at both high (> 140 ng ml^{-1}) and low (< 49 ng ml^{-1}) drug levels. Other evidence[34,35] suggests that clinical responses occur only when the plasma levels exceed 120 ng ml^{-1}. However, a different statistical interpretation[36] of these data suggests that they support the curvilinear response proposed by Åsberg. High circulating nortriptyline levels are associated with some electrocardiographic abnormalities.[37]

Further evidence has been presented that nortriptyline obeys two-compartment model kinetics in the body.[38] This suggests that varied dose-response relationships reported for this agent may need to be reconsidered, since levels of drug in the tissue compartment may be more closely related to pharmacologic effects than circulating drug levels. Evaluation of factors that may contribute to variations in circulating tricyclic antidepressant levels showed that black patients had 50% higher nortriptyline levels than white patients receiving the drug.[24] This may explain the more rapid response to tricyclic treatment by black patients. Decreased rates of nortriptyline metabolism by black patients may also result in treatment failure and increased side effects in this population.

Studies in twins have shown that the extent of binding of nortriptyline to plasma proteins may be influenced by both genetic and environmental factors, with variance between individuals within pairs being greater in dizygotic than in monozygotic twins.[39] Steady-state plasma levels of most tricyclic antidepressants appear to vary considerably among subjects, but remain constant for the same subject, after single and multiple doses.[40]

Nortriptyline crosses the placenta rapidly to enter foetal circulation.[41] Although the infant can metabolize the drug effectively, it does so at a reduced rate, yielding a plasma $t_{0.5}$ of 56 h compared with 17 h in the parent (Figure 2.3). A report that tricyclic antidepressants may have teratogenic properties[42] has not been substantiated in two retrospective studies.[43,44] Kinetic experiments in dogs on three closely related tricyclic antidepressants showed that their rate of elimination could be related to lipophilicity and metabolic route.[45]

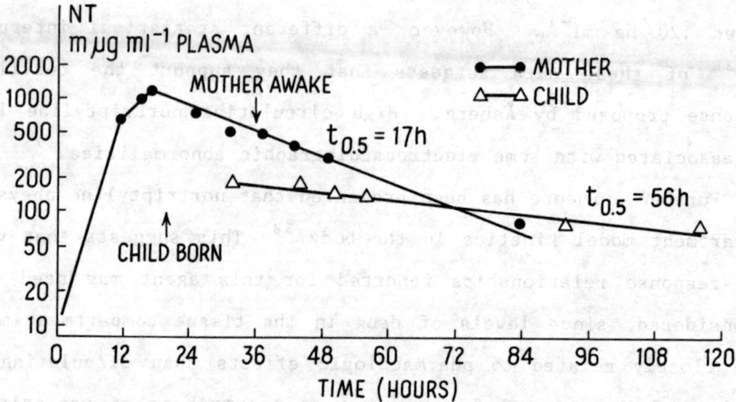

Figure 2.3 Disappearance of nortriptyline from plasma of an intoxicated mother and her newborn infant. Reproduced by permission from *J. Pediatr.*, 1972, <u>80</u>, 496.

Eighty percent of nortriptyline urinary excretion products was accounted for by the metabolite, 10-hydroxynortriptyline, and the disappearance rate of drug from plasma was determined mainly by conversion into this metabolite.[46] It appears that for 'fast' metabolizers the rate-limiting step for plasma drug clearance is the rate of blood flow through the liver.

Plasma clearance rates of nortriptyline are similar from single and repeated doses, and steady-state plasma levels can be predicted from single-dose data.[47] However, large individual variability may occur.[48-50] In 17 volunteers (mean age 25.5 yr) who received a single 75 mg p.o. dose, nortriptyline $t_{0.5}$ varied between 14 and 51 h (mean 26) while the plasma clearance ranged from 16 to 115 l h⁻¹ (mean 54).[49] The same dose administered to a group of 20 depressed elderly patients (mean age 81 yr) yielded significantly prolonged $t_{0.5}$ values (23.5-79 h, mean 45 h) and reduced plasma clearance values (8-38.5 l h⁻¹, mean 20 l h⁻¹). However, conflicting results were reported later,[50] which suggested poor correlation between age and nortriptyline elimination. As nortriptyline is primarily metabolized by hepatic demethylation and hydroxylation, its clearance is unaltered in chronic renal failure.[50]

Most of the tricyclic antidepressants appear to induce hepatic drug-metabolizing enzymes to a small extent in man.[51,52] However, their metabolism appears to be unaltered by the benzodiazepines, and it is suggested that when tranquilizing drugs are required to supplement tricyclic antidepressants the benzodiazepines should be given preference over barbiturates and phenothiazines.[53-55]

Imipramine

The systemic availability of p.o. imipramine is poor and erratic. Availability is reduced, in part, by first-pass metabolism, but the extent of the first-pass effect appears unrelated to drug $t_{0.5}$ or clearance in individual subjects.[56] It has been estimated that 30-77% of orally dosed drug may be removed by first-pass hepatic clearance.[57]

Portal-vein catheterization studies in patients showed that imipramine is absorbed rapidly after p.o. doses.[58] Levels of drug in portal and cubital veins are compared in Figure 2.4. Drug appeared in the portal circulation 10 min after dosing. Peak portal-vein values were obtained within 30 and 40 min, while portal and cubital levels converged to similar values by 80 min.

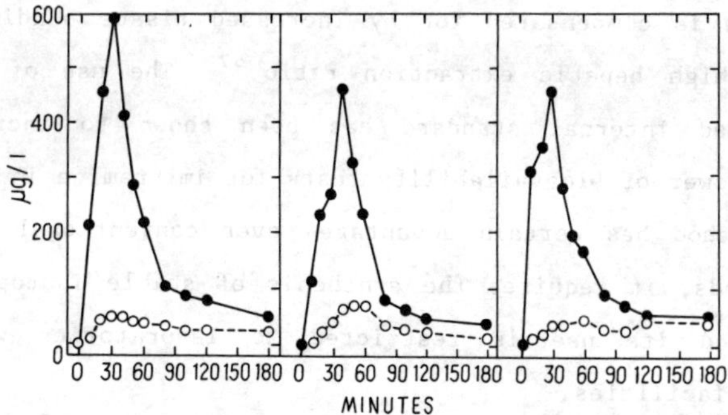

Figure 2.4 Concentrations of imipramine in plasma in the portal (•) and cubital (o) veins in three subjects after single doses of imipramine hydrochloride 0.5 mg kg^{-1} body weight. Reproduced by permission from *Clin. Pharmacol. Ther.*, 1976, *19*, 584.

Studies in rats showed that ^{14}C-imipramine is poorly absorbed from the stomach, and that blood and tissue levels of ^{14}C are closely related to the rate of stomach emptying.[59] This may partially explain the wide variation in circulating levels of imipramine in man, in whom gastric emptying is known to be extremely variable.[60] After p.o. administration of imipramine 10 mg kg^{-1} b.i.d. for 3 weeks to rats, biliary excretion for 50 min after dosing was decreased to 16% of that after a single dose. Drug absorption was also slowed, while the rate of 2-hydroxylation and 10-hydroxylation, but not demethylation, was decreased relative to controls.[61] Reduced biliary excretion of drug is thought to be due to slower absorption and also a reduced rate of drug metabolism, which may result from product inhibition.

Thioridazine has been shown to reduce biliary and urinary excretion of radioactivity after p.o. doses of ^{14}C-imipramine to rats.[62] These effects were attributed to thioridazine reducing absorption of imipramine owing to delayed stomach emptying. Diazepam, on the other hand, had little or no effect on imipramine pharmacokinetics in this species.

Rat-liver perfusion studies suggest that hepatic metabolism and biliary elimination of imipramine are not linearly related to dose size, even within the therapeutic range. However, reduced metabolism at high doses is compensated for by increased tissue binding, which maintains a high hepatic extraction ratio.[57] The use of a stable isotope-labeled internal standard has been shown to increase the statistical power of bioavailability tests for imipramine in humans.[63] While the method has certain advantages over conventional bioavailability methods, it requires the synthesis of stable isotope-labeled compounds, and its use is restricted to laboratories with mass spectrometry facilities.

Steady-state levels of imipramine varied considerably following repeated doses to patients.[64] Patients with steady-state levels less than 50 ng ml^{-1} reached this value within one week of dosing, while those with levels greater than this reached steady-state in 2-3 weeks;

steady-state levels appeared to be age-dependent in both men and women. Considerable variations in circulating levels of imipramine, and also its active metabolite desipramine, have been reported also by Gram et al.[65] Although regressions were not attempted in their studies, 11 of 12 patients who responded satisfactorily (Hamilton Rating Scale < 8) had plasma levels of imipramine > 45 ng ml^{-1} and desipramine > 75 ng ml^{-1}; 12 unresponsive patients (Hamilton Rating Scale $\geq$ 8) had lower plasma concentrations.

Another report supports the concept that while the relationship between plasma levels of nortriptyline, and therapeutic effects is curvilinear, the relationship for imipramine is linear, with optimum response occurring in the drug concentration range 150-240 ng ml^{-1}.[66]

Comparisons of the pharmacokinetics of imipramine, nortriptyline, and antipyrine in man have shown that imipramine has a higher clearance, shorter $t_{0.5}$, and a smaller apparent distribution volume than nortriptyline.[67] There was a significant correlation between the clearances of the two compounds. There was also a positive correlation between imipramine and antipyrine clearances.

Butriptyline

The p.o. bioavailability of butriptyline from a sustained-release formulation (75 mg tablet) has been compared with that from conventional tablets (3 x 25 mg).[68] In 14 healthy male subjects, the sustained-release tablet yielded an average peak plasma butriptyline concentration of 20.3 ng ml^{-1} at 7.5 h, compared with 46.5 ng ml^{-1} at 2.6 h from conventional tablets. Differences in both C_{max} and T_{max} were statistically significant. The half-value duration (HVD), defined as the time span during which the plasma butriptyline concentration exceeded half the maximum concentration,[69] averaged 6.8 h for conventional tablets and 17.4 h for the sustained-release formulation, thus confirming prolonged absorption from the latter. Overall bio-

availability was similar from the two formulations. The terminal
$t_{0.5}$ of <u>ca</u>. 20 h also was formulation independent.

Protriptyline

Unlike imipramine protriptyline undergoes relatively minor first-
pass metabolism, accounting for 10-25% of a p.o. dose. Protriptyline
has a longer biological $t_{0.5}$ than amitriptyline and nortriptyline,
ranging from 54 to 92 h in normal individuals.[70] Protriptyline
appears similar to imipramine in that there appears to be no upper
limit to plasma levels for optimal therapeutic efficacy.[71] In patients receiving chronic protriptyline, steady-state plasma levels of
drug varied more than 3-fold from 113 to 376 ng ml^{-1},[72] whereas the
volume of distribution showed little intersubject variation. Elimination $t_{0.5}$ values varied over a wide range, from 54 to 198 h.

Other Tricyclic Antidepressants

Despite its similar chemical structure, the plasma $t_{0.5}$ of
desmethylimipramine is considerably shorter and the plasma clearance
about twice that for nortriptyline[73] (Figure 2.5). This may be due to

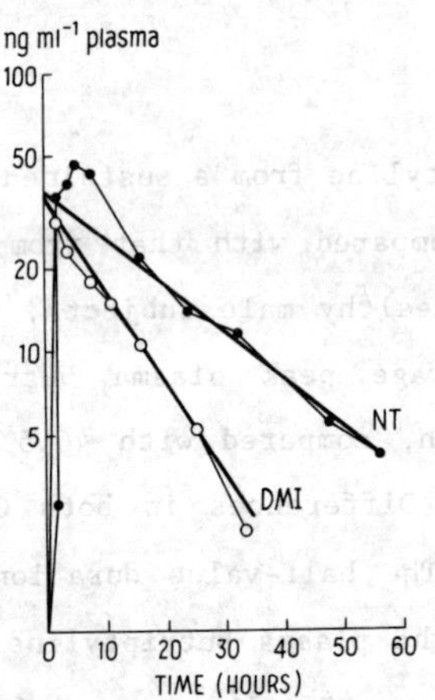

Figure 2.5   Log plasma concentrations of desmethylimipramine and nortriptyline against time in a human
subject after single doses (1 mg kg^{-1}). Each circle
is the average of triplicate estimations. Reproduced
by permission from <u>Eur. J. Clin. Pharmacol</u>., 1972, <u>5</u>,
1.

lower plasma-protein binding and larger distribution volumes associated with desmethylimipramine.

In two parallel groups of healthy subjects receiving 75 and 150 mg p.o. doses of desipramine hydrochloride, average peak plasma concentrations of desipramine were 30.7 and 60.9 ng ml^{-1}, respectively, both achieved at <u>ca</u>. 6 h postdose.[74] There were no statistically significant differences in the $t_{0.5}$ values between the two dose groups, the mean values being 19.7 and 18.4 h, respectively.

The imipramine analogue lofepramine was shown to undergo considerable first-pass metabolism to form desmethylimipramine after p.o. doses,[75] the bioavailability of unchanged drug being less than 10% of the dose. Despite extensive first-pass hepatic clearance, absorption of drug is rapid with peak levels appearing within 1 h of dosing. As with other tricyclic antidepressants, lofepramine appears to distribute extensively into tissues.

The isoquinoline analogue nomifensine is absorbed rapidly after p.o. dosing.[76] The pharmacokinetics of nomifensine were studied in healthy volunteers who received the drug as single p.o. doses (75 and 150 mg) and as an i.v. infusion (75 mg).[77] After p.o. doses peak serum concentrations were reached at 1-1.5 h. Elimination $t_{0.5}$ values averaged 1.8 and 2.5 h for the p.o. and i.v. doses, respectively, although large individual differences in serum levels were noted. After both p.o. and i.v. infusion doses, the maximum pharmacologic effect, as determined by pharmaco-EEG and psychometric tests, occurred between 4 and 6 h postdose. The pharmacodynamic results correlated better with free nomifensine serum concentrations than with total (conjugated plus unconjugated) concentrations.

Unlike most other tricyclic antidepressants, nomifensine has a relatively short biological $t_{0.5}$. It appears to have a large distribution volume of almost 6 l kg^{-1}, but this value was calculated assuming complete absorption following p.o. doses.[75]

Doxepin also has a short biological $t_{0.5}$ relative to most other tricyclic antidepressants.[78] This compound undergoes considerable (55-87%) first-pass metabolism, while disappearance of drug from blood is biphasic with a terminal $t_{0.5}$ value of <u>ca</u>. 17 h. Circulating levels of the metabolite desmethyldoxepin are initially lower than those of the parent compound, but the metabolite has a more prolonged $t_{0.5}$ of 50 h. The longer duration of desmethyldoxepin in the body compared with that of the parent drug is consistent with the concept that secondary amines tend to have longer biological $t_{0.5}$ values than tertiary amines. The tricyclic agent, chlorprothixene, is extensively distributed in the body and has an overall distribution volume in man approaching 1000 l and a biological $t_{0.5}$ of 8-12 h.[79]

The psychotropic agent viloxazine is rapidly absorbed after a single 100 mg p.o. dose.[80] As shown in Figure 2.6, where each blood and c.s.f. concentration represent data from one patient, the elimina-

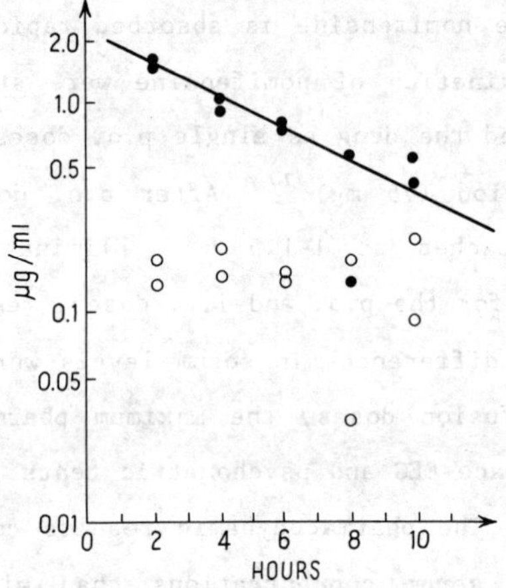

Figure 2.6   Concentrations of viloxazine in blood (●) and c.s.f. (o) after a single p.o. dose of 100 mg. Reproduced by permission from <u>Eur. J. Clin. Pharmacol.</u>, 1980, <u>17</u>, 179.

tion $t_{0.5}$ of viloxazine in blood was 4.5 h. In contrast, viloxazine concentrations in c.s.f. were virtually unchanged during 10 h. However, no accumulation of drug in blood or c.s.f. was observed after chronic administration of viloxazine, 150 mg d^{-1}, for 4 weeks.

A 75 mg p.o. dose of dothiepin yielded mean peak concentrations in blood and plasma of 36 and 47 ng ml^{-1}, respectively, at <u>ca</u>. 3 h.[81] Fitting individual data to a triexponential curve yielded an average elimination $t_{0.5}$ value of 22 h. As with other tricyclic antidepressants, considerable interindividual variations were observed in plasma dothiepin concentrations, probably due to variability in first-pass metabolism. After p.o. administration of dothiepin, blood levels of two metabolites, dothiepin S-oxide and northiaden, were measurable and reached peak values of 81 and 10 ng ml^{-1}, respectively, at 5 h. Dothiepin S-oxide was eliminated at a similar rate to the parent drug while northiaden was more slowly eliminated, the respective mean $t_{0.5}$ values being 19 and 33 h.

Antipsychotic Agents

Chlorpromazine

The bioavailability of p.o. dosed chlorpromazine is generally poor. Although the compound is extensively metabolized, first-pass metabolism may not be an important factor owing to its long elimination $t_{0.5}$. Bioequivalency problems with commercial chlorpromazine formulations have been aggravated by the absence of sensitive and specific assays at low drug and metabolite concentrations. A method of combining clinical and kinetic data has been proposed.[82] However, a pharmacological method using pupilometry has been shown to be extremely sensitive and to correlate well with circulating levels of unchanged drug.[83]

Two computerized methods, MULTIFIT, based on a time domain, and PLTEST, based on frequency response, were compared in obtaining an appropriate pharmacokinetic model relating chlorpromazine-induced changes in rectal temperature[84] and miotic response[85] in rabbits. Both methods appear to be useful for quantitative analysis of chlorpromazine bioavailability and pharmacokinetics, particularly in the case of low drug levels.

The biological availability of chlorpromazine after single p.o. doses to volunteers ranged from 10 to 69%, and averaged 32% relative to i.m. doses.[86] The metabolite chlorpromazine sulphoxide was found after p.o., but not i.m., doses, suggesting pre-systemic formation of this metabolite.

The absorption of liquid suspensions of chlorpromazine hydrochloride was similar to a new palatable embonate salt of this drug in schizophrenic patients.[87] Concomitant antacid administration resulted in lower plasma chlorpromazine levels,[88] and reduced enteral absorption appeared to be due to absorption of chlorpromazine into the antacid gel rather than a pH effect. Plasma levels of chlorpromazine are reduced by 40% and the area under the plasma level curve by 27%, when co-administered with lithium.[89] While former theories are proposed to explain this interaction, the precise mechanism is not known The extent of the interaction may explain inadequate therapeutic response to chlorpromazine in the presence of lithium, and the sudden onset of chlorpromazine toxicity in some patients after withdrawal of concurrent lithium therapy.

Plasma levels of chlorpromazine following single p.o. doses to healthy volunteers have been described by a two-compartment open model with zero-order absorption following a lag time.[90] The use of zero-order input provided superior description of the data compared to first-order input. The mean α and β $t_{0.5}$ values were 1.6 and 18 h, respectively.

Children need larger doses of chlorpromazine than adults to achieve the same plasma level of drug, but optimum plasma levels of chlorpromazine in children (40-80 ng ml^{-1}) are lower than in adults (50-300 ng ml^{-1}). While good correlations were obtained between the antipsychotic effect of chlorpromazine and drug levels both in the c.s.f. and in plasma in patients after 2 weeks of treatment, correlations between drug levels and effect were reduced after 4 weeks. In another study plasma levels in patients correlated well with peripheral autonomic measures, but central measures were inconsistent.[92]

Chlorpromazine and many of its metabolites are sequestered by erythrocytes, and it is important that whole blood rather than plasma be used to determine circulating levels of these compounds.[93,94] Erythrocytes have been shown also to influence the binding of chlorpromazine to albumin, although binding to plasma proteins does not appear significantly to influence the overall elimination of drug from the body.[95] No differences could be detected in plasma chlorpromazine clearances in control and cirrhotic subjects, and susceptibility of cirrhotics to this drug may be due to increased sensitivity of cerebral neurones rather than impaired metabolism.[96] Wide individual variations in plasma levels of chlorpromazine have been reported in patients,[92,97] and studies after chronic dosing to children and adult patients suggest that chlorpromazine induces its own metabolism.[98,99]

Rapid placental transfer of chlorpromazine occurs in the goat, with foetal plasma levels approaching 50% of maternal values within 10 min of the mother receiving an i.v. dose.[100] The foetal:maternal plasma ratio remained constant at <u>ca</u>. 0.5 for 1 h, whereas foetal: maternal concentration ratios in the liver, kidney, heart, and brain all approached unity. There was a marked effect of the drug on foetal heart rate.

Levomepromazine

Single p.o. doses (25 mg kg^{-1}) of levomepromazine in the rat were rapidly absorbed, and the average t_{max} was 1.4 h.[101] Large interindividual variations in blood levels were observed. Oral bioavailability, compared with an intraarterial (i.a.) reference dose (10 mg kg^{-1}), averaged 28% in 5 rats. Mean distribution volume and total body clearance after i.a. doses were 16.6 l kg^{-1} and 12.3 ml min^{-1}, respectively.

Elimination $t_{0.5}$ values of levomepromazine after p.o. and i.a. doses were similar, and averaged 6.1 h. Blood levels of two major nonpolar metabolites, N-monodesmethyl levomepromazine and levomepromazine sulfoxide, were 179% and 65%, respectively, of the levomepromazine levels after p.o. dosing. However, the respective metabolite concentrations averaged only 15% and 25% of the levomepromazine levels following i.a. administration, as shown by the dose-normalized AUC values in Figure 2.7. These results suggest that the metabolites were formed predominantly before reaching the systemic circulation.

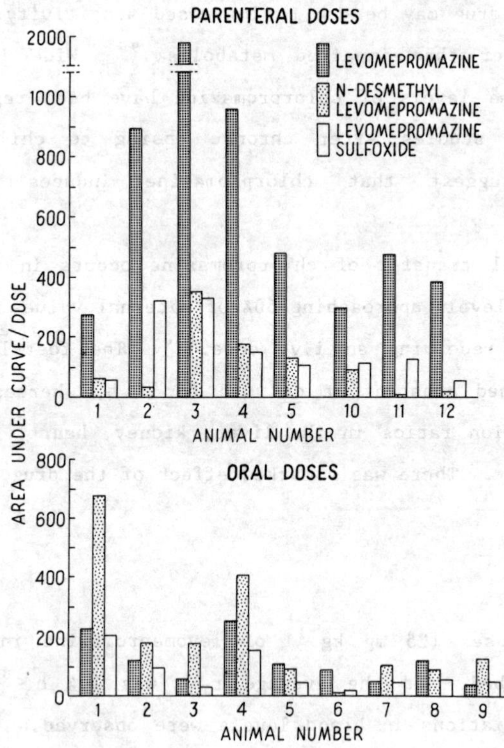

Figure 2.7 Area under blood concentration curves of levomepromazine and metabolites, divided by the administered dose of levomepromazine. Reproduced by permission from *Acta Pharmacol. Toxicol.*, 1982, **50**, 148.

Trifluoperazine

Twenty-four hour urinary excretion of parent drug and the sulphoxide metabolites of chlorpromazine and thioridazine was independent of dose in patients, whereas excretion of trifluoperazine and its sulphoxide metabolite was highly dose-dependent.[102] However, 24 h urinary excretion of combined drug and metabolite accounted for < 10% of the dose. Studies in rats confirmed the minor contribution of renal mechanisms to trifluoperazine elimination with > 90% of absorbed compound appearing as faecal metabolites, due partly to biliary excretion.[103] The distribution of trifluoperazine in the rat is similar to that of chlorpromazine. Drug accumulates in liver, lung, and, to a lesser extent, brain tissue. As with other phenothiazines, no sulphoxide metabolite of trifluoperazine was found in the brain. This is contrary to postulated catalytic sulphoxidation in brain tissue.[104]

Fluphenazine

After i.m. injection of ^{14}C-fluphenazine decanoate and ^{14}C-fluphenazine enanthate as solutions in sesame oil to Sprague-Dawley rats, similar peak brain concentrations of fluphenazine were reached at 4 h and 24 h, respectively.[105] There were no apparent differences in brain levels of total radioactivity from the two esters.

Binding of fluphenazine to normal human serum was studied *in vitro* by equilibrium dialysis at an initial fluphenazine concentration of 24.4 ng ml^{-1}.[106] As shown in Figure 2.8, the free fraction of fluphenazine increased progressively with age, from *ca.* 6% at 25-29 yr to *ca.* 8% at 72-88 yr. Fluphenazine serum binding decreased also in an equimolar mixture of the drug with thioridazine.

Methotrimeprazine

Presystemic metabolism may be the cause of high circulating levels of the sulphoxide metabolite of p.o. methotrimeprazine.[107]

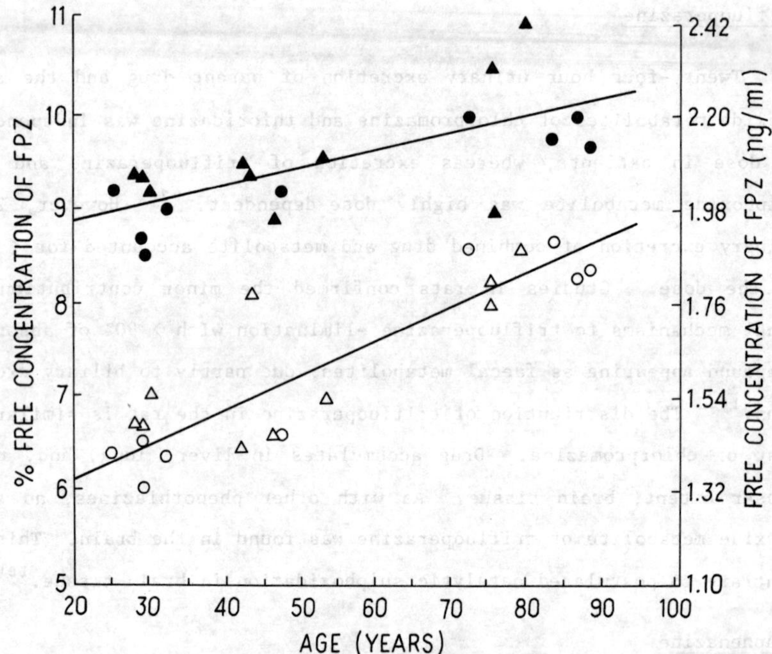

Figure 2.8   Age versus free fluphenazine (FPZ) concentration in human serum samples. o male, Δ, female, ●
male with thioridazine, ▲ female with thioridazine.
Reproduced by permission from the Brit. J. Clin.
Pharmacol., 1982, 9, 432.

Plasma levels of the metabolite were higher than those of unchanged
drug following p.o. doses, but were undetected in plasma after i.m.
doses. The overall distribution volume of methotrimeprazine was 23-42
1 mg^{-1} and the biological $t_{0.5}$ was 15-30 h.   The apparent $t_{0.5}$
of the sulphoxide was ca. 30% shorter than that of the parent drug,
although this value varied considerably between individuals. Following p.o. dosage of tablet and syrup formulations of levomepromazine,
the biological $t_{0.5}$ of unchanged drug ranged from 16.5 to 77.8 h.[108]
The ratio of total clearance to the absorbed fraction was calculated
by means of equation 2.3, and was shown to vary 13-fold between

$$\frac{Cl}{F_{p.o.}} = \frac{D}{AUC}$$

(2.3)

individuals. In this equation $Cl/F_{p.o.}$ is the total drug clearance divided by the absorbed fraction, D is the administered dose, and AUC represents the area under the plasma drug-level curve during one dosage interval. The considerable variation in $Cl/F_{p.o.}$ values may thus be due to changes in drug $t_{0.5}$, distribution, or the percentage of dose absorbed.

Butaperazine

Considerable individual differences were observed in drug blood-levels in patients receiving butaperazine in five different dosage forms.[109] Highest levels were obtained from a liquid concentrate, although there was little difference in clinical efficacy between the concentrate and tablet formulations. Patients responding to the drug generally had higher blood-levels than nonresponders.

Thioridazine

Thioridazine is well absorbed from the GI tract.[110] The drug distributes extensively into tissues, yielding highest concentrations in the lung, liver, adrenals, and spleen.[111-113] Thioridazine and its principal metabolites are extensively bound to plasma proteins.[111,112] While the total concentration of thioridazine in c.s.f. was only 1% of that in serum, the unbound drug concentration in c.s.f. was nearly twice that in serum.[114] Other drugs that compete with thioridazine for serum protein binding sites *in vitro* include propranolol and the tricyclic antidepressants amitriptyline, nortriptyline, and clomipramine.[115] The major psychoactive metabolites of thioridazine, formed primarily via sulfoxidation, are mesoridazine (side-chain sulfoxide) and sulforidazine (side-chain sulfone) as well as several other compounds.[116-119] Unchanged thioridazine constitutes approximately 20% or less of circulating levels of drug-derived material in plasma, the ring sulfoxide and side-chain sulfoxide (mesoridazine) being the major plasma metabolites.[116] Plasma concentrations of these compounds are proportional to single doses up to 100 mg thioridazine.[120] However, the mesoridazine:thioridazine concentration ratio decreases substantially with multiple drug administration, suggesting that Michaelis-Menten kinetics are involved in the metabolism of thioridazine to mesoridazine.[121]

Plasma concentration ratios of mesoridazine, and also the ring sulfoxide, to those of thioridazine were significantly higher in alcoholics than in nonalcoholic patients.[122] The authors suggest that alcoholics with minor liver dysfunction have induced metabolizing capacity whereas those with more advanced deterioration of liver function have decreased metabolizing capacity.

Approximately 90% of a p.o. dose of ^{35}S-thioridazine in man was metabolized prior to excretion.[110] Total recovery of radioactivity was 30% in the urine and 50% in the feces. Similarly, after parenteral doses of ^{14}C-thioridazine in the rat[123] and dog,[124] approximately 15 and 20-25%, respectively, of the administered radioactivity was excreted in 168 h urine. The terminal $t_{0.5}$ for thioridazine and its active metabolites in psychiatric patients is <u>ca</u>. 16 h, with considerable intersubject variation.[125] Elimination of thioridazine is slower at night than at other times, and the serum $t_{0.5}$ of the drug and also drug levels increase with age.[125] The elimination of thioridazine appears not to be influenced by other medication.

<u>Thiothixene</u>

Poor correlations were obtained between circulating plasma levels of both thiothixene and thioridazine and clinical effects in schizophrenic or paranoic patients.[126] Drug plasma levels were closely related to dose size, although levels of thiothixene declined with repeated doses because of induction of drug-metabolizing enzymes. Reduced plasma levels of thiothixene with repeated doses was confirmed in another study in schizophrenic patients.[127] However, in this study, therapeutic effect was associated with peak plasma levels occurring between 10 and 22.5 µg ml^{-1}; these levels were obtained from widely varying doses.

Haloperidol

In patients with paranoid schizophrenia, the bioavailability of haloperidol from p.o. solutions was less than that from an i.m. dose, resulting in significantly lower plasma concentrations after the p.o. doses, with larger interindividual fluctuation.[128] The disposition of i.v. administered haloperidol was studied in rhesus monkeys using a radioimmunoassay.[129] The elimination $t_{0.5}$ values in two animals were 16 and 7.6 h, similar to reported values in man. The drug was eliminated almost entirely by metabolism, with only 0.01% of the dose excreted unchanged in 24 h urine.

After rapid i.v. injection into patients, serum concentrations of unchanged haloperidol declined biexponentially, indicating two-compartment model kinetics.[130] The overall distribution volume, $V_{d(extrap)}$, varied between 1200 and 2000 l, confirming extensive tissue sequestration, and the terminal $t_{0.5}$ varied between 12.6 and 22.0 h. With an elimination $t_{0.5}$ of this duration, it is clear that a period of at least 3-5 days should be allowed before a steady-state dose-response relationship can be established with this drug.[131]

In 22 schizophrenic patients aged 22-79 yr who received 3-45 mg haloperidol daily for 6 m, serum concentrations of both free and total haloperidol correlated significantly with daily dose.[132] The percent free haloperidol, which averaged 12.5%, was constant in the tested range of steady-state concentrations, and was unrelated to age. *In vitro* data suggest that thioridazine and oleic acid may enhance the percent of unbound haloperidol in normal human serum.

The tissue distribution characteristics of haloperidol,[133] moperone,[134] and trifluperidol[135] have been shown to be dose-dependent in rats. Initial uptake into the brain is rapid for all three compounds, and brain levels of drug can exceed blood levels by a factor of ten. Haloperidol and trifluperidol are metabolized slowly in the liver whereas breakdown of moperone is rapid and extensive.

Droperidol

Droperidol is rapidly absorbed after i.m. injection, and plasma profiles of unchanged drug obey two-compartment model kinetics. The plasma elimination $t_{0.5}$ is <u>ca</u>. 130 min with little individual variation. Like haloperidol, droperidol has a distribution volume considerably larger than total body weight and is extensively metabolized.[136] Some of the problems associated with analysis of data based on total radioactivity measurements with these types of compounds have been described.[137]

Sulpiride

The pharmacokinetics of the new antipsychotic agent sulpiride were studied in 6 subjects after receiving single 100 mg i.v. and p.o. doses on separate occasions.[138] The mean serum $t_{0.5}$ after i.v. administration, determined by two-compartment model analysis, was 5.3 h and systemic clearance was 415 ml min^{-1}. Seventy percent of the i.v. dose was recovered unchanged in 36 h urine. In contrast, the p.o. dose was slowly absorbed, reaching peak serum levels at 3-6 h, and only 15% of the dose was recovered in urine as unchanged sulpiride. The p.o. bioavailability of sulpiride is 27%. As hepatic metabolism appears to play a relatively minor role in the elimination of sulpiride, low bioavailability is believed to reflect incomplete GI absorption.

Sedatives, Hypnotics, and Tranquilizers

Barbiturates

Despite their extensive use, <u>in vivo</u> absorption and distribution characteristics of most barbiturates are poorly documented.

Phenobarbital

Phenobarbital is administered both p.o. and i.m., but neither of these routes has been shown to be quantitatively superior to the other. Previous studies relating derived barbiturate substituent constants R_m and absorption characteristics were expanded to describe correlations between chromatographic R_m values and <u>in situ</u> gastric absorption rate constants k_a.[139] Absorption constant-substituent relationships are described in the form of equations 2.4 and 2.5, where a and b are constants. Correlation coefficients of actual versus calculated k_a and Δk_a values were +0.998 and +0.999,

$$\log k_a = a + bR_m \tag{2.4}$$

$$\Delta \log k_a = b\Delta R_m \tag{2.5}$$

respectively. Similar expressions are derived relating R_m values to concentrations required to elicit pharmacologic effects. The chromatographic system utilized in this study is less cumbersome than previous bulk-phase partition procedures, although both methods may be of general application in examining drug absorption behaviour.

The bioavailability characteristics of p.o. phenobarbital have been studied in terms of <u>in vitro</u> release of free acid and the sodium salts from compressed tablets.[140] The sodium salt is released faster than the free acid into water but considerably more slowly into 0.1N HCl, even in the presence of a surface active agent. Although surfactants increase the aqueous solubility of barbiturates, they tend to inhibit transfer of drug from aqueous to lipoidal solvents and may retard drug availability <u>in vivo</u>.[141-143] Others have shown absorption of p.o. dosed phenobarbital to be largely independent of the dosage form.[144] An average p.o. dose of 2.9 mg kg^{-1} phenobarbital yielded a mean serum C_{max} of 5.5 µg ml^{-1} at 2.3 h, and an overall bioavailability of <u>ca</u>. 95%.[145]

As indicated above, the relative absorption efficacy of phenobarbital from p.o. and i.m. doses is uncertain. Following single injections into the deltoid muscle of adult human volunteers, the bioavailability of phenobarbital was 80% of that from an equivalent p.o. dose.[146] Incomplete absorption of i.m. phenobarbital, a phenomenon not noted previously in infants,[147] may be due to precipitation of drug at the injection site and/or its slow release from that site, giving rise to low and possibly undetectable circulating drug levels.

Intramuscular doses (<u>ca</u>. 10 mg kg^{-1}) of phenobarbital sodium appeared to be more rapidly absorbed than phenobarbital acid, peak plasma barbiturate concentration in 12 infants being achieved at 0.9 and 5.8 h, respectively.[148] However, no significant differences were observed in the mean peak concentrations after dosing the sodium salt and the acid (16.2 and 13.8 μg ml^{-1}, respectively), or in the respective AUC values.

After 10 mg kg^{-1} i.m. doses to very young infants, absorption of phenobarbital was rapid with peak blood levels of about 13 μg ml^{-1} occurring between 45 and 120 min postdose.[149] The average c.s.f. to blood concentration ratio was 0.49. Similar peak values were obtained after equivalent p.o. doses although the time of peak blood levels varied between 1 and 6 h.[150] These results indicate that phenobarbital is absorbed faster from i.m. than from p.o. doses in young children, who have a smaller muscle mass than adults.

The effect of activated charcoal on serum levels of p.o. administered phenobarbital was examined using a randomized crossover design in 5 healthy subjects.[151] As shown in Figure 2.9, the absorption of a 200 mg p.o. dose of phenobarbital was almost completely prevented when 50 g of activated charcoal was ingested within 5 min. Inhibition was less when charcoal was given 1 h after the phenobarbital dose, the mean serum AUC of phenobarbital being 53% of the control value.

Ethanol has been shown to increase the absorption of phenobarbital from the peritoneal cavity of the rat, but appeared to have no effect on pentobarbital transport.[152]

Other studies in rats indicate that the absorption of phenobarbital, and a number of other drugs, from the lung can be faster than from the small intestine.[153] Comparison of chloroform:water partitioning, aqueous diffusion coefficients, and absorption rates suggests that absorption in the lung occurs across a lipid-pore membrane. In

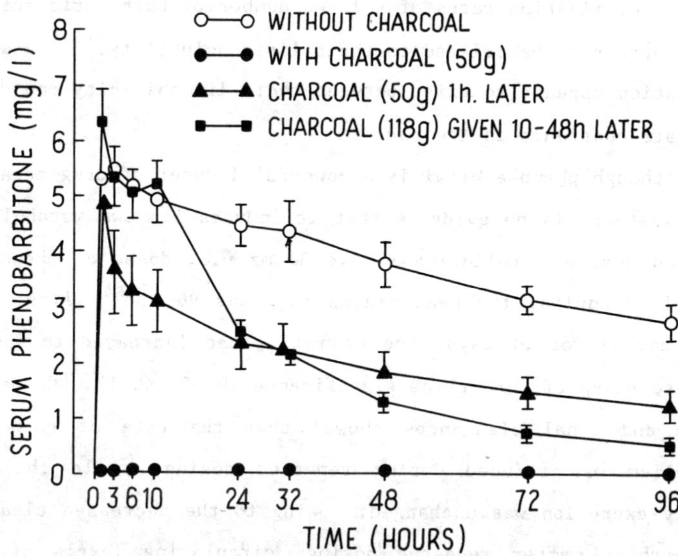

Figure 2.9   Effect of activated charcoal on serum phenobarbitone concentration. Phenobarbitone 200 mg was ingested in a crossover study without or with activated charcoal. Mean ± SEM in five volunteers. Reproduced by permission from <u>Eur. J. Clin. Pharmacol.</u>, 1980, <u>17</u>, 51.

extending previous studies,[154] serum levels of phenobarbital have been described in terms of two-compartment model kinetics after i.v. doses to neonates, 1-12 month-old babies, and infants.[155] Distribution volumes, and also the microscopic distribution rate constants, k_{12} and k_{21}, were similar in the three age groups, but the elimination $t_{0.5}$ in neonates (119 ± 16 h) was significantly longer than in babies (63 ± 5 h) and in infants (69 ± 3 h). Near the time of peak plasma concentration after administering i.m. phenobarbital, the c.s.f.:plasma barbiturate concentration ratio was 0.4-0.5.[148] In another study employing 17 infants,[156] a linear relationship was observed between plasma and brain tissue levels of phenobarbital. The mean brain: plasma phenobarbital ratio was 0.71. The blood-brain barrier to some barbiturates in rats was not affected by ethanol, even in intoxicating amounts.[152]

The elimination rates of a large number of barbituric acid derivatives appear to be related to their lipid solubility.[157] However, no correlation appears to exist between their lipophilicity and distribution rate constants in the rat.

Although phenobarbital is a powerful inducer of drug metabolizing enzymes, there is no evidence that it induces its own metabolism with repeated dosing. Following single 30 mg p.o. doses of phenobarbital to healthy adults, the mean plasma $t_{0.5}$ was 96 h.[158] After repeated daily dosing for 21 days, the mean $t_{0.5}$ had increased to 150 h; the increase being of borderline significance ($0.05 < p < 0.1$). Comparison of plasma and renal clearances showed that the rate of phenobarbital metabolism was reduced during repeated dosing, while the rate of urinary excretion was unchanged. Owing to the decreased clearance of phenobarbital after repeated dosing, circulating levels of drug at steady-state were greater than those predicted from first-dose kinetics. This is illustrated for three individuals in Figure 2.10.

Following repeated daily doses to neonates at a level of 5 mg kg^{-1} d^{-1} for four weeks, the plasma $t_{0.5}$ of phenobarbital decreased from an initial value of 115 h to 67 h.[159] Differences in phenobarbital metabolism autoinduction in the two populations were probably related to the higher dose used and the initially immature conditions of enzyme systems in neonates.[160] Immature hepatic metabolism of phenobarbital in the newborn has been demonstrated by Boréus et al.,[161] who obtained a mean plasma drug $t_{0.5}$ of 79 h in nursing mothers compared to 111 h in their infants during the first week of life. Infants and children also exhibit a lower phenobarbital plasma level:dosage ratio than adults, and a linear correlation was established between this ratio and age for children between 2 m and 6.5 yr.[162] The elimination $t_{0.5}$ of phenobarbital in infants averaged 64 h with a range of 37–131 h.[148]

Multiple doses of charcoal between 10 and 48 h after administering phenobarbital caused a decrease in phenobarbital $t_{0.5}$ from 110

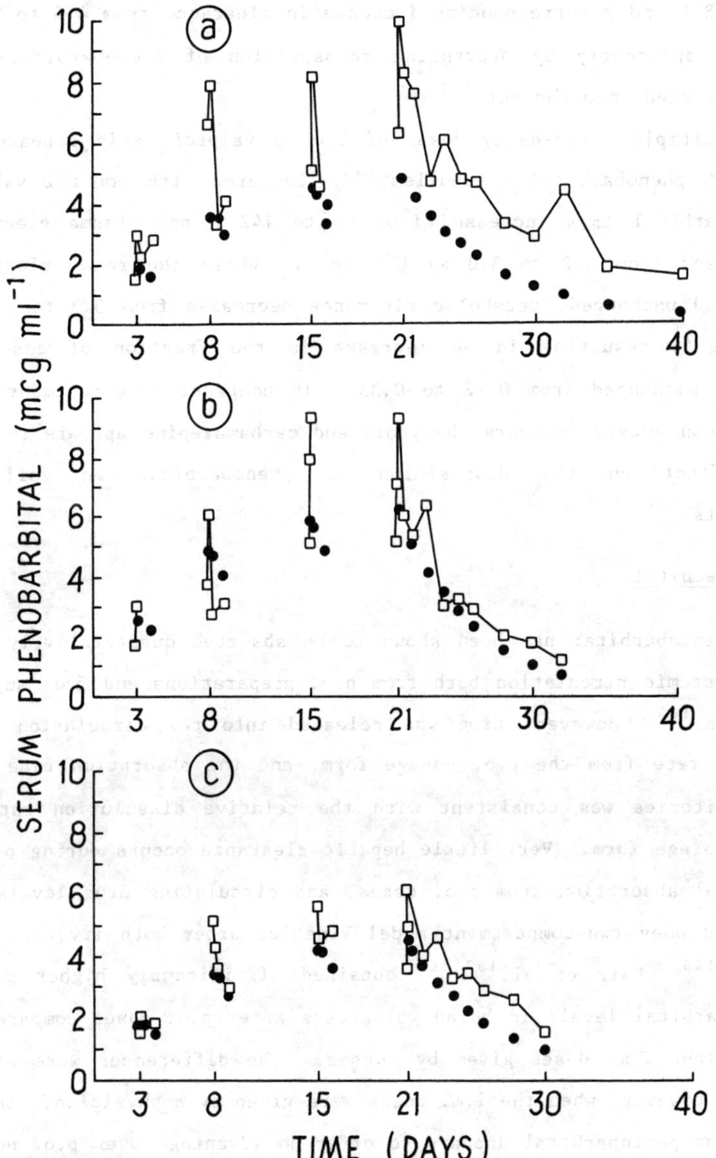

Figure 2.10 Serum levels (□) of phenobarbital in subject 1 (a), subject 2 (b), and subject 3 (c) during Days 3, 8, 15 and after the final dose of a 30 mg daily repeated-dose regimen. Solid circles(●) indicate predicted values based on single-dose data. Reproduced by permission from J. Clin. Pharmacol., 1979, 19, 282.

to 19.8 h and a corresponding increase in clearance from 4.6 to 23 ml min^{-1}, apparently by preventing reabsorption of phenobarbital that was secreted into the gut.[151]

Multiple twice-daily doses of 250 mg valproic acid appeared to inhibit phenobarbital metabolism.[163] Compared with control values, phenobarbital $t_{0.5}$ increased from 96 to 142 h and plasma clearance decreased from 4.2 to 3.0 ml h^{-1} kg^{-1}. While the renal clearance remained unchanged, metabolic clearance decreased from 3.3 to 2.0 ml h^{-1} kg^{-1}, resulting in an increase in the fraction of dose excreted unchanged from 0.22 to 0.33. In contrast, pretreatment with the known enzyme inducers phenytoin and carbamazepine appears to have no effect on the disposition of phenobarbital in epileptic patients.[164]

Pentobarbital

Pentobarbital has been shown to be absorbed quantitatively into the systemic circulation both from p.o. preparations and from suppositories.[165] However, drug was released into the circulation at a faster rate from the p.o. dosage form, and the absorption rate from suppositories was consistent with the relative dissolution rate of this dosage form. Very little hepatic clearance occurs during pentobarbital absorption from p.o. doses, and circulating drug levels appear to obey two-compartment model kinetics after both i.v. and p.o. doses.[166] Nair et al.[167,168] obtained significantly higher plasma pentobarbital levels in human volunteers after p.o. doses compared to equivalent i.m. doses given by nurses. The differences were attenuated, however, when the i.m. doses were given by a physician. Intramuscular pentobarbital appears to offer no advantage over p.o. doses. The absorption of p.o. doses of pentobarbital is delayed, but not reduced, in the presence of food.[169]

Pentobarbital appears to distribute evenly between red blood cells, plasma water, and plasma proteins.[166] The binding of pentobarbital and other barbiturates to human serum albumin is pH dependent; the binding is associated predominantly with the ionized species.[170] Induced pentobarbital narcosis by various drugs seems to be associated with displacement from serum proteins rather than a synergistic action on the c.n.s. or inhibition of metabolism.[171]

Binding of pentobarbital to plasma proteins is reduced by salicylate, while binding to red cells is unaffected.[172] The protein binding of pentobarbital, and also phenytoin[173] and thiopental,[174] to plasma proteins is reduced in uraemia,[175] although ratios of red cell : plasma concentrations of pentobarbital and phenytoin were similar in normal and uraemic subjects.

Studies in rats showed that lung tissue and blood concentrations of pentobarbital, hexobarbital, and thiopental were unrelated. Differences in the $t_{0.5}$ values in lung tissue and serum, and also considerable tissue retention of pentobarbital, support the postulate that these barbiturates have peripheral effects in the lungs.[176]

The plasma $t_{0.5}$ of pentobarbital ranged from 18 to 48 h (mean 27 h) in normal individuals, and from 10 to 38 h (mean 21 h) in uraemic patients.[177] It is suggested that altered clearances of pentobarbital in uraemia are related to reduced apparent distribution volumes rather than accelerated metabolism. Pentobarbital elimination kinetics are independent of renal function in the dog.[178] Pentobarbital metabolism is inhibited by ethanol[179] and halothane,[180] and is induced by haloperidol and promethazine.[181]

Amylobarbital

Kojima has shown that the presence of food can delay the GI absorption of amylobarbital in rats.[182] The distribution and elimination of amylobarbital were shown to be dose-dependent over the dose range 3.2-6.5 mg kg^{-1} in man.[183] However, there was no change in the plasma clearance rate with different doses. The decay in amylobarbital serum concentrations was biphasic over 48 h after i.v. injection, and positive correlations were obtained between the terminal serum decay rates and rates of excretion of hydroxyamylobarbital.[184] The rates of oxidative metabolism of amylobarbital correlated well with those of glutethimide and sulphinpyrazone in man,[185] but none of these correlated well with that of antipyrine.

There was no evidence of induction of amylobarbital hydroxylation in 16 newborn children of mothers who had been receiving chronic barbiturate therapy.[186]   Plasma $t_{0.5}$ values in seven babies ranged from 17 to 49 h, comparable with values reported previously in babies of mothers who had received only one dose of amylobarbital. Some evidence of genetic control has been demonstrated over the rate of amylobarbital metabolism in monozygotic twins.[187]   A high correlation between the distribution volume of amylobarbital and the amount of adipose tissue suggested extensive uptake of the unionized lipid-soluble fraction of amylobarbital into adipose tissue.

Studies in dogs have shown that metabolism of amylobarbital is a saturable process and is essentially zero-order over a dose range of 5-40 mg kg^{-1}.[188]   The rate of metabolism was markedly increased by chronic administration of phenobarbital and was reduced by SKF 525-A. The pharmacokinetic behaviour of amylobarbital was sensitive to body pH and observed changes appeared to be a function of relative concentrations of ionized and unionized drug. The degree of ionization and protein binding also influenced the extent of amylobarbital excretion in saliva.[189]

Hexobarbital

Hexobarbital obeys two-compartment model kinetics in man after i.v. infusion.[190]   Although the overall distribution volume $V_{d,ss}$ was relatively constant (1.0 ± 0.12 1 kg^{-1}) the biological $t_{0.5}$ varied from 160 to 441 min. Differences in the duration of pharmacological activity of (+) and (-) enantiomers of hexobarbital, and also the influence of caffeine on the pharmacological response to the racemic mixture, may be due to response changes within the c.n.s. rather than to differences in rates of drug clearance or distribution.[191,192] However differences have been reported also between the elimination kinetics of the two isomers and differences in their depressive activities have been associated with pharmacokinetic effects.[193] McCarthy and Stitzel[194] showed that the two isomers $\underline{d}$- and $\underline{l}$-hexobarbital are handled differently by the hepatic microsomal system of the rat, rabbit, and mouse, and the isomers are also affected differently by enzyme inducing agents.

Hepatic clearance of hexobarbital is significantly reduced in patients with acute hepatitis and recovery of drug-metabolizing capacity is delayed relative to recovery from the disease.[195] The elimination $t_{0.5}$ of hexobarbital is approximately 6 h in normal individuals, but this value increases to 8 h and 17 h in patients with compensated and decompensated liver cirrhosis, respectively.[196] The degree of binding by hexobarbital to plasma proteins was similar in healthy individuals (42-52%) and in cirrhosis patients (36-59%) despite reduced serum albumin levels in cirrhosis. Ethanol is capable of inducing the metabolism of hexobarbital and some other drugs, but it has an inhibitory effect while still present in the cell.[197]

Other Barbiturates

Secobarbital is absorbed faster than heptobarbital after p.o. doses to non-fasted subjects, although both compounds are absorbed at a slower rate than ethinamate and methaqualone.[198] Secobarbital is cleared from the blood at about one-third the rate of heptobarbital. Observed $t_{0.5}$ values were 28.9 and 9.7 h for secobarbital and heptobarbital, respectively. The longer $t_{0.5}$ of secobarbital is consistent with prolonged activity of this barbiturate.[199,200] The pharmacokinetics of secobarbital were dose-dependent in the dog and the rabbit.[201] In the latter species, levels of drug in the liver, and to a lesser extent in brain and fat, were higher than those in plasma. After reaching peak levels at about 10 min after i.v. injection, the decline of secobarbital in brain tissue was biphasic and the terminal rate was slower than that in plasma. The mean elimination $t_{0.5}$ of secobarbital was decreased to 11 h in drug abuse patients receiving repeated doses of secobarbital and amylobarbital, whereas the $t_{0.5}$ of amylobarbital was essentially unchanged at 14-16 h.[203]

The plasma $t_{0.5}$ of cyclobarbital in four of six human volunteers was between 8 and 11 h, an appropriate value for drugs used in the treatment of insomnia.[204] In the two other subjects, however, the $t_{0.5}$ was 15-17 h, which may create a substantial risk of residual drug effects during the morning after dosing. The elimination kinetics of this barbiturate need to be studied in larger and varied populations.

Although the elimination of butobarbital followed first-order kinetics in humans, excretion of its 3'-hydroxy and 3'-oxo metabolites appeared to follow capacity-limited kinetics, at least during the initial days of excretion.[205] The elimination $t_{0.5}$ of butobarbital decreased to <u>ca</u>. 20-25% of the original value of <u>ca</u>. 30 h during repeated administration to human volunteers, presumably due to enzyme induction.[206]

Saidman and Eger[207] described a computer model to evaluate the influence of site of administration, blood flow, and hepatic metabolism on blood and brain levels of centrally acting drugs, with particular reference to thiopental. Hepatic clearance, rather than placental uptake, is a principal factor in preventing foetal narcosis from mothers receiving thiopental.[208] This appears to be due to liver uptake rather than metabolism due to the immaturity of oxidative drug-metabolizing enzymes in the foetus and newborn.[209]

The dose of thiopental necessary for induction of anesthesia was lower in elderly than in young men, average values being 4.14 and 6.22 mg kg^{-1}, respectively.[210] Increased sensitivity to thiopental in elderly patients is probably related to a prolonged elimination

$t_{0.5}$, 13 h compared with ca. 7 h in the young. Nonetheless, no correlation was observed between dose or concentration of thiopental and its effect on cardiac function.

Uraemic rats had higher tissue levels of ^{14}C after doses of ^{14}C-thiopental, and also higher relative levels of free thiopental in plasma compared to control animals despite normal plasma total protein and albumin levels.[211] Reduced binding to plasma proteins appears to accelerate drug distribution and to increase drug levels in brain and cardiac tissue.

The Benzodiazepines

The benzodiazepines are used for a variety of effects including sedation, hypnosis, anxiety, muscle relaxation and anticonvulsant activity. They particularly dominate in the area of anxiety and their use has increased dramatically during the review period. Various members of this class of compounds will be considered in the approximate order that they are used.

Diazepam

Absorption of p.o. dosed diazepam is generally reported to be good and bioavailability does not vary markedly from different commercial products.[212] Intramuscular dosing of diazepam generally results in faster absorption than p.o. dosing although variation in absorption rates can occur depending on the injection site.[213]

In a study using 37 individuals aged 19-79 yr, the absorption of diazepam was rapid and was not influenced by sex, age, or Billroth gastrectomy.[214] A 5 mg tablet administered upon fasting yielded a mean plasma peak concentration of 157 ng ml^{-1} at 0.9 h postdose. There were no significant differences in drug plasma levels and bioavailability when a single 10 mg dose of diazepam was given by i.v. or i.m. injection, and as a p.o. tablet or rectal solution.[215] However, the absorption rate was significantly greater from the rectal solution than from the tablet and the i.m. dose (Figure 2.1), the respective

mean T_{max} values being 17, 52, and 95 min. Relatively low bioavail-

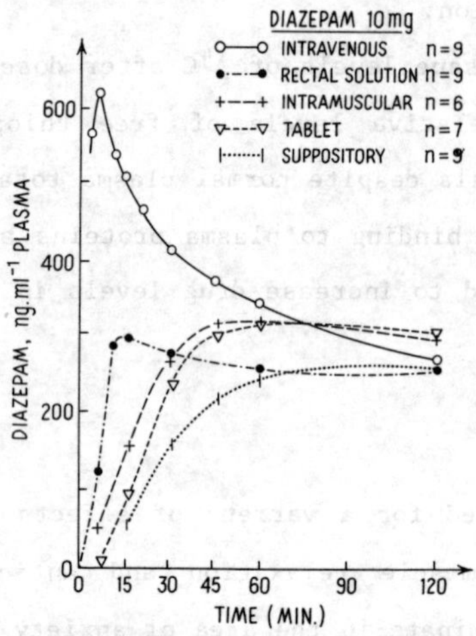

Figure 2.11 Mean plasma concentrations of diazepam on
linear scale after single i.v., i.m., p.o., and rectal
administration of 10 mg diazepam in different dosage
forms, to healthy human subjects. Reproduced by permission from Int. J. Pharmaceut., 1980, 5, 127.

ability was obtained from diazepam suppositories,[215] with considerable

variation in absorption characteristics between different formula-

tions.[216] A single dose of a 15 mg controlled release diazepam cap-

sule yielded essentially the same extent of absorption and elimination

characteristics as conventional tablets (5 mg, t.i.d.),[217] as shown in

Figure 2.12. In addition, no difference in mean steady-state concen-

trations of diazepam or N-desmethyldiazepam was observed between the

two treatments during multiple dosing.

The influence of stomach emptying rate on the absorption of p.o.

dosed diazepam has been studied in patients. Metaclopramide caused

faster absorption and higher circulating levels of diazepam while

morphine, pethidine, and atropine caused levels of diazepam to be

lower and delayed.[218] Oral diazepam gave rise to higher circulating

levels of drug compared to i.m. dosage in normal pregnant women,[219]

whereas patients with pre-eclampsia, who had been receiving diazepam

previously, had relatively high diazepam levels from the i.m. route.

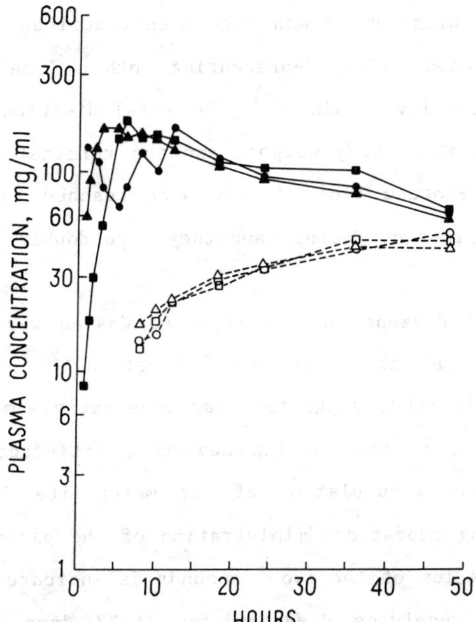

Figure 2.12 Mean plasma diazepam (closed symbols) and N-desmethyldiazepam (open symbols) concentrations for 11 subjects after 5 mg diazepam t.i.d. (circles), after a single 15 mg diazepam dose in the CR formulation to fasted subjects (triangles), and after a single 15 mg diazepam in the CR formulation to fed subjects (squares). Reproduced by permission from J. Pharmacokin. Biopharm., 1981, 9, 679.

This was thought to be due to reduced gastric motility and secretion resulting from previous diazepam doses inhibiting the absorption of orally dosed drug. Reports on the influence of alcohol on diazepam absorption from p.o. doses are conflicting. One study indicates that diazepam absorption is delayed but not significantly reduced due to alcohol,[220] while another shows generally increased diazepam levels due to interaction with a variety of alcoholic beverages.[221] Diazepam absorption is delayed by antacid preparations, and also by food.[222] However, the extent of absorption, as reflected in the area under the plasma profile, was unchanged by the antacid and was increased by 26% due to food. Diazepam is absorbed rapidly after rectal administration to children, and this dosage route is recommended for treatment.[223]

Blood levels of diazepam in man have been described in terms of a three-compartment open model, representing both a 'shallow' and a 'deep' compartment after i.v. dosing.[224] The total distribution volume varied from 160 to 205% of body weight, and the terminal elimination $t_{0.5}$ was 21-37 h. Plateau blood levels were reached by about the seventh day of multiple p.o. dosing, and they were double those after the initial dose.

Plasma levels of diazepam during repeated dosing were described adequately by linear two-compartment model kinetics.[225] Plasma profiles obtained in this study suggested that once-daily administration of a total daily dose in the evening may be a satisfactory dosage regimen. Considerable accumulation of the metabolite N-desmethyl-diazepam occurs during repeated administration of the parent drug.[226] The relative accumulation of the two compounds is indicated in Figure 2.13. In patients receiving diazepam for 18-22 days, metabolite levels were 2- to 3-fold higher compared to those of the parent drug and had not reached a plateau level during that period. On discontinuation of therapy, diazepam and metabolite levels in plasma

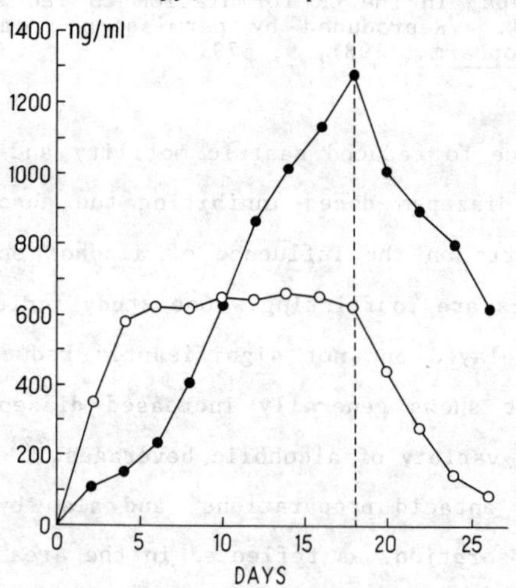

Figure 2.13 Plasma diazepam (o——o) and N-desmethyl-diazepam (●——●) following 10 mg i.v. every 4 hours. Broken line indicates when therapy was discontinued. Reproduced by permission from Brit. J. Anaesthesia, 1976, 48, 1087.

declined with $t_{0.5}$ values of 2-4 and 4-8 days, respectively. Accumulation of N-desmethyldiazepam in plasma during chronic diazepam dosage has been confirmed in another study, which suggested also that the $t_{0.5}$ of parent drug increased significantly from 34 h to 53 h after repeated dosing.[227] Other studies have shown, on the other hand, that diazepam can induce its own metabolism after repeated doses.[228,229] Increased plasma levels of N-desmethyldiazepam after repeated diazepam dosing may be due to saturation of tissues with this metabolite.[230]

Diazepam has been shown to be rapidly taken up by, and also cleared from, the c.n.s. after i.v. injection into rats.[231] Although both diazepam and N-desmethyldiazepam levels in c.s.f. are in equilibrium with free plasma levels after single drug doses,[232] levels of the metabolite in c.s.f. increase during repeated dosing to produce levels significantly higher than those in plasma (Figure 2.14).[233] The clinical significance of N-desmethyldiazepam accumulation is uncertain.

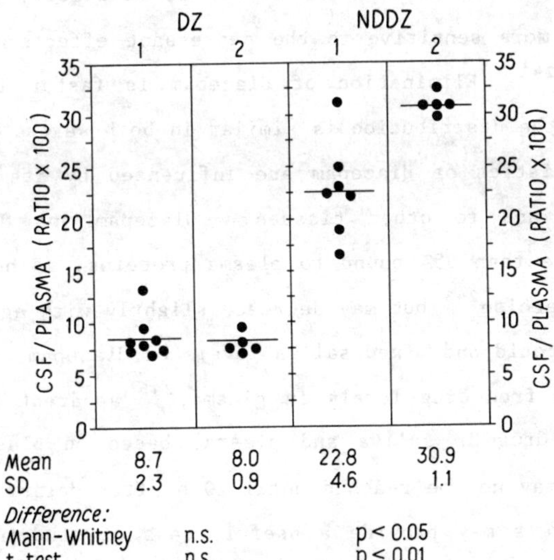

Figure 2.14   Comparison of c.s.f.:plasma ratios of diazepam (DZ) and N-desmethyldiazepam (NDDZ) in acutely treated patients (Group 1) and in long-term plus acutely treated patients (Group 2). Reproduced by permission from *Acta Pharmacol. Toxicol.*, 1975, <u>37</u>, 17.

Biotransformation of diazepam was inhibited, and c.s.f. levels were increased, when the drug was administered with ethanol to rats.[234] Brain levels of unchanged drug were approximately six times higher in ethanol-treated rats than in animals receiving only diazepam. This is probably a causative factor in diazepam potentiation by ethanol.

In chronic alcoholics, circulating levels of diazepam are low because of impaired absorption after p.o. doses,[235] and also of increased metabolism or altered distribution after i.v. doses.[236] Reported elevation of plasma diazepam levels at 6 h following i.v. injection[237] appears to be due to enterohepatic cycling of drug induced by food ingestion.[238]

Evidence has been presented that circulating levels of diazepam decrease with age.[239] The effect appears to be due to an increased distribution volume, which more than compensates for an increased diazepam elimination $t_{0.5}$ in the elderly.[240] Interpretation of these data in terms of therapeutic effect is difficult, however, as the elderly are more sensitive to the depressant effects of diazepam than the young.[241] Elimination of diazepam is faster in men than women, although the distribution is similar in both sexes.[242] Distribution characteristics of diazepam are influenced by its binding to plasma proteins and to other tissues. Diazepam and N-desmethyldiazepam are more than 95% bound to plasma proteins. Binding is not influenced by exercise[243] but may decrease slightly with age.[244]

Although parotid and mixed saliva levels of diazepam are reported to be similar to free drug levels in plasma,[245] apparent equilibrium between unbound drug in saliva and plasma, based on plasma protein binding of 98%, may not be reached until 20 h after dosing. Nonetheless, saliva levels may provide a useful means of studying diazepam binding to plasma proteins.[246]

Diazepam binding to plasma proteins is reduced by circulating free fatty acids,[247] and is also reduced in alcoholic patients.[248] In the latter case the degree of binding was related to the concentration of plasma albumin.

Diazepam plasma binding exhibits diurnal variation,[249] the free fraction being highest between 11:00 p.m. and 8:00 a.m. and lowest at 9:00 a.m. Reciprocal variations in plasma diazepam concentration were observed as a result of tissue and vascular redistribution of the drug. It has been reported that the percent of diazepam free in plasma was significantly greater in contraceptive-treated females (1.99%) than in contraceptive-free females (1.67%) or in males (1.46%), probably due to reduced plasma albumin concentrations during estrogen and progestogen therapy.[250] A small i.v. dose of heparin (100 units) significantly reduced plasma protein binding of diazepam, chlordiazepoxide, and oxazepam, resulting in a 150-250% rise in drug free fraction.[251] This effect was probably related to activation of lipoprotein lipase by heparin, thus elevating the plasma levels of free fatty acids which in turn displace the benzodiazepines from albumin. These changes occurred within 90 sec of the heparin dose, and returned to baseline after 30 to 45 min. Plasma binding of diazepam is not significantly altered in hyperthyroidism.[252]

Protein binding of diazepam is reduced in uraemic patients due to decreased binding affinity rather than depleted binding sites.[253] Binding to plasma proteins in uraemic plasma returns to normal after charcoal treatment. In patients with severe renal insufficiency, the unbound fraction of plasma diazepam after a single dose was significantly increased to ca. 7%.[252] The mean volume of distribution of unbound diazepam decreased to 57 1 kg^{-1}, compared with 157 1 kg^{-1} in healthy volunteers, while intrinsic clearance was not significantly changed. In another study, plasma binding of diazepam was found to be reduced in nephrotic and uraemic patients as well as in transplant recipients relative to controls, although only the nephrotic patients had reduced plasma albumin concentrations.[254]

Diazepam crosses the human placenta rapidly, achieving distribution equilibrium between mother and foetus within 5-10 min after a 20-30 mg i.v. dose.[255] In general levels of unchanged drug and N-desmethyldiazepam in foetal and cord blood exceed those in maternal blood.[259] As protein-binding of diazepam in foetal blood is only 86%, compared to > 95% in maternal blood, the possibility of active placental transfer of drug from mother to foetus has to be considered.[259]

Placental transfer of both diazepam and desmethyldiazepam is <u>ca</u>. 4-fold greater than the more water soluble clorazepate.[260] However it may vary under different conditions, being far less during uterine contractions than during relaxation.[261] Diazepam and N-desmethyldiazepam are stored in foetal tissues, giving rise to prolonged blood levels and possibly toxic effects in the newborn for several days after parturition.[262]

Diazepam and/or metabolites can be transferred from the mother to the baby in maternal milk,[263,264] but only a small fraction of the dose ingested by the mother reaches the infant by this route.[265] Interestingly, the pharmacokinetics of diazepam in the mother may change dramatically during the immediate postnatal period;[266] the elimination $t_{0.5}$ increasing to 24-114 h, compared with a normal value of 18-44 h. The prolonged $t_{0.5}$ appears to be related to changes in the distribution of diazepam, and not to a reduction in elimination as the total plasma clearance (18 - 43 ml min^{-1}) is similar to normal values.

The clinical pharmacokinetics of diazepam have been reviewed by Mandelli et al.[267] Several reports have indicated positive relationships between circulating levels of diazepam, and also of N-desmethyldiazepam, and clinical and toxic effects.[268-273] There is some evidence however, that clinical effects may be related to the rate of absorption of both diazepam and oxazepam rather than to circulating drug levels.[274] Considerable differences in diazepam blood levels occur between individuals.[275]

Diazepam is eliminated almost entirely by biotransformation. After a 10 mg i.v. dose, mean plasma clearance of diazepam was 23.4 ml min^{-1} in 6 healthy male subjects and 14.0 ml min^{-1} in 5 females on oral contraceptives, probably due to impaired drug metabolism.[276] Large interindividual variations in diazepam disposition were observed, and were attributed to differences in plasma protein binding and intrinsic clearance. Slight decreases in diazepam plasma binding and total clearance were observed in the elderly.[277]

The metabolism of diazepam can be inhibited by high concentration of N-desmethyldiazepam. In 6 healthy subjects who received 0.1 mg kg^{-1} i.v. diazepam with and without pretreatment with metabolite (20 mg d^{-1} for 1 week), mean diazepam plasma clearance decreased and elimination $t_{0.5}$ increased in the presence of high N-desmethyldiazepam plasma levels that averaged 671 ng ml^{-1}.[278] The respective mean values were 9.1 ml min^{-1} and 65.8 h compared with the control values of 11.5 ml min^{-1} and 38.5 h. Impairment of diazepam clearance appeared to be dependent on metabolite plasma concentration, which at least partially explained conflicting results reported by others.[279] In the latter study, the presence of N-desmethyldiazepam in plasma averaging 481 ng ml^{-1} was shown to have no influence on diazepam pharmacokinetics.

Concomitant treatment with cimetidine (1000 mg d^{-1}) and diazepam resulted in a nearly 40% increase in the average steady-state plasma concentration of diazepam.[280,281] A corresponding decrease in diazepam clearance was observed, approximately 11-14 ml min^{-1} compared with 20 ml min^{-1} in controls. Furthermore, a prolonged $t_{0.5}$ of N-desmethyldiazepam suggested that the elimination of the metabolite was also impaired by cimetidine. Ethanol also inhibits intrinsic hepatic clearance of diazepam. In 6 healthy male volunteers who received 10 mg i.v. doses of diazepam, mean total and free plasma levels of diazepam were higher, and those of metabolite lower, when alcohol was administered concurrently, with blood alcohol maintained at 800-1000 mg l^{-1}.[282] On the other hand, diazepam metabolism was induced in epileptic patients receiving carbamazepine and other antiepileptic drugs.[283] Serum N-desmethyldiazepam concentrations following a 10 mg i.v. dose of diazepam were higher in epileptic patients than in normal volunteers, and the respective diazepam clearances were 3.1 and 1.2 l h^{-1}. The $t_{0.5}$ of diazepam was accordingly shortened in the patients to <u>ca</u>. 13 h compared to 34 h in normals.

In the dog, a 2 mg kg^{-1} i.v. dose of diazepam yielded plasma drug levels that declined triexponentially.[284] The mean elimination $t_{0.5}$ of parent compound ws 3.2 h, while those of two metabolites, N-desmethyldiazepam and oxazepam, were 3.6 and 5.7 h, respectively. Similar elimination characteristics were observed after p.o. doses, which yielded an absolute bioavailability of 74-100%.

The plasma $t_{0.5}$ of diazepam,[285] and N-desmethyldiazepam,[286] were increased several-fold in patients with cirrhosis or fibrosis, compared with normal controls. Plasma clearance of drug did not correlate with standard liver function tests. The biological $t_{0.5}$ of diazepam is about 30 h in full-term human newborns, but may increase to 70-80 h in premature newborns. The $t_{0.5}$ may be significantly reduced in the newborn of mothers receiving phenobarbital, presumably as a result of induction of foetal drug-metabolizing enzymes.[287] Induction of hepatic microsomal enzymes has also been demonstrated following repeated dosing of bromazepam to rats.[288]

Biliary excretion of diazepam was measured in five patients with T-tube drainage. Only 0.3 - 0.4% of chronic diazepam doses was excreted via this route. Negligible biliary excretion of diazepam and N-desmethyldiazepam has been reported following single i.v. doses of labelled drug.[289] Secretion of diazepam into the gut via gastric juices is inferred in a study by Kortilla et al.[290] who showed that circulating levels of i.v. diazepam were increased when subjects ate shortly after dosing.

Oxazepam

Oxazepam differs from most other benzodiazepines in that it has no active metabolites.[291] After p.o. dosing as tablets or suspension, peak oxazepam blood levels were observed within 1-2 h.[292] The drug has a relatively short elimination $t_{0.5}$ of 4-8 h compared to diazepam.

No accumulation of unchanged drug or conjugate was observed in blood after multiple doses of oxazepam every 4 h.[293] This may be due to enzyme induction, as accumulation might be expected for a drug administered at dosage intervals similar to its biological $t_{0.5}$. Equal i.v. doses of the succinate half-esters of (+)- and (-)-oxazepam to mice resulted in blood-levels of (+)-oxazepam ca. 4-fold higher than those obtained for (-)-oxazepam,[294] the racemic mixture yielding intermediate levels. After p.o. dosing to mice and rats, no differences were observed in blood levels of the two stereoisomers, and the difference in levels after i.v. doses was attributed to a possible stereospecific esterase in the blood or liver.

The clinical pharmacokinetics of lorazepam and oxazepam have been reviewed.[295] The mean elimination $t_{0.5}$ of oxazepam increased to 25 h in patients with renal insufficiency, and 33 h in patients on haemodialysis.[296] Nonetheless, intrinsic clearance of oxazepam was similar in normal and uraemic individuals, the mean values being 2.0 - 2.9 1 h^{-1} kg^{-1}. Other investigators[297] also have shown similar concentrations of free oxazepam in plasma of healthy volunteers and patients with chronic renal failure following repeated daily administration of 10 mg oxazepam. Therefore, it was suggested that no dosage adjustment of oxazepam is necessary in patients with renal disease.[296,297] The elimination rate, apparent distribution volume, and blood:plasma ratio of oxazepam, and also the urinary excretion of oxazepam glucuronide, were unaffected by acute viral hepatitis and cirrhosis.[298]

Unlike that of diazepam, the elimination $t_{0.5}$ of oxazepam (5-8 h) is shorter in pregnant women than in non-pregnant women. Oxazepam crosses the placenta, and an umbilical cord:maternal vein drug concentration ratio of 1.35 was reported.[299] The elimination $t_{0.5}$ of oxazepam (22 h) in the newborn is 3-4 times longer than in the mother.

Lorazepam

The pharmacokinetics of lorazepam have been studied after i.v.[300,301] and p.o.[302] doses. After i.v. doses, plasma lorazepam levels decreased biexponentially and were described in the form of equation 2.6 where C is the plasma drug level at time t after dosing,

$$C = Ae^{-\alpha t} + Be^{-\beta t} \qquad (2.6)$$

α and β are hybrid rate constants, and A and B are intercepts on the ordinate at zero time. Lorazepam had a terminal plasma $t_{0.5}$ of 14 h, an overall distribution volume of 1.1 - 1.3 l kg^{-1}, and a total clearance of 1.1 ml min^{-1} kg^{-1}. The elimination $t_{0.5}$ of lorazepam glucuronide was almost identical to that of the parent drug, suggesting that its apparent elimination rate may be limited by its rate of formation. Bioavailability of lorazepam is similar after p.o. and i.m. administration and absorption kinetics from both routes are dose-independent. Of a p.o. dose of lorazepam, 88% was recovered in urine, of which 86% was lorazepam glucuronide. After chronic dosing for 26 weeks there was no evidence that lorazepam stimulated or inhibited its own metabolism.[303]

Circulating lorazepam is approximately 80% bound in serum.[304] The unbound fraction is generally similar to the c.s.f.:serum concentration ratio, suggesting that access to the c.s.f. is restricted to unbound lorazepam.[305]

Kinetic parameters obtained from a single dose of lorazepam may accurately predict steady-state values after repeated dosing, and there is no evidence of hepatic enzyme induction.[306] However, correlations between predicted and observed steady-state values for particular individuals may be poor. Two independent studies have shown that the pharmacokinetics of lorazepam are not significantly influenced by age.[307,308] The elimination $t_{0.5}$ of lorazepam is increased from a normal value of 22 h to 47 h in cirrhosis.[308] This appears to be due to increased distribution of drug into extravascular sites because of decreased binding to plasma proteins, rather than to impaired hepatic clearance.

The elimination rate of lorazepam is unchanged after single doses in renal impairment.[309] In two patients with chronic renal failure, no impairment of lorazepam excretion was observed after a single 2.5 mg p.o. dose; the $t_{0.5}$ values were 10 and 12 h.[310] However, after administering 4 or 5 doses at 12 h intervals, the $t_{0.5}$ increased to 32 and 70 h, indicating impaired excretion of drug. N-desmethyldiazepam, unlike the parent drug, is removed efficiently by dialysis.[309]

Nitrazepam

Nitrazepam, one of the oldest benzodiazepines, is widely used as a hypnotic world-wide, except in the United States where it is not available. Nitrazepam is rapidly absorbed after p.o. doses but its overall systemic availability, ca. 50-90%, is somewhat less than that of diazepam.[311] Reduced absorption of nitrazepam may be due to acid degradation in the stomach.[311] Nitrazepam is 85-90% bound in plasma and the free fraction equilibrates with c.s.f. Drug concentrations are lower in saliva.[312,313] There is no significant correlation between nitrazepam plasma levels and clinical or side effects.[312] The elimination $t_{0.5}$ of nitrazepam has been variously reported to be 21 h after i.v. doses, and 25-50 h after p.o. doses.[313-315] The pharmacokinetics of nitrazepam show considerable age dependency. Two-compartment model analysis of plasma data following p.o. doses yielded mean β-phase $t_{0.5}$ values of 29 h and 40 h, and overall apparent distribution volumes, $V_{d\beta}$, of 2.4 and 4.8 1 kg^{-1} in young and geriatric subjects, respectively.[315] The longer $t_{0.5}$ and the larger apparent distribution volume in geriatric patients had the effect of producing similar plasma clearances in the two age groups. A comparison of the plasma nitrazepam profiles in young and old subjects is shown in Figure 2.15. Unlike diazepam, nitrazepam appears not to induce its own metabolism with repeated dosing. Nitrazepam crosses the placenta freely, and the efficiency of transfer increases with advancing pregnancy.[316]

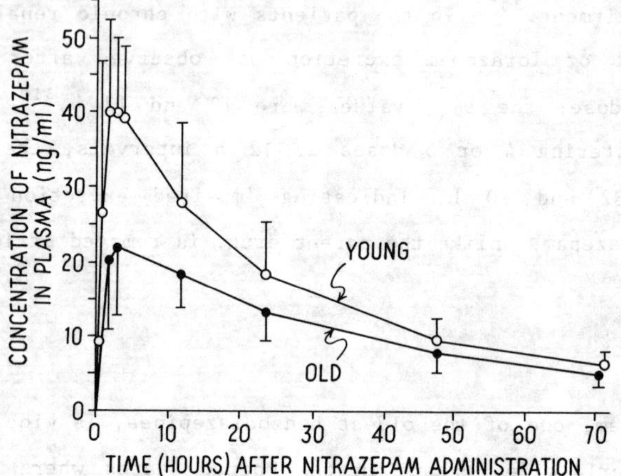

Figure 2.15 Plasma concentration of nitrazepam (ng ml^{-1}; mean ± SD) in sick geriatric patients and healthy volunteers after a single 5 mg p.o. dose. Reproduced by permission from *Eur. J. Clin. Pharmacol.*, 1979, 15, 163.

Flunitrazepam

The pharmacokinetics of flunitrazepam were studied in 12 patients undergoing otologic operations.[317] After a single i.v. dose of 14-33 μg kg^{-1}, the average elimination $t_{0.5}$ was 25 h and the serum clearance was 94 ml min^{-1}. A similar study[318] in 20 patients, aged 19-79 yr, showed that age has no effect on flunitrazepam disposition kinetics, although the sedative effect appeared to increase in patients aged over 60 yr. No correlation was found between serum drug concentration or $t_{0.5}$ and sedation. After p.o. administration of a 2 mg tablet, peak plasma flunitrazepam levels of 10-15 ng ml^{-1} were reached at 2 h postdose.[319] The terminal $t_{0.5}$ ranged from 20 to 36 h and was thus similar to that observed after i.v. doses. Repeated daily administration of a 2 mg tablet for 28 days yielded virtually no accumulation of flunitrazepam or metabolites, and no changes in the onset and depth of sleep in patients.

Flurazepam

Flurazepam hydrochloride has been shown to be rapidly and completely absorbed in the dog and man.[320] Elimination is also rapid and due solely to biotransformation. After both single and chronic doses of flurazepam the major component present in blood is the pharmacologically active metabolite N-dealkylflurazepam.[321]

In 26 healthy 19 to 85 yr old subjects who received a single 15 mg p.o. dose of flurazepam, the average plasma concentration of N-dealkylflurazepam reached a peak of 10-15 ng ml^{-1} between 4 h and 29 h postdose.[322] Large intersubject variability in elimination rate was also observed; the $t_{0.5}$ of the metabolite ranged from 37 to 289 h, and tended to increase with age. Repeated nightly dosing for 15 nights resulted in extensive accumulation of metabolite, the mean accumulation ratio in 18 subjects being 7.5. N-dealkylflurazepam is extensively (96-97%) bound to plasma proteins. The fraction unbound appears to increase with age, possibly because of lower plasma albumin concentrations in the elderly.

Prazepam

Rapid dealkylation of prazepam to form N-desmethyldiazepam occurs after p.o. dosing. Considerable biotransformation occurs during the first-pass.[323,324]. After a 30-mg p.o. dose of prazepam, N-desmethyldiazepam was the only major drug-related substance found in plasma.[325] The average peak metabolite concentrations were 342 and

265 ng ml^{-1} at 3-4 h after prazepam administration to male and female volunteers, respectively, suggesting a larger volume of distribution in women. The plasma concentration of N-desmethyldiazepam was approximately 1.6 times that in whole blood, and 10 times that in milk of healthy lactating women.[325] The mean elimination $t_{0.5}$ of metabolite, independent of sex, was 60 h and remained unchanged after repeated dosing of prazepam, 60 mg d^{-1}, for 3 days. However in two groups of subjects, 22-42 yr and 62-85 yr, the mean $t_{0.5}$ increased with age in men, from 62 to 128 h, but appeared to be independent of age in women.[326]

Prazepam inhibits drug-metabolizing enzymes as measured by antipyrine $t_{0.5}$ values in man, yet has the opposite effect on microsomal proteins in the rat.[327] It appears also to induce its own metabolism in rats, but has little induction effect in man.

Temazepam

Temazepam circulates predominantly as unchanged drug after single p.o. and rectal doses, and is excreted partially unchanged in the urine.[328] Temazepam is readily absorbed from p.o. solutions[328] and capsules.[329-331] A mean peak plasma level of 670 ng ml^{-1} was obtained 45 min after a 20 mg p.o. dose, and concentrations subsequently declined with a $t_{0.5}$ of 5-10 h. Plasma concentrations of temazepam have been described by a triexponential function.[330] Mean $t_{0.5}$ values of the absorption, distribution, and elimination phases were 13 min, 50 min, and 8 h, respectively. Considerable species differences are reported in the disposition of temazepam. Whereas in man 80% of the dose is excreted in urine and 12% in faeces, in the rat 15% appears in urine and 78% in faeces.[332]

The pharmacokinetics and pharmacodynamics of temazepam were compared with those of nitrazepam in 16 healthy young volunteers.[333] Temazepam exhibited a mean plasma $t_{0.5}$ of 12-14 h, approximately one-half that of nitrazepam, and produced psychomotor effects that were of lower magnitude and shorter duration than those of nitrazepam. After single and multiple daily p.o. doses of 20 mg temazepam, Ochs et al.[334] reported average elimination $t_{0.5}$ values of 9-10 h, total clearance of 2.3 ml min^{-1} kg^{-1}, and virtually no accumulation of drug after 7 consecutive doses. Following a single 30 mg p.o. dose to 32 healthy volunteers (24-84 yr), neither the $t_{0.5}$ nor the clearance of temazepam was significantly related to age.[335] However, the fraction of temazepam unbound in plasma, normally averaging 2.6% over the concentration range of 160-4160 ng ml^{-1}, tended to increase with age.

Clorazepate

The antianxiety agent clorazepate is almost completely transformed to N-desmethyldiazepam before reaching the systemic circulation, and as such serves as yet another prodrug for this active metabolite.[336] No significant differences were observed in clorazepate or N-desmethyldiazepam blood levels following p.o. doses of mono- and di-potassium salts of clorazepate to dogs.[337] Both salts were absorbed rapidly, yielding peak drug levels at <u>ca</u>. 1 h. These levels then declined with a $t_{0.5}$ of 1-2 h. Absorption of clorazepate, as reflected in circulating metabolite levels, was equivalent from slow-release and fast-release dosage forms. The serum N-desmethyldiazepam $t_{0.5}$ was unchanged after 14 days of clorazepate treatment.[338]

In healthy volunteers, N-desmethyldiazepam was completely bioavailable from p.o. and i.m. doses of 20 mg clorazepate compared to the same dose given intravenously.[339] The peak plasma concentration of N-desmethyldiazepam after p.o. dosing averaged 356 ng ml^{-1} at 0.9 h, higher and achieved more rapidly than that of 290 ng ml^{-1} at 2.7 h after the i.m. dose.

Although reduced systemic availability of N-desmethyldiazepam has been reported from single p.o. doses of clorazepate at elevated gastric pH,[340-343] steady-state plasma N-desmethyldiazepam concentrations during chronic clorazepate therapy, 7.5 mg nightly for 30 nights, were not influenced by concurrent antacid administration.[344] However, absorption of clorazepate is reduced in elderly patients, and in patients following Billroth gastrectomy.[345] The mean apparent volume of distribution of N-desmethyldiazepam increased significantly to 159 l in obese patients, reflecting the lipophilic nature of this compound.[346] Consequently, a lower peak plasma concentration of 149 ng ml^{-1} was observed in the obese compared with 249 ng ml^{-1} in controls, while the peak time was virtually unchanged at 1.5 h. Plasma clearance was identical in the two subject groups, $\underline{ca}$. 13 ml min^{-1}. However, the large distribution volume in obese subjects resulted in a prolonged $t_{0.5}$ of 154 h compared to 57 h in controls.

Tobacco smoking appears to induce hepatic enzymes governing metabolism of N-desmethyldiazepam. After a 20 mg p.o. dose of clorazepate, the mean peak plasma N-desmethyldiazepam concentration and elimination $t_{0.5}$ were 413 ng ml^{-1} and 55 h, respectively, in 6 healthy non-smokers, but these values decreased to 245 ng ml^{-1} and 30 h, respectively, in 6 smokers.[347] Accordingly, the sedative effect of N-desmethyldiazepam was also less potent in the smokers. The plasma $t_{0.5}$ of i.m. injected clorazepate decreased from a normal value of 2 h to 1.3 h in pregnant women, while the $t_{0.5}$ of N-desmethyldiazepam increased from 68 to 188 h.[348] Peak plasma levels of both compounds were lower in pregnant females than in non-pregnant females, probably due to increased body weight and greater distribution volume in pregnancy. N-desmethyldiazepam crosses the human placenta at a faster rate than clorazepate, and is also transferred to the neonate in human milk.[349]

Chlordiazepoxide

Although chlordiazepoxide is frequently dosed i.m. for rapid effect, two independent studies have shown that absorption of drug from i.m. injection sites is slower than after p.o. doses and may give rise to lower and less reproducible blood levels.[350-353] Circulating levels of the active metabolite, desmethylchlordiazepoxide, also peak significantly earlier following p.o. doses. Representative chlordiazepoxide blood levels following p.o. and i.m. doses are given in Figure 2.16.

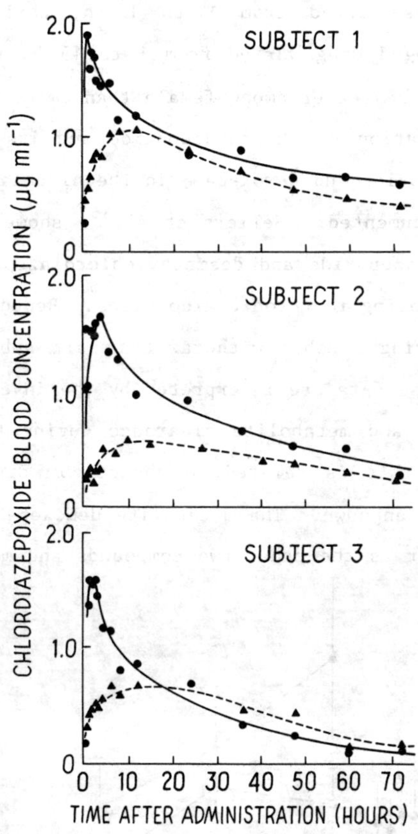

Figure 2.16. Chlordiazepoxide blood concentrations during 72 h following p.o. (● —— ●) and i.m. (▲ -- ▲) administration of 50 mg to three healthy subjects. Reproduced by permission from New Engl. J. Med., 1974, 291, 1116.

Overall absorption of chlordiazepoxide was not reduced, but the rate of drug absorption and desmethylchlordiazepoxide formation were reduced, when drug was administered with a $Mg(OH)_2$,$Al(OH)_3$ antacid.[354] Certain subjective effects of chlordiazepoxide were avoided when the absorption rate was reduced.

Previous studies relating chlordiazepoxide blood levels at specific times after dosing with clinical effects[355] have been criticized by Greenblatt et al.,[356] who demonstrated widely varying absorption and biotransformation rates of this drug among individuals. Peak blood level times varied from 1 to 12 h, while biological $t_{0.5}$ values for unchanged drug varied from 1 to 15 h. Variation in these parameters was much greater among female than among male subjects.

Slow accumulation of chlordiazepoxide and its metabolites, desmethylchlordiazepoxide and demoxepam, in the circulation with repeated doses is well documented. Sellers et al.[357] showed that circulating levels of chlordiazepoxide and desmethylchlordiazepoxide may decrease with continuous dosing to chronic alcoholics. Reduced levels of these two compounds during alcohol withdrawal in six subjects is shown in Figure 2.17. These data are interpreted by the investigators in terms of increased drug and metabolite clearance during the dosing period, although whether this is related to changes in distribution or biotransformation is unknown. The metabolite demoxepam was not affected in the same manner as the other two compounds and mean levels of this

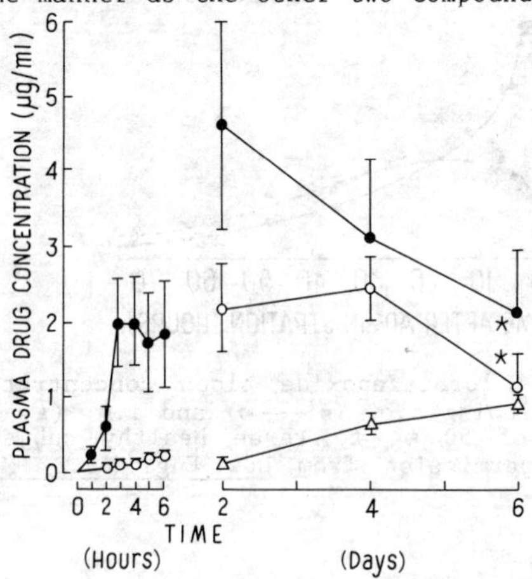

Figure 2.17   Plasma chlordiazepoxide (●) and metabolite concentrations (desmethylchlordiazepoxide o; demoxepam Δ) during alcohol withdrawal in six chronic alcoholics. Chlordiazepoxide dose 25 mg administered orally at 06.00 h, 12.00 h, 18.00 h, and 24.00 h, each day. Reproduced by permission from <u>Brit. J. Clin. Pharmacol.</u>, 1978, <u>6</u>, 370.

metabolite continued to increase during the sampling period. The clinical pharmacokinetics of chlordiazepoxide have been reviewed.[358]

Several approaches have been used to model the pharmacokinetics of chlordiazepoxide. Typically, plasma concentration-time curves were described by a biexponential expression consistent with a two-compartment model after i.v. doses to healthy male volunteers.[359] Mean $t_{0.5}$ values of distribution and elimination phases were 0.25 h and 9.4 h, respectively, while mean volumes of the central compartment (V_1) and the overall distribution volume ($V_{d\beta}$) were 18% and 31%, respectively, of body weight. Drug absorption from i.m. doses was comparatively slow, and adequate description of resulting plasma levels of chlordiazepoxide required incorporation of a two-compartment 'muscle model' which included precipitated and solubilized drug in muscle tissue. Distribution volumes of chlordiazepoxide were significantly larger in female subjects than in males, suggesting more extensive drug distribution among females.[360] Chlordiazepoxide is taken up by red cells to only a limited extent. During repeated p.o. doses the mean absorption $t_{0.5}$ of chlordiazepoxide was 12.3 min and bioavailability was complete.[361] Multiple regression analysis showed that circulating levels of p.o. dosed drug and its metabolite desmethylchlordiazepoxide were negatively correlated with subject weight. Lower levels of metabolite were associated with increasing age, while lower levels of both drugs were observed in females.[362]

Kaplan et al.[363] derived a six-compartment open model to describe the pharmacokinetics of chlordiazepoxide hydrochloride and metabolites. Pharmacokinetic parameters were obtained by separately administering each compound, and excellent agreement was obtained between actual and theoretical plasma levels for all compounds after chlordiazepoxide dosage. Subsequent studies[364,365] confirmed that the kinetics of the lactam metabolite fitted a two-compartment model and showed also that its elimination rate was slow relative to chlordiazepoxide. The disposition and elimination kinetics of chlordiazepoxide are variable amongst subjects, and are affected by a variety of conditions. The elimination $t_{0.5}$ is longer in young women than in men. The elimination rate and plasma clearance of chlordiazepoxide may be reduced in women taking oral contraceptives.[366] The clearance of chlordiazepoxide is also reduced in acute alcoholism[367] and in patients with liver disease.[368] However, changes in plasma clearance of chlordiazepoxide, and other benzodiazepines, in liver disease do not correlate well with conventional liver-function tests.

The mean elimination $t_{0.5}$ from an i.v. dose (0.6 mg kg^{-1}) of chlordiazepoxide was 7.1 h, but this was prolonged to 11.8 h when the drug was given with a concurrent p.o. dose of ethanol.[369] Ethanol reduced the mean plasma clearance of total and unbound chlordiazepoxide from 26.6 and 468 ml min^{-1}, respectively, in the controls to 16.6 and 264 ml min^{-1}. In addition, plasma levels of N-desmethylchlordiazepoxide were also higher and declined more slowly in the presence of alcohol. Morgan et al.[370] studied the chronic effect of alcohol on chlordiazepoxide disposition in 5 normal volunteers and in 15 patients with alcoholic hepatitis. Following a 25 mg i.m. dose of chlordiazepoxide hydrochloride, plasma clearance in the patients was approximately one-half of that in normals, while the average $t_{0.5}$ was nearly 2.5 times longer. Increased disappearance rates of chlordiazepoxide and its metabolites were observed after a single pretreatment dose to mice.[371] Increased clearance was insufficient to explain observed tolerance, and the possibility of altered drug distribution between blood and brain tissue cannot be excluded.

Chlordiazepoxide has been shown to cross the human placenta and may have adverse effects on the foetus.[372]

Other Benzodiazepines

The bioavailability of clobazam from p.o. tablets has been shown to be dose-proportional.[373] Peak plasma concentrations following

10, 20, and 40 mg doses to healthy adults were 206, 473, and 945 ng ml^{-1}, respectively, occurring between 1.8 and 2.5 h. The mean plasma $t_{0.5}$ of clobazam was <u>ca</u>. 18 h regardless of the dose. Co-administration of food with clobazam reduced the rate but not the extent of clobazam absorption.[374] A 20 mg dose of clobazam given after a standard breakfast yielded a decreased mean peak plasma concentration of 333 ng ml^{-1} at a prolonged peak time of 2.5 h, compared with 465 ng ml^{-1} at 1.7 h after dosing in the fasting state. However, food had no influence on the AUC and the elimination $t_{0.5}$ of the drug, nor did it affect plasma concentrations of desmethylclobazam, a major metabolite of clobazam.

Bromazepam appears to be efficiently absorbed from p.o. doses in man.[375] Intact drug is eliminated with a $t_{0.5}$ of <u>ca</u>. 12 h but only 2% intact drug is recovered in urine. Major urinary metabolites are the glucuronide conjugates of 3-hydroxybromazepam and a 3-hydroxybenzoylpyridine derivative.

The clearance of clonazepam is increased by phenobarbital pretreatment, but its apparent distribution is unaltered.[376] Decreased clonazepam levels by anticonvulsants may thus be attributable to enzyme induction.

After a 0.88 mg p.o. dose of ^{14}C-triazolam, approximately 85% of the dose was absorbed.[377] The mean peak plasma concentration of 8.8 ng ml^{-1} was reached at 1.3 h. Triazolam was <u>ca</u>. 89% bound to serum proteins in the concentration range of 20-1000 ng ml^{-1}. Nearly 85% of the administered radioactivity was recovered in urine, primarily as α-hydroxytriazolam and 4-hydroxytriazolam. The elimination $t_{0.5}$ of triazolam averaged 2.3 h, while that of the metabolites was <u>ca</u>. 4 h.

Other Sedatives and Hypnotics

Equivalent p.o. and i.v. doses of chlormethiazole base to healthy volunteers indicated a mean systemic bioavailability of 10% and plasma clearance of 15.1 ml min^{-1} kg^{-1}.[378] In patients with alcoholic cirrhosis of the liver, almost complete bioavailability was observed while mean clearance of chlormethiazole decreased to 10.8 ml min^{-1} kg^{-1}. The marked increase in chlormethiazole bioavailability in patients was due primarily to saturation of first-pass effect in the cirrhotic liver. Cumulative urinary excretion of unchanged chlormethiazole was less than 0.1% of p.o. and i.v. doses in both subject groups.

Both methohexitone[379] and chlormethiazole[380] have been shown to obey multicompartment kinetics following i.v. infusion. The terminal methohexitone $t_{0.5}$ was relatively short (70-125 min) in healthy volunteers. The terminal chlormethiazole $t_{0.5}$ in eight aged subjects, on the other hand, varied between 5.1 and 15.3 h; this value being significantly longer than that reported in young adults.

The clinical pharmacokinetics of hypnotic drugs have been reviewed by Breimer,[381] while Chang and Chiou[382] have illustrated some practical shortcomings in the indirect method of monitoring drug levels in blood through saliva, with special reference to tranquillizers.

Methaqualone was absorbed more efficiently from a preparation containing this drug together with diphenhydramine than from a tablet containing methaqualone alone.[383] On the other hand p.o. doses of a preparation containing methaqualone, carbromal, and benactyzine hydrochloride administered in the evening to healthy subjects resulted in lower serum levels of methaqualone than when this drug was administered alone, although with considerable individual variation.[384]

Different blood levels of methaqualone, obtained from various p.o. dosage forms, appeared to correlate well with clinical effects and also with _in vitro_ dissolution rates. Methaqualone obeys two-compartment model kinetics after single and repeated p.o. doses[385,386] and has a biological $t_{0.5}$ of 20-40 h. Steady-state circulating drug levels were obtained within one week of repeated dosing and steady-state levels were predictable from single-dose pharmacokinetic parameter values.[385] The drug readily crossed the blood-brain barrier[387] and c.s.f. levels were similar to levels of unbound drug in serum. These observations were obtained from single determinations, however, and the actual kinetics associated with methaqualone transfer between serum and c.s.f. were not studied. The pharmacokinetics of the non-barbiturate hypnotic, ethchlorvynol, have been described in man in terms of the two-compartment open model,[388] and slow disappearance of drug was shown to be due largely to extensive tissue distribution.

The absorption of chloral hydrate and its betaine complex was studied in 9 healthy male subjects following equivalent p.o. and rectal doses of chloral hydrate (500 mg) and chloral betaine (881.5 mg).[389] According to cumulative urinary excretion of the metabolite, trichloroacetic acid, absorption was more efficient from the p.o. dose, with 17-19% recovery in 24 h urine compared with 10-12% of the rectal dose. No statistically significant difference was observed between the absorption of chloral hydrate and its betaine complex administered via the same route. Interactions between chloral hydrate and ethanol have been studied from the point of view of metabolism,[390] haemodynamics,[391] and clearance.[392] A detailed study[393] of the pharmacokinetics of chloral hydrate, trichloroethanol, and their metabolites has demonstrated that microscopic rate constants and apparent distribution volumes are complex functions of protein binding, red cell:plasma partition coefficients, the true volume of plasma or blood, and haematocrit. This excellent study illustrates the complexity of definitive pharmacokinetic analysis and causes one to question the validity of many pharmacokinetic constants in the literature.

Anticonvulsants

High interest in the dose-response relationships of this group of drugs is reflected in the appearance of numerous review articles on

their absorption, distribution,[394] metabolism, excretion,[395] pharmacodynamic and pharmacokinetic relationships,[396] clinical pharmacokinetics,[397] and interactions with other anticonvulsants or other
drugs.[398]   Routine monitoring of anticonvulsant blood levels in
patients continues to draw attention. Relationships between circulating levels of many anticonvulsant drugs and clinical effects have been
established with reasonable accuracy,[399,400] although considerable
variation in circulating drug levels may occur due to formulation
effects, particularly during combination therapy.[401,402] Although
the monitoring of anticonvulsant blood levels may be useful in situations of inadequate dosing or overdosing,[403] it does not replace
clinical observations in the majority of cases.[404]

Phenytoin

Reports on the bioavailability of phenytoin from different
formulations and under various circumstances are conflicting.[405] Systemic availability may vary between tablets and capsules,[406,407]
among encapsulated formulations,[408] between solid formulations and
suspensions,[409,410] between tablets containing phenytoin calcium
and phenytoin acid,[411] and between formulations containing the sodium
salt and the free acid.[412] Area analysis showed that the overall
bioavailability of a brand of phenytoin capsules varied from 58 to 86%
after single p.o. doses, compared with i.v. administered drug. The
bioavailability increased to between 72 and 106% after repeated
doses.[413]

In other instances only small differences were observed between
different phenytoin products. For example, equivalent bioavailability
was obtained from capsules and an aqueous solution of phenytoin,
although initial plasma levels were higher from the solution.[414] No
differences were reported in the bioavailability of phenytoin from
capsules and tablets from the same manufacturer, estimated from
circulating levels of phenytoin or urinary excretion of the major

metabolite 5-(p-hydroxyphenyl)-5-phenylhydantoin (HPPH).[415] Simi-larly, only small differences were reported in the bioavailability of phenytoin from some commercial formulations.[416,417] Comparison of a capsule and 4 commercial tablets of phenytoin sodium in 20 patients showed only slight changes in serum phenytoin concentrations due to formulations at dose levels of 150 - 400 mg daily.[418]

In 6 healthy male subjects who received single p.o. doses of 400, 800, and 1600 mg phenytoin, peak serum concentrations of 3.9, 5.7, and 10.7 mg l^{-1}, respectively, were achieved at 8.4, 13.2, and 31.5 h postdose.[419] The mean percent absorbed ranged from 92% of the 400 mg dose to 78% of the 1600 mg dose, although the difference was not statistically significant. It was suggested that prolonged and nearly complete absorption of large phenytoin doses was due to slow dissolution and continued absorption from the colon. Only small differences were reported in phenytoin absorption in the presence and absence of antacids,[420] but postprandial administration of phenytoin caused increased absorption.[421] The food-related increase in phenytoin absorption is not due to inhibition of metabolism as the serum level of HPPH is also increased. Absorption of phenytoin from i.m. injections may be prolonged over several days.[422] Pharmacokinetic inter-pretation of plasma data indicated that prolonged absorption may be due to precipitation and redissolution of drug at the injection site.

Oral administration of phenytoin to infants after delivery results in poor absorption of drug into the circulation.[423] In 21 infants who received 15 - 20 mg kg^{-1} phenytoin intravenously, a mean plasma level of 14.5 ± 3.0 µg ml^{-1} was achieved. After p.o. doses of up to 12 mg kg^{-1} d^{-1} however, no phenytoin could be detected in plasma.

In vitro experiments using everted rat intestinal segments showed that phenytoin absorption may be impaired by kaolin, dimethicone, and calcium citrate.[424] Apparent zero-order disappearance of a phenytoin suspension from rat intestinal segments was attributed to rate-limiting dissolution of suspended particles rather than to saturation of absorption processes.[425] Three independent studies have shown that phenytoin serum levels exhibit twin peaks following single p.o. and i.m. doses.[422,426,427] Although the second peak has not been explained, its occurrence appears to coincide with an increased rate of urinary excretion of HPPH,[422] and may reflect extra-vascular concentration (and release). Errors introduced when assuming linear pharmacokinetics for phenytoin are discussed by Jusko et al.,[428] who examined the bioavailability of p.o. phenytoin products using classical linear methods and also a nonlinear method based on equation 2.7 which incorporates both nonlinear (metabolism) and linear (renal excretion) elimination components.

$$C_{int} = \lim_{t \to \infty} \int_{o}^{t} \left[\frac{Cl_R}{V_d} \cdot C_p + \frac{V_{max}C_p}{K_m + C_p} \right] dt \qquad (2.7)$$

In this equation C_{int} is a parameter related to drug bioavailability, Cl_R is renal clearance of drug, V_d is the apparent distribution volume, C_p is the plasma level of drug at time t, and V_{max} and K_m are Michaelis-Menten type constants. Comparison of the two methods indicated that the linear calculation may underestimate true drug bioavailability depending on dose size and the magnitude of the absorption rate compared with V_{max} and K_m.

The influence of saturable phenytoin kinetics on dose-response relationships is discussed by Martin et al.,[429] who describe methods to calculate phenytoin dosage to achieve required steady-state drug levels, and also clinical implications of changes in drug bioavailability, drug interactions, and hepatic disease. Other studies have reported poor relationships between serum anticonvulsant levels and the degree of seizure control, particularly with minor seizures, but better relationships were observed with major seizures.[430,431] Although serum-levels of phenytoin vary between subjects,[432,433] dosage and serum-levels associated with clinical toxicity are consistent within the same individual.[434]

Evidence has been presented of meaningful drug level-response relationships for phenytoin, particularly during adjuvant drug therapy,[435] in patients presenting management problems,[436] in mentally retarded patients,[437] and in patients with generalized epileptic seizures.[438] Matzke et al.[439] reported plasma concentrations of phenytoin in a patient following a massive overdose that were in good agreement with analog computer simulations based on published values of V_{max} and K_m, 9 mg kg^{-1} d^{-1} and 7 mg 1^{-1}, respectively.[440] Nonetheless, Vozeh et al.[441] reported that a Bayesian feedback prediction method, which uses both feedback and population information concerning phenytoin clearance and its inter- and intraindividual variability, allows better prediction than methods that use less population information.[440,442,443]

In 19 children aged 2 m to 20 yr who took a fixed phenytoin dose of 4 - 17.9 mg kg^{-1} d^{-1} for more than 10 days, little fluctuation in serum phenytoin concentrations was observed.[444] Variations in concentration were inversely related to the average concentration. As previously described by Wagner,[445] this phenomenon is consistent with nonlinear elimination kinetics.

Circulating phenytoin is extensively bound to plasma proteins. The fraction unbound averaged 11% in young epileptics (18 - 33 yr) and increased to 13% in elderly patients (62 - 87 yr) who also had decreased concentrations of plasma albumin.[446] Casto et al.[447] demonstrated a good correlation between the concentration of free phenytoin in plasma and phenytoin concentration in urine (Figure 2.18). The correlation was not influenced by age, urine pH, or urine flow. Binding of phenytoin to plasma proteins decreased to 74% in uraemic patients[448] due to decreased phenytoin-albumin association constant, typically from 4.1 x 10^3 to 1.8 x 10^3 M^{-1}.[449] Phenytoin binding to plasma albumin is decreased also in the presence of salicylate, but appears not to be affected by the cations ouabain or EDTA.[450,451] Aspirin induced an increase in free phenytoin fraction and a decrease in total serum phenytoin, but did not alter free serum phenytoin concentration.[452,453]

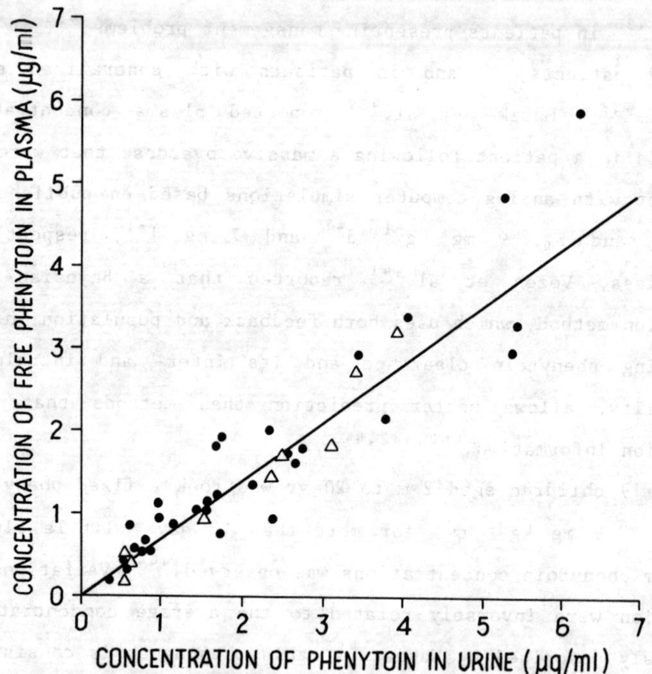

Figure 2.18   Correlation of urine and plasma free phenytoin concentrations. Linear regression equation: C_{pf} = 0.70 C_u - 0.003; r^2 = 0.876.   Triangles indicate patients $\leq$ 12 yr old. Reproduced by permission from Clin. Pharmacol. Ther., 1982, 32, 628.

Plasma phenytoin levels are higher in female subjects receiving p.o. contraceptives than in matched untreated subjects.[454] They are reduced after pretreatment with folic acid[455] and valproic acid,[456,457] but are not significantly affected by smoking.[458] Both folic acid and valproic acid increased the clearance of phenytoin, but only valproic acid displaced phenytoin from binding to plasma proteins. Competition between valproic acid and phenytoin for plasma-protein binding sites has been demonstrated in dogs, although the degree of binding in dogs is less than in man.[459]

The degree of toxic manifestations appears to be inversely proportional to the degree of binding of phenytoin to serum proteins,[460,461] and a positive relationship has been demonstrated between circulating free drug and its concentration in c.s.f. in man.[462] The circulating unbound fraction of phenytoin is between two and four times greater than normal in uraemic plasma.[463]

Although phenytoin is cleared from the body almost entirely by metabolism, plasma clearance of unchanged drug from patients with acute viral hepatitis is unaltered.[464] This finding is explicable in terms of decreased binding to plasma proteins in acute viral hepatitis resulting in exposure of an increased concentration of unbound drug to the liver. Protein binding of phenytoin is reduced in uraemia resulting in lower plasma levels of total drug and an increased apparent volume of distribution.[465] The binding of phenytoin to serum albumin was decreased to _ca_. 80% in a patient with dialysis encephalopathy.[466] Increased binding after haemodialysis appeared to be related to reduced circulating levels of dialysible metabolites rather than to changes in circulating free fatty acids. In a study involving 29 patients, the cerebral uptake of phenytoin and phenobarbital was slower than that of the benzodiazepines clonazepam and diazepam.[467] Once equilibrium was established, circulating levels of unbound phenytoin correlated well with drug levels in brain tissue and c.s.f.[468-470] Barth et al.[471] reported a twofold variation in the unbound phenytoin fraction in normal individuals and, relating their observations to previous studies, concluded that measuring total circulating phenytoin levels is an adequate drug monitoring procedure in most cases. However in hepatic and renal diseases and some other cases, it is desirable to monitor the unbound, active drug in plasma. These authors, and others,[472-474] advocate the use of salivary drug levels for phenytoin monitoring. However, Ayers and Burnett[475] provide a word of caution regarding the use of this methodology with some p.o. formulations.

Conrad et al.[476] suggested that species differences in phenytoin tolerance may be partially explained in terms of differences in protein binding of phenytoin and HPPH. Phenytoin was more extensively bound to human plasma proteins than those of the rat at all plasma concentrations studied, and the free drug concentration in rat plasma was approximately 1.6 times that in human plasma. The reverse was true of HPPH, where the free metabolite concentration in human plasma was approximately 1.4 times that in rat plasma.

Plasma concentrations of phenytoin and also phenobarbital are reduced, and the free fraction of phenytoin is increased, in pregnancy.[477,478] Reduction of phenytoin binding correlated with gestational age, from 91% in nonpregnant women to 87% during the third trimester.[478] Reduced circulating drug levels were attributed to possible fluid retention, and also foetal and placental tissue volumes. However reduction in phenytoin levels may be due also to an increased rate of plasma drug clearance.[479]

Phenytoin and phenobarbital freely cross the placental barrier.[480,481] In 6 full-term newborn infants born to epileptic mothers, the equilibrium cord:maternal plasma concentration ratio of these anticonvulsants was approximately unity, compared with a higher ratio of ca. 1.7 for valproic acid.[481] The newborn appears to be able to metabolize phenytoin at about the same rate as adults.[482] Michaelis-Menten elimination kinetics of phenytoin were observed in the newborn, with apparent zero-order kinetics occurring at plasma phenytoin concentrations of 2 - 10 μg ml^{-1}, which is similar to the concentration range at which transition from first-order to zero-order kinetics occurs in adults.[483]

Reviews have been published on the metabolism and the pharmaco-kinetics of phenytoin.[484] At therapeutic doses, the elimination of phenytoin is nonlinear due to saturable hepatic metabolism. Data in the rat showed that increasing i.v. doses from 10 to 50 mg kg^{-1} were associated with a four-fold increase in mean apparent $t_{0.5}$, from 64 to 267 min.[485] The amount excreted as conjugates of HPPH averaged 59% for the 10 mg kg^{-1} dose and 39% for the 50 mg kg^{-1} dose.

The decline in serum phenytoin concentrations with time can generally be described by equation 2.8. Metabolism of phenytoin to

$$\frac{dC}{dt} = - \frac{V_{max} \cdot C}{K_m + C} \tag{2.8}$$

HPPH is age-dependent: children metabolize at a faster rate than adults.[485-488] The value of V_{max} was 17.9 mg kg^{-1} d^{-1} in children under 1 yr of age and decreased to 9.6 mg kg^{-1} d^{-1} at 16 - 22 yr.[489] Similar decreases in metabolic capacity with increasing age were reported in another study,[490] in which 40 children (8 - 33 months) and 21 adults (18 - 66 yr) had mean V_{max} values of 20.4 and 8.7 mg kg^{-1} d^{-1}, respectively. However, after correcting for differences in the ratio of liver:body weight, V_{max} was 0.4 mg per g of liver d^{-1} in both age groups. Values of K_m in the children and adults were similar, averaging 7.5 and 9.4 mg l^{-1}, respectively. Further studies in 92 adult epileptic patients showed a continued decrease in V_{max} with age, the respective mean values being 7.5, 6.6, and 6.0 mg kg^{-1} d^{-1} in the 20 - 39, 40 - 59, and 60 - 79 yr age groups.[491] Again, K_m was not affected by age, the overall mean being 5 - 6 µg ml^{-1}. Using equation 2.9, where C_{ss} is the steady-

$$\text{Dose (mg kg}^{-1} \text{ d}^{-1}) = \frac{V_{max} \cdot C_{ss}}{K_m + C_{ss}} \tag{2.9}$$

state concentration, it was estimated that the elderly (60 - 79 yr) required 21% less phenytoin per day than the 20 - 39 yr group to maintain a steady-state concentration of 15 µg ml^{-1}. Bach et al.[492] reported an age-related decrease in free phenytoin clearance, from 569 ml min^{-1} in young subjects (mean age 28.8 yr) to 309 ml min^{-1} in the elderly (mean age 83.5 yr), although no significant difference in total phenytoin clearance was observed between the two age groups. In this study, little or no correlation between liver volume and phenytoin clearance was observed. Marked fluctuations have been demonstrated in phenytoin clearance rates in newborn and in young infants.[493] For infants in the first week of life, plasma phenytoin $t_{0.5}$ was prolonged and variable (21 ± 12 h). In older infants the $t_{0.5}$ was 7.6 ± 3.5 h. In premature infants the $t_{0.5}$ was increased to 75 ± 65 h. The apparent drug distribution volume (ca. 0.8 l kg^{-1}) was similar in all age groups. In another study 11 children aged between 6 m and 7 yr had phenytoin $t_{0.5}$ values ranging from 1.2 to 16.1 h, while the overall drug distribution volume varied from 0.27 to 1.0 l kg^{-1}.[494]

The saturable nature of phenytoin metabolism, and wide individual differences in the values of the Michaelis-Menten constants V_{max} and K_m, may give rise to variable accumulation of drug in the body with repeated dosing.[495,496] Repeated administration of phenytoin to healthy individuals gave rise to plasma level-time data that was adequately described by a one-compartment open model with zero-order input and Michaelis-Menten elimination, as described by equation 2.10

$$\frac{dC}{dt} = \frac{k_O}{V_d} - \frac{V_{max}C}{V_d(K_m + C)} \tag{2.10}$$

where k_O is the rate of phenytoin administration.[497] In five individuals V_{max} and K_m varied from 5.3 to 8.4 mg kg^{-1} d^{-1} and from 0.83 to 4.18 mg l^{-1}, respectively. Various methods have been proposed to determine the Michaelis-Menten constants for phenytoin,[498] and these parameters appear to be unaffected by metabolite feed-back inhibition.[499]

In normal subjects, 52 - 94% of dosed phenytoin is recovered as HPPH. The renal clearance of this metabolite is similar to the GFR when corrected for protein binding, suggesting elimination only by filtration.[500] While plasma levels of conjugated HPPH reach plateau values after 4 days of repeated dosing to normal individuals, plasma levels of this metabolite accumulate to ten times normal values in uraemic individuals, and accumulation persists after 15 days of repeated doses.

Neither polyuria nor oliguria appears likely to influence phenytoin serum concentrations in the short term.[501] High circulating levels of HPPH in renal failure could cause accumulation of phenytoin, owing to product inhibition of metabolism.[502,503] This theory is not supported however by the observation that plasma $t_{0.5}$ of phenytoin in uraemic subjects was actually reduced relative to that in normals. Increased drug clearance in uraemic patients was attributed to induction of metabolizing enzymes, but it could be explained equally well by the same argument as that used in the case of viral hepatitis.[464] In spite of reduced protein binding in uraemia, phenytoin is not appreciably cleared from the circulation by haemodialysis.[504]

As suggested in two recent reviews,[505,506] the most important drug interactions concerning phenytoin include those that result in inhibition of phenytoin metabolism. In 9 nonepileptic patients who received phenytoin, 200 - 300 mg d^{-1} for 2 - 4 m, the average steady-state serum phenytoin concentration was 5.7 mg 1^{-1}.[507] Serum phenytoin increased to 9.1 mg 1^{-1} following coadministration of cimetidine, 1 g d^{-1}, for 3 weeks, but returned to 5.8 mg 1^{-1} within 2 weeks of withdrawal of cimetidine (Figure 2.19). Thus, the metabolism of phenytoin was probably inhibited by cimetidine. Furthermore, phenytoin is an inducer of hepatic microsomal enzymes. The mean clearance of antipyrine in these patients was 0.67 and 1.61 ml min^{-1} kg^{-1}, respectively, before and after repeated doses of phenytoin.[507] Induction by phenytoin was partially antagonized by cimetidine, which subsequently decreased the antipyrine clearance to 1.01 ml min^{-1} kg^{-1}.

In 11 male alcoholics with no evidence of chronic liver disease, the mean total clearance of phenytoin was 0.023 l kg^{-1} h^{-1} during alcohol ingestion but increased to 0.033 l kg^{-1} h^{-1} during alcohol withdrawal.[508] It was postulated that alcohol inhibited phenytoin metabolism but induced hepatic enzymes, thereby leading to increased phenytoin clearance on cessation of drinking.

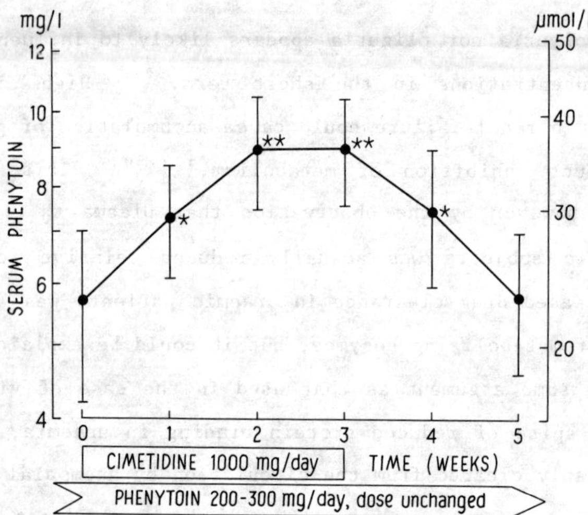

Figure 2.19   Effect of cimetidine on serum phenytoin concentration in 9 patients after 2 to 4 months on phenytoin (mean ± SEM). Asterisk indicates significant difference (p < 0.05*; <0.01**) from values at 0 and 5 weeks. Reproduced by permission from Eur. J. Clin. Pharmacol., 1981, 21, 215.

The metabolism of phenytoin is decreased after pretreatment with disulphiram,[509] and with SKF-525A, but is accelerated by phenobarbital pretreatment.[510] The hepatic clearance of phenytoin may increase in infectious mononucleosis.[511] Clearance of phenytoin and some other anticonvulsants increases moderately during pregnancy, but returns to normal after delivery.[512] The increase in clearance, which may explain previous reports of reduced anticonvulsant levels in pregnant women, appears to be due to increased hepatic metabolism.

Mephenytoin

Marked stereoselective differences in the metabolism of racemic mephenytoin have been observed in man.[513] In 7 subjects who received 23 μmol kg^{-1} of racemic mephenytoin containing ^{14}C and and ^{3}H labeled enantiomers, the major urinary metabolites were 3-methyl-5-(4-hydroxyphenyl)-5-ethylhydantoin (4-OH-M) and 5-phenyl-5-ethylhydantoin (PEH). Approximately 91% of the 4-OH-M was formed from S-mephenytoin and was rapidly excreted with a mean $t_{0.5}$ of 3.8 h.

In contrast, R-mephenytoin appeared to contribute more extensively to the demethylated product PEH which was excreted relatively slowly.

Ethosuximide

Ethosuximide is rapidly absorbed following p.o. doses and distributes freely into body tissues It is cleared slowly from the body and has a plasma $t_{0.5}$ of <u>ca</u>. 50 - 60 h in man.[514] As a consequence of slow clearance, drug accumulates in the body during multiple dosing, and steady-state plasma levels are not reached until the ninth day of a once-daily dosage regimen.

Typically, in 6 normal subjects receiving ethosuximide 250 mg twice daily for 10 days, the average $t_{0.5}$ was 53.7 h.[515] Continued administration of ethosuximide with concomitant carbamazepine (200 mg d^{-1}) for 18 days resulted in a reduced ethosuximide $t_{0.5}$ of 44.6 h, probably due to induction of ethosuximide metabolism by carbamazepine. Similar induction effects by primidone and valproic acid have also been reported.[516] Metabolic clearance of ethosuximide appeared to be greater in children (under 10 yr) than in young adults (16 - 34 yr), as indicated by a lower plasma concentration:dose ratio in the former group.[516]

Extended studies under carefully controlled conditions have confirmed that circadian rhythm influences steady-state ethosuximide levels in rhesus monkeys.[517] During long-term i.v. infusion plasma levels of drug show two minima, between 12.00 and 14.00 h, and between 20.00 h and midnight. Although the influence of circadian rhythm on ethosuximide levels was limited, ongoing studies indicated that similar variations with valproic acid and clonazepam may have therapeutic significance.

Considerable species differences have been demonstrated in the elimination rate of ethosuximide. The serum $t_{0.5}$ of ethosuximide is <u>ca</u>. 17 h in the dog, 10 h in the rat, and only 1 h in the mouse.[518] Ethosuximide is negligibly bound to plasma proteins and rapidly enters the c.s.f. from the circulation in dog, reaching equilibrium 20 - 30

min after dosing. Dose-dependent elimination kinetics for ethosuximide are suggested by the demonstration of a nonlinear relationship
between plasma levels and dose increments.[519] This is illustrated in
Figure 2.20 for two patients receiving between 10 and 50 mg kg^{-1}
ethosuximide daily.

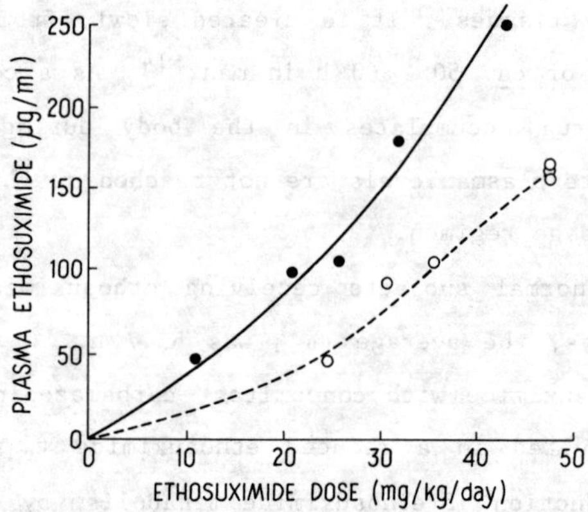

Figure 2.20 Curvilinear relation between steady-state
plasma ethosuximide levels and drug dose in two
patients. Reproduced by permission from Clin. Pharmacokin., 1979, 4, 38.

While similar nonlinearity in the case of phenytoin is due to
saturable elimination kinetics,[520] there is as yet no evidence that a
similar explanation obtains for ethosuximide.

The low protein binding of ethosuximide is associated with ready
passage of this compound across the placenta and into breast milk, the
concentration ratio of ethosuximide in breast milk and human serum
approaching unity.[521] Following ethosuximide therapy to the mother
during the last trimester of pregnancy, the concentration of transplacentally acquired ethosuximide in the neonate declined with a
$t_{0.5}$ of 41 h; this value being similar to that reported previously
in children.

Methsuximide

Methsuximide is readily absorbed and rapidly distributed through-out the body after p.o. doses and the drug freely crosses the blood-brain barrier.[522] The N-demethylated metabolite is formed rapidly _in vivo_, and it is cleared from the body slower than the parent compound in some cases.[523] The contribution of this metabolite to the anti-epileptic effect of methsuximide is not known.

Methsuximide obeyed two-compartment kinetics following i.v. dosing to dogs, while blood levels of desmethylmethsuximide were described by single-compartment kinetics.[524] Plasma levels of both compounds following i.v. doses of methsuximide were described by the kinetic model shown in Figure 2.21, where A's represent the amount of drug in the first or second body compartment, M is the amount of metabolite in its body compartment, the C's and V's refer to concentration and volume terms, while the k's are first-order rate constants. A typical plasma profile obtained after administering i.v. methsuximide is shown in Figure 2.22. The plasma metabolite $t_{0.5}$

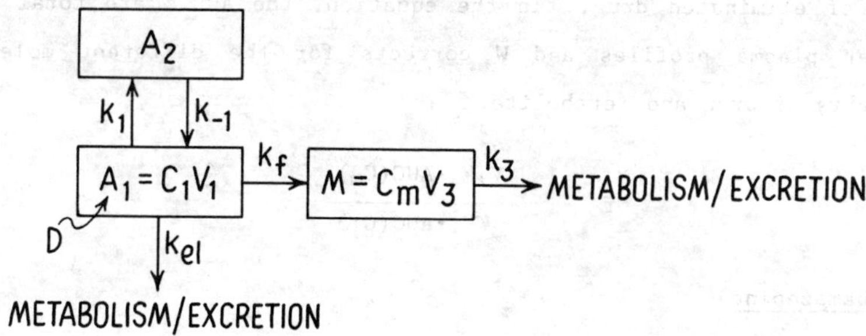

Figure 2.21 Pharmacokinetic model describing plasma levels of methsuximide and its major metabolite N-desmethyl methsuximide in the dog following i.v. methsuximide. Reproduced by permission from _J. Pharm. Sci._, 1977, **66**, 688.

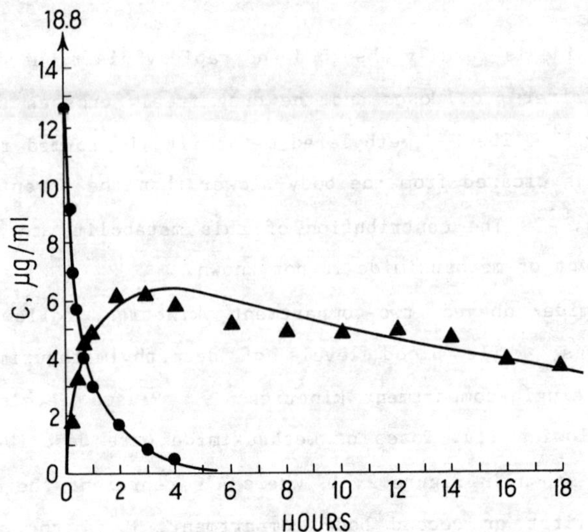

Figure 2.22   Methsuximide -●- and N-desmethyl
methsuximide -▲- plasma levels after a 250 mg i.v.
injection of methsuximide to a dog.   Reproduced by
permission from J. Pharm. Sci., 1977, 66, 688.

was ca. 15 h, compared to 1 - 3.5 h for the parent drug, and it is

suggested that pharmacological effects after repeated methsuximide

doses may be due primarily to the active metabolite which accumulates

during repeated doses.   Values of k_f, calculated from the relation-

ship shown in equation 2.11, showed that the metabolite accounted for

40% of eliminated drug.   In the equation, the AUC's are total areas

under plasma profiles and W corrects for the different molecular

weights of drug and metabolite.

$$k_f = \frac{V_3 k_3 \cdot AUC(C_m)}{WV_1 \cdot AUC(C_1)} \qquad (2.11)$$

Carbamazepine

Carbamazepine is generally reported to be well absorbed following

p.o. doses of tablets and solutions[525,526] but may be variable

from different formulations,[527,528] and also from different dose

sizes of the same dosage form.[529]   The bioavailability of carbamazepine from a 500 mg dose was 20% less compared to a 200 mg dose in healthy volunteers. Bioavailability data in one study have suggested that carbamazepine absorption is inversely related to particle size.[530] Carbamazepine absorption is increased somewhat in the presence of food, but the overall pharmacokinetics of the drug appear to be dose-independent. The elimination $t_{0.5}$ of 30 - 35 h after single doses was considerably reduced, and observed plasma levels were lower than predicted values after repeated dosing, indicating possible induction of drug-metabolizing enzymes.[531,532]

Studies in rhesus monkeys have yielded absolute carbamazepine bioavailability of greater than 80% from i.m. doses.[533] Absorption was rapid, with peak plasma drug levels occurring within 1 h. Despite a twofold difference in bioavailability between different parenteral formulations, the mean elimination $t_{0.5}$ and plasma clearance in the monkey were independent of formulation and averaged <u>ca</u>. 1.1 h and 5 1 h^{-1}, respectively.

In 91 patients receiving chronic carbamazepine there was no significant correlation between steady-state drug levels and the daily drug dosage.[534] There was, however, a good correlation ($r = + 0.64$, p < 0.001) between plasma levels of carbamazepine and its pharmacologically active metabolite carbamazepine-10,11-epoxide, which is less bound to plasma proteins than the parent drug. The epoxide:carbamazepine ratios in serum vary considerably among young adult patients and also at different times of the day in the same patient.[535] Parent drug and metabolite were present in c.s.f. at concentrations from 19 to 34% and 26 to 71% of the respective serum levels. In another study the mean brain:plasma ratio of carbamazepine in patients undergoing unilateral temporal lobectomy was 1.4 while the equivalent ratio of the epoxide metabolite ranged from 0.6 to 1.5.[536,537] The ratio for carbamazepine was similar in patients receiving the drug alone or in combination with other anticonvulsants, but the ratio for the epoxide metabolite was increased in patients on combined treatment.

This observation was interpreted as a possible explanation for the enhanced effect often obtained by combining carbamazepine with other antiepileptic drugs. The elimination $t_{0.5}$ of carbamazepine is shorter, and total clearance of drug is 5 - 10 times higher, in neonates and children compared to adults.[538] Poor correlations were found between dosage and circulating carbamazepine levels in children.[539] In children receiving combination therapy circulating levels of epoxide were significantly higher than those in children receiving carbamazepine alone, suggesting that other drugs induce the rate of metabolism of carbamazepine to the epoxide.

The extent of carbamazepine binding to serum or plasma proteins appears to be similar in healthy subjects[540] and in epileptic patients.[541] The mean free fraction of carbamazepine was 0.23 - 0.24 while that of carbamazepine-10,11-epoxide was 0.32. Plasma protein binding of carbamazepine was independent of age and other concurrently administered anticonvulsants.[541] The data demonstrated also that saliva concentrations of carbamazepine and the epoxide are good indicators of respective free concentrations in plasma. Carbamazepine penetrates not only into saliva[542] but also into bile.[543,544] Although the bile:plasma concentration ratio in humans was 0.62 (range 0.24 - 0.82), only 1% of administered drug was recovered in 72 h bile. This precludes any significant enterohepatic circulation of carbamazepine.[543]

Carbamazepine crosses the placental barrier rapidly[545] yielding foetal:maternal plasma level ratios between 0.5 and 0.8. Carbamazepine-10,11-epoxide is also present in foetal plasma and tissue. However, recovery from tissues was poor and metabolite levels were not determined. The concentration of carbamazepine in breast milk was 60% of total plasma levels.[544]

The pharmacokinetics of carbamazepine have been shown to exhibit both time and dose dependence. The mean elimination drug $t_{0.5}$ in human volunteers was reduced from 38 h following single p.o. doses to

21 h following repeated doses.[546] Although steady-state circulating drug levels were poorly predicted from single dose data, they were adequately predicted when correction was made for the increased elimination rate constant. In the same study, the elimination rate constant of carbamazepine increased while the absorbtion rate constant decreased with increasing dose size. In another study the elimination $t_{0.5}$ of carbamazepine decreased from a mean value of 50 h following a 200 mg dose, to 28 h following a 900 mg dose.[547] These authors observed a weak negative correlation between drug distribution volume and dose size. Pitlick et al.[548] formalized the time-dependency of carbamazepine elimination rate constant and fitted observed elimination rate changes to equation 2.12, where k_{el}^{o} and k_{el}^{∞} are elimination rate constants at t_o and t_{∞}, respectively, and k_i is a first-order rate constant. Application of this model to evaluate

$$k_{el}(t) = k_{el}^{\infty} - (k_{el}^{\infty} - k_{el}^{o})e^{-k_i t} \qquad (2.12)$$

k_{el} resulted in close agreement between calculated and observed carbamazepine levels during repeated doses.

Other studies have shown that the time course of induction may be complex, discontinuous, and prolonged for 14 - 22 days after initiation of therapy.[549] Induction may be increased in the presence of other anticonvulsant agents.[550] The elimination rate of carbamazepine-10,11-epoxide, which has similar anticonvulsant properties to the parent drug, may also be induced.[551] In 13 healthy male subjects who received 100 mg carbamazepine twice daily for 28 d, significant decreases in plasma levels of carbamazepine were observed, while plasma epoxide concentrations were unchanged.[552] Similar findings were reported in epileptic patients. In a study employing tetra-deuterium-labeled carbamazepine in children,[553] autoinduction was shown to occur rapidly and was complete within 1 m of daily drug treatment. The mean clearance of carbamazepine was 0.028 1 kg^{-1} h^{-1} before treatment but increased to 0.036 1 kg^{-1} h^{-1} on day 2 of therapy. A maximum clearance value of ca. 0.056 1 kg^{-1} h^{-1} was reached within 2 - 4 weeks of treatment, while continued treatment for 4 m resulted in no further increase in carbamazepine clearance.

The rate of carbamazepine metabolism in newborns was, like phenytoin, similar to or greater than that in adults.[554] It is possible, however, that the increased rate of drug metabolism in newborns may have resulted from enzyme induction via the mother.

Although the monkey has been proposed as a suitable model for evaluating carbamazepine as an anticonvulsant,[555] the pharmacokinetics of carbamazepine in this species are different from those in man.[556] After zero-order infusion into monkeys carbamazepine levels in blood declined according to Michaelis-Menten kinetics as indicated in Figure 2.23. Using this method of analysis, elimination $t_{0.5}$ values,

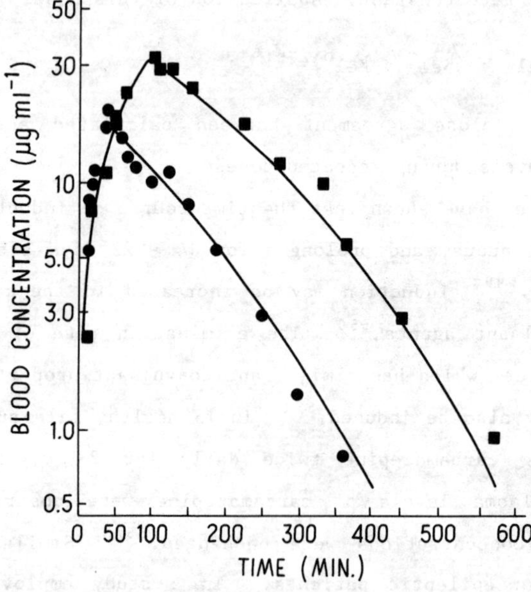

Figure 2.23   Semi-logarithmic plots of blood concentration versus time for zero-order i.v. infusion of carbamazepine in a monkey. Doses were 160 mg during 45 min (●——●) and 335 mg during 90 min (■——■). Reproduced by permission from <u>Res. Comm. Chem. Path. Pharmacol.</u>, 1975, <u>10</u>, 303.

$0.693/(V_{max}/K_m)$, of <u>ca</u>. 60 min were obtained. These values are somewhat shorter than those reported in this species assuming first-order kinetics[554] and considerably shorter than values reported in man.

Carbamazepine was shown to accelerate its own metabolism in adult and immature rats after repeated administration, as demonstrated by a reduction in drug $t_{0.5}$ and a 50% increase in clearance.[557] Repeated doses of carbamazepine to rats also shortened pentobarbital sleeping time and significantly decreased pentobarbital brain levels.

Carbamazepine induces the rate of clonazepam metabolism in monkeys[558] and in man.[559] In monkeys premedication with carbamazepine caused a reduction in carbamazepine elimination $t_{0.5}$ from a normal range of 5.2 - 12.2 h to 3.7 - 7.7 h, while in man the mean induced $t_{0.5}$ of carbamazepine was 23 h compared with a normal value of 32 h.

Oxcarbazepine

Orally dosed oxcarbazepine was rapidly absorbed and converted to its active metabolite, 10,11-dihydro-10-hydroxy-carbamazepine, which showed higher and more prolonged plasma concentrations than parent drug.[560] In urine, <u>ca</u>. 2 - 8% of the dose was excreted as conjugated oxcarbazepine and 30 - 50% of dose as free or conjugated metabolite. A second urinary metabolite, 10,11-dihydro-<u>trans</u>-10,11-dihydroxy-carbamazepine, accounted for 2 - 6% of the dose.

Valproic Acid

The clinical pharmacokinetics of valproic acid have been reviewed.[561] Valproic acid has been shown to be equally bioavailable after p.o. doses of valproic acid in capsules and a syrup,[562] and of valproic acid in capsules or valproate sodium in dragées.[563] Compared with i.v. drug, p.o. doses of sodium valproate to man are 86 - 100% bioavailable from solutions and 68 - 100% bioavailable from conventional and enteric-coated tablets.[562,564-566] Although circulating levels of valproic acid are dose-related, they vary among individuals.[567] Rectal absorption of valproic acid from aqueous enema was comparable to absorption from p.o. doses.[568,569] Steady-state levels of valproate can be predicted with some accuracy from single-dose data, but correlations between plasma levels and dosage are variable.[570] The percentage of circulating valproate bound to plasma proteins varies from 90% in man, 80% in the dog, and 65% in the rat, to 12% in the mouse.[571] In all species the calculated hepatic extraction ratios are smaller than the free drug fraction, indicating restrictive and liver blood-flow independent metabolism.

The valproate free fraction increases markedly in patients with impaired renal function.[572] Serum protein binding of valproic acid is also drug concentration dependent, the free fraction increasing from only 6% at 64 mg 1^{-1} to 14% at 125 mg 1^{-1}.[573] Valproic acid is displaced from serum albumin by salicylates, resulting in a 3- to 4-fold increase in the steady-state free fraction in serum.[573] On the other hand, valproic acid tends to displace diazepam from plasma protein binding sites,[574] but appears to have no effect on the plasma protein binding of phenobarbital and carbamazepine.[575]

Transfer of valproate to the mouse brain occurs rapidly, and concentrations of drug in brain tissue are 20 - 25% of those in serum.[576] In epileptic patients, levels of valproic acid in c.s.f. were one-tenth of those in plasma.[577] In a pregnant rhesus monkey given a single 50 mg kg^{-1} i.v. dose of sodium valproate, the drug rapidly crossed the placental barrier.[578] Valproic acid concentration in foetal blood exceeded that in maternal blood within 15 min of dosing and the terminal foetal:maternal concentration ratio was <u>ca.</u> 1:3.

Although valproic acid is cleared predominantly by metabolism, hepatic clearance is restricted and independent of liver blood flow.[563] Following i.v. administration, valproic acid blood levels decline biexponentially, with initial and terminal phase $t_{0.5}$ values of <u>ca</u>. 1 and 12 h, respectively.[563,565] The volume of distribution at steady state and the total clearance averaged 12.6 l and 51 ml min^{-1}, respectively. The mean terminal $t_{0.5}$ after a 900 - 1000 mg p.o. dose was 8 - 9 h, but increased to 10 - 15 h after repeated dosing twice daily for 5 d. This change was explained in terms of the inhibitory effect of valproic acid on drug metabolism. Autoinhibition was reflected also in the dose-related decline in intrinsic clearance, which averaged 89 and 72 ml h^{-1} kg^{-1} after a 4 d treatment with 500 and 1000 mg d^{-1}, respectively.[579] In contrast to earlier findings under steady-state conditions,[580-582] no diurnal oscillation in valproic acid disposition was observed following a single dose in rhesus monkeys.[583]

Concomitant anticonvulsant therapy with carbamazepine and phenytoin facilitates elimination of valproic acid, probably due to induction of hepatic microsomal enzymes. This led to lower serum levels[584,585] and increased intersubject variation in the plasma clearance of valproic acid.[586] The elimination $t_{0.5}$ of valproate increased to 19 h in patients with cirrhosis and acute hepatitis.[587]

<u>Dipropylacetamide</u>

The effect of food on the bioavailability of valproic acid from a single 600 mg p.o. dose of dipropylacetamide was evaluated in 6 healthy male volunteers using a randomized crossover design.[588] Administration of dipropylacetamide after a standard meal resulted in a prolonged absorption lag time of 2.3 h, compared with 0.6 h when the drug was given under fasting conditions. Slower gastric emptying of the postprandial dose of dipropylacetamide apparently caused an increased drug exposure to metabolizing enzymes, resulting in a 19% increase in the bioavailability of valproic acid. The elimination $t_{0.5}$ of valproic acid, approximately 13 - 15 h, appeared to be unaffected by food.

Clonazepam

Following simultaneous 3 mg kg^{-1} p.o. and i.v. administration of ^{14}N- and ^{15}N-clonazepam in the rat, clonazepam bioavailability was estimated to be 7.2%.[589] Approximately 40% of the dose was metabolized in the intestinal wall while an additional 11% was metabolized presystemically in the liver. The elimination $t_{0.5}$ was 70 min. On the other hand clonazepam was well absorbed from p.o. doses in man.[590] Doses ranging from 0.028 to 0.11 mg kg^{-1} resulted in serum drug levels between 13 and 72 ng ml^{-1}. The drug has a $t_{0.5}$ of ca. 30 h and is cleared almost entirely by metabolism. Although clonazepam is extensively metabolized, its long $t_{0.5}$ excludes the possibility of a significant first-pass effect after p.o. doses.

Other antiepileptic agents appear to induce clonazepam metabolism. Nineteen days of pretreatment with phenytoin (4.3 mg kg^{-1} d^{-1}) and also phenobarbital (1.4 mg kg^{-1} d^{-1}) caused increases in mean clonazepam clearance from 0.10 to 0.14 l kg^{-1} h^{-1} and from 0.09 to 0.12 l kg^{-1} h^{-1}, respectively.[591] Serum levels of clonazepam were reduced by concomitant phenytoin therapy due, apparently, to increased metabolism to the 7-amino metabolite.[592] The volume of distribution of clonazepam (3.2 - 3.8 l kg^{-1}) and its protein binding (85 - 88%) were unaffected by the enzyme inducers.

In both slow and rapid acetylators, only ca. 0.5% of a 2 mg p.o. dose of clonazepam was recovered unchanged in 96 h urine.[593] However, urinary recovery of the sequential metabolites 7-aminoclonazepam and 7-acetamidoclonazepam were determined by the acetylator phenotype. The respective values were 22.7% and 1.5% of the dose in slow acetylators and 13.6% and 3.9% of the dose in rapid acetylators.

Primidone

Following a single 30 mg kg^{-1} p.o. dose to dogs primidone was absorbed rapidly, reaching peak serum concentrations at 2 h postdose.[594]   The $t_{0.5}$ of primidone was 5 h while that of phenylethyl-malonamide, which reached a peak concentration at 6.5 h, was 7.5 h. After repeated doses the concentration of primidone in c.s.f. was <u>ca.</u> 80% of that in plasma, and was believed to reflect the free drug concentration in plasma.

Primidone has a relatively short elimination $t_{0.5}$ of <u>ca.</u> 8 h in man and steady-state levels are reached within 48 h of commencement of a multiple-dose regimen.[595]   Plasma levels of major metabolites of primidone, phenobarbital and phenylethylmalonamide, are as high as those of the parent drug after multiple dosing.

The plasma $t_{0.5}$ of primidone in young children (4.5 to 11 h) is similar to that in adults.[596]   Primidone is excreted largely as unchanged drug in children, with only 5% appearing in urine as the metabolite phenobarbital.   The rate of primidone metabolism to form phenobarbital varies considerably, and it is suggested that consequent variations in circulating phenobarbital levels may be of clinical significance.

Primidone was shown to be dialyzable.[597]   In uraemic patients on chronic haemodialysis, the mean $t_{0.5}$ of primidone after single 250 or 500 mg p.o. doses given 2 h before haemodialysis was 5.1 h.   The dialysis clearance (CL_{dp}), calculated using equation 2.13, averaged 97.7 ml min^{-1}.

$$CL_{dp} \;=\; Q_d \cdot C_{do}/C_{pi} \hspace{3cm} (2.13)$$

This clearance value was considerably greater than the metabolic clearance of 30 ml min^{-1} for primidone.   In equation 2.13, Q_d is the dialyzate flow, C_{do} is the dialyzate drug concentration, and C_{pi} is arterial plasma concentration.

The metabolism of primidone is enhanced by concurrent use of other antiepileptic drugs. Following a 250 mg p.o. dose of primidone, the $t_{0.5}$ averaged 15.2 h in 10 control patients and 8.3 h in 9 patients who were also on phenytoin and/or carbamazepine.[598]   The metabolites phenobarbital and phenylethylmalonamide appeared in serum of patients on combination therapy more rapidly than in those on primidone alone. In contrast no differences were observed in pharmacokinetic parameters between normal subjects who received phenylethylmalonamide as a single 400 mg p.o. dose and patients receiving chronic antiepileptic therapy.[599] Phenylethylmalonamide was rapidly and almost completely absorbed from the GI tract and was eliminated predominantly unchanged in urine. Its mean $t_{0.5}$ in man was approximately 20 h.

References

1. J.M. Van Rossum, *Psychiatria Neurlogia Neurochirurgia*, 1973, 76, 217.

2. J.F. Gram and J.B. Winslows, *Commun. Psychopharmacol.*, 1979, 2, 373.

3. S.C. Risch, L.Y. Huey, and D.S. Janowsky, *J. Clin. Psychiat.*, 1979, 40, 58.

4. G.E. Schumacher and J. Weiner, *Amer. J. Hosp. Pharm.*, 1974, 31, 59.

5. T.B. Cooper, *Clin. Pharmacokin.*, 1978, 3, 14.

6. *Ciba Foundation Symposium*, London, July 3-5, 1979.

7. S. Kaumeier, *Int. J. Clin. Pharmacol.*, 1978, 16, 27.

8. A.H. Glassman and J.M. Perel, *Clin. Pharmacol. Ther.*, 1974, 16, 198.

9. G. Burrows, B.A. Scoggins, L.R. Turecek, and B. Davies, *Clin. Pharmacol. Ther.*, 1974, 16, 639.

10. M. Åsberg, *Clin. Pharmacol. Ther.*, 1974, 16, 215.

11. D. Luchins and J. Ananth, *J. Nerv. Ment. Dis.*, 1976, 162, 430.

12. J.M. Petit, D.G. Spiker, J.F. Ruwitch, V.E. Ziegler, A.N. Weiss, and J.T. Biggs, *Clin. Pharmacol. Ther.*, 1977, 21, 47.

13. D. Sharples, *J. Pharm. Pharmacol.*, 1976, 28, 100.

14. D.G. Spiker, A.N. Weiss, S.S. Chang, J.F. Ruwitch, and J.T. Biggs, *Clin. Pharmacol. Ther.*, 1975, 18, 539.

15. A. Jorgensen, *Eur. J. Clin. Pharmacol.*, 1977, 12, 187.

16. A. Jorgensen and V. Hansen, *Eur. J. Clin. Pharmacol.*, 1976, 10, 337.

17. H.J. Rogers, P.J. Morrison, and I.D. Bradbrook, *Brit. J. Clin. Pharmacol.*, 1978, 6, 181.

18. V.E. Ziegler, J.T. Biggs, A.B. Ardekani, and S.H. Rosen, *J. Clin. Pharmacol.*, 1978, 18, 462.

19. W.A. Garland, B.H. Min, and D.J. Birkett, *Res. Comm. Chem. Path. Pharmacol.*, 1978, 22, 475.

20. A.A. Jeffrey and P. Turner, *Brit. J. Clin. Pharmacol.*, 1978, 5, 268.

21. D. DeMaio, F. Drago, P. Nielsen, V. Ascalone, and M. Cisternino, *Arzneim.-Forsch.*, 1980, 30, 335.

22. G. Alvan, O. Borga, M. Lind, L. Palmer, and B. Sievers, *Eur. J. Clin. Pharmacol.*, 1977, 11, 219.

23. M. Gibaldi, *J. Pharm. Sci.*, 1975, 64, 1036.

24. B. Alexanderson, O. Borga, and G. Alván, *Eur. J. Clin. Pharmacol.*, 1973, 5, 181.

25. L.F. Gram and K.F. Overø, Clin. Pharmacol. Ther., 1975, 18, 305.

26. B. Alexanderson, O. Borgå, and G. Alván, Eur. J. Clin. Pharmacol., 1973, 5, 181.

27. M. Rowland, J. Pharm. Sci., 1972, 61, 70.

28. G. Alván, Eur. J. Clin. Pharmacol., 1973, 5, 236.

29. S. Dawling, P. Crome, and R. Braithwaite, Eur. J. Clin. Pharmacol., 1978, 14, 445.

30. S.A. Montgomery, R. McAuley, D.B. Montgomery, R.A. Braithwaite, and S. Dawling, Clin. Pharmacokin., 1979, 4, 129.

31. P. Kragh-Sørensen, Chr. E. Hansen, P. Chr. Baastrup, and E.F. Hvidberg, Psychopharmacologia, 1976, 45, 305.

32. V.E. Ziegler, P.J. Clayton, J.R. Taylor, B.T. Co, and J.T. Biggs, Clin. Pharmacol. Ther., 1976, 20, 458.

33. M. Åsberg, B. Crönholm, F. Sjöqvist, and D. Tuck, Brit. Med. J., 1971, iii, 331.

34. R.A. Braithwaite, R. Goulding, G. Theano, J. Bailey, and A. Coppen, Lancet, 1972, i, 1297.

35. G.D. Burrows, B. Davies, and B.A. Scoggins, Lancet, 1972, ii, 619.

36. M. Gruvstad, Lancet, 1973, i, 95.

37. V.E. Ziegler, B.T. Co, and J.T. Biggs, Amer. J. Psychiat., 1977, 134, 441.

38. K.F. Overø, L.F. Gram, and V. Hansen, Eur. J. Clin. Pharmacol., 1975, 8, 343.

39. B. Alexanderson and O. Borgå, Eur. J. Clin. Pharmacol., 1972, 4, 196.

40. J.P. Tillement, Thérapie, 1973, 28, 249.

41. F. Sjöqvist, P.G. Bergfors, O. Borgå, M. Lind, and H. Ygge, J. Pediatr., 1972, 80, 496.

42. W.G. McBride, Med. J. Australia, 1972, No. 1, 492.

43. G.S. Rachelefsky, J.W. Flynt, A.J. Ebbin, and M.G. Wilson, Lancet, 1972, i, 838.

44. P. Banister, C. Dafoe, E.S.O. Smith, and J. Miller, Lancet, 1972, i, 838.

45. K.F. Overø, J. Pharm. Pharmacol., 1973, 25, 957.

46. B. Alexanderson and O. Borgå, Eur. J. Clin. Pharmacol., 1973, 5, 174.

47. B. Alexanderson, Eur. J. Clin. Pharmacol., 1972, 4, 82.

48. S. Dawling, P. Crome, R.A. Braithwaite, and R.R. Lewis, Eur. J. Clin. Pharmacol., 1980, 18, 147.

49. S. Dawling, P. Crome, and R. Braithwaite, Clin. Pharmacokin., 1980, 5, 394.

50. S. Dawling, K. Lynn, R. Rosser, and R. Braithwaite, Brit. J. Clin. Pharmacol., 1981, 12, 39.

51. K. O'Malley, M. Browning, I. Stevenson, and M.J. Turnbull, Eur. J. Clin. Pharmacol., 1973, 6, 102.

52. K. O'Malley, P.R. Sawyer, I.H. Stevenson, and M.J. Turnbull, Brit. J. Pharmacol., 1972, 44, 372P.

53. G. Silverman and R.A. Braithwaite, Brit. Med. J., 1973, iii, 18.

54. G. Silverman and R.A. Braithwaite, Brit. Med. J., 1972, iv, 111.

55. V.R. Gauch and J. Modestin, Arzneim.-Forsch., 1973, 23, 687.

56. L.F. Gram and J. Christiansen, Clin. Pharmacol. Ther., 1975, 17, 555.

57. A.R. Beaubien and A.P. Pakuts, Drug Metab. Dispos., 1979, 7, 34.

58. H. Dencker, S.J. Dencker, A. Green, A. Nagy, Clin. Pharmacol. Ther., 1976, 19, 584.

59. A.R. Beaubien, L.F. Mathieu, J. Pharm. Pharmacol., 1976, 28, 451.

60. R.C. Heading, J. Nimmo, L.F. Prescott, and P. Tothill, Brit. J. Pharmacol., 1973, 47, 415.

61. A.R. Beaubien, L.F. Mathieu, J.A. Huddleston, and H.F. James, Arch. Int. Pharmacodyn. Ther., 1977, 225, 6.

62. A.R. Beaubien, L.F. Mathieu, and B.B. Coldwell, J. Pharm. Pharmacol., 1975, 27, 484.

63. H.d'A. Heck, S.E. Buttrill, N.W. Flynn, R.L. Dyer, M. Anbar, T. Cairns, S. Dighe, and B.E. Cabana, J. Pharmacokin. Biopharm., 1979, 7, 233.

64. L.F. Gram, I. Sondergaard, J. Christiansen, G.O. Petersen, P. Bech, N. Reisby, I. Ibsen, J. Ortmann, A. Nagy, S.J. Dencker, O. Jacobsen, and O. Krautwald, Psychopharmacology, 1977, 54, 255.

65. L.F. Gram, N. Reisby, I. Ibsen, A. Nagy, S.J. Dencker, P. Bech, G.O. Petersen, and J. Christiansen, Clin. Pharmacol. Ther., 1976, 19, 318.

66. J.M. Perel, R.L. Stiller, and A.H. Glassman, Comm. Psychopharmacol., 1978, 2, 429.

67. L.F. Gram, P.B. Andreasen, K.F. Overø, and J. Christiansen, Psychopharmacology, 1976, 50, 21.

68. J. Bourgouin, M.-A. Gagnon, R. Elie, D. Dvornik, R. Gonzalez, and M. Kraml, Biopharm. Drug Dispos., 1981, 2, 123.

69. J. Meier, E. Nüesch, and R. Schmidt, Eur. J. Clin. Pharmacol., 1974, 7, 429.

70. V.E. Ziegler, J.T. Biggs, L.T. Wylie, W.H. Coryell, K.M. Hanifl, D.J. Hawf, and S.H. Rosen, Clin. Pharmacol. Ther., 1978, 23, 580.

71. J.T. Biggs and V.E. Ziegler, Clin. Pharmacol. Ther., 1977, 22, 269.

72. J.P. Moody, S.F. Whyte, A.J. MacDonald, and G.J. Naylor, Eur. J. Clin. Pharmacol., 1977, 11, 51.

73. B. Alexanderson, Eur. J. Clin. Pharmacol., 1972, 5, 1.

74. D. Weiner, D. Garteiz, M. Cawein, T. Dusebout, G. Wright, and R. Okerholm, J. Pharm. Sci., 1981, 70, 1079.

75. G.P. Forshell, B. Siwers, and J.R. Tuck, Eur. J. Clin. Pharmacol., 1976, 9, 291.

76. L. Vereczkey, G. Bianchetti, S. Garattini, and P.L. Morselli, Psychopharmacologia, 1975, 45, 225.

77. B. Saletu, J. Grünberger, L. Linzmayer, and K. Taeuber, Int. Pharmacopsychiat., 1982, 17, 43.

78. V.E. Ziegler, J.T. Biggs, L.T. Wylie, S.H. Rosen, D.J. Hawf, and W.H. Coryell, Clin. Pharmacol. Ther., 1978, 23, 573.

79. J. Raaflaub, Experientia, 1975, 31, 557.

80. O. Elwan and H.K. Adam, Eur. J. Clin. Pharmacol., 1980, 17, 179.

81. K.P. Maguire, G.D. Burrows, T.R. Norman, and B.A. Scoggins, Brit. J. Clin. Pharmacol., 1981, 12, 405.

82. G.M. Simpson, E. Varga, M. Reiss, T.B. Cooper, P.E. Bergner, and J.H. Lee, Clin. Pharmacol. Ther., 1974, 15, 631.

83. V. Smolen, H. Murdock, W. Stoltman, J. Clevenger, L. Combs, and E. Williams, J. Clin. Pharmacol., 1975, 15, 734.

84. V.F. Smolen, A.K. Jhawar, W.A. Weigand, R.M. Paeline, and P.B. Kuehn, J. Pharm. Sci., 1976, 65, 1600.

85. P.B. Kuehn, A.K. Jhawar, W.A. Weigand, and V.F. Smolen, J. Pharm. Sci., 1976, 65, 1593.

86. S.G. Dahl and R.E. Strandjord, Clin. Pharmacol. Ther., 1976, 21, 437.

87. S.F. Cooper, J.M. Albert, J. Hillel, and G. Caille, Curr. Ther. Res., 1973, 15, 73.

88. W.E. Fann, J.M. Davis, D.S. Janowsky, H.J. Sekerke, and D.M. Schmidt, J. Clin. Pharmacol., 1973, 13, 388.

89. L. Rivera-Calimlim, B. Kerzner, and F.E. Karch, Clin. Pharmacol. Ther., 1978, 23, 451.

90. L.R. Whitfield, P.N. Kaul, and M.L. Clark, J. Pharmacokin. Biopharm., 1978, 6, 187.

91. B. Wode-Helgodt, S. Borg, B. Fryö, and G. Sedvall, Acta Psychiat. Scand., 1978, 58, 149.

92. J.E. March, D. Danato, P. Turano, and W.J. Turner, J. Med., 1972, 3, 146.

93. P.N. Kaul, M.K. Ticku, and M.L. Clark, J. Pharm. Sci., 1972, 61, 1753.

94. I. Hahn, G. Krieglstein, J. Krieglstein, and K. Tschentscher, Arch. Pharmakol., 1973, 278, 35.

95.   S.H. Curry, J. Pharm. Pharmacol., 1972, 24, 818.

96.   J.D. Maxwell, M. Carrella, J.D. Parkes, R. Williams, G.P. Mould, and S.H. Curry, Clin. Sci., 1972, 43, 143.

97.   G. Sakalis, S.H. Curry, G.P. Mould, and M.H. Lader, Clin. Pharmacol. Ther., 1972, 13, 931.

98.   P.N. Kaul, L.R. Whitfield, and M.L. Clark, J. Pharm. Sci., 1976, 65, 694.

99.   L. Rivera-Calimlim, PH.H. Griesbach, and R. Perlmutter, Clin. Pharmacol. Ther., 1979, 26, 114.

100. B.M. Boulos, L.E. Davis, S.D. Larks, G.G. Larks, C.R. Sirtori, and C.H. Almond, Arch. Int. Pharmacodyn. Ther., 1971, 194, 403.

101. P.-A. Hals and S.G. Dahl, Acta Pharmacol. Toxicol., 1982, 50, 148.

102. N.R. West, M.P. Rosenblum, H. Sprince, S. Gold, D.H. Boehme, and W.H. Vogel, J. Pharm. Sci., 1974, 63, 417.

103. N.R. West and W.H. Vogel, Arch. Int. Pharmacodyn. Ther., 1975, 215, 318.

104. P.C. Borg and G.C. Cotzias, Proc. Nat. Acad. Sci. U.S.A., 1962, 48, 617.

105. A.C. Altamura, R. Whelpton, and S.H. Curry, Biopharm. Drug Dispos., 1979, 1, 65.

106. F.J. Rowell, S.M. Hui, A.F. Fairbairn, and D. Eccleston, Brit. J. Clin. Pharmacol., 1980, 9, 432.

107. S.G. Dahl, Clin. Pharmacol. Ther., 1976, 19, 435.

108. S.G. Dahl, R.E. Strangjord, and S. Sigfusson, Eur. J. Clin. Pharmacol., 1977, 11, 305.

109. G.M. Simpson, R. Lament, T.B. Cooper, J.H. Lee, and R.B. Bruce, J. Clin. Pharmacol., 1973, 13, 288.

110. S. Eiduson and E. Geller, Biochem. Pharmacol., 1963, 12, 1429.

111. K. Zehnder, F. Kalberer, W. Kreis, and J. Rutschmen, Biochem. Pharmacol., 1962, 11, 535.

112. E.C. Dinovo, R.O. Bost, I. Sunshine, and L.A. Gottschalk, Clin. Chem., 1978, 24, 1828.

113. A. Hupf and H. Eckert, Triangle, 1976, 10, 113.

114. G. Nyberg, R. Axelsson, and E. Mårtensson, Eur. J. Clin. Pharmacol., 1981, 19, 139.

115. G. Nyberg and E. Mårtensson, Arch. Pharmacol., 1982, 319, 189.

116. E. Mårtensson, G. Nyberg, and R. Axelsson, Curr. Ther. Res., 1975, 18, 687.

117. H. Freeman, H. Rivera, M. Oktem, and N. Oktem, Curr. Ther. Res., 1969, 11, 263.

118. H. Haase, M. Bergener, and H. Hasselmeijer, Med. Welt., 1967, 18, 542.

119. N. Petrilowitsch, Int. Pharmaco.-Psychiat., 1968, 1, 230.

120. M.G. Choc and R.G. Lehr, Sandoz, Inc., 1983, Report
      DM-1-11/14/83.

121. M.G. Choc, R.G. Lehr, and R.J. DiSerio, Sandoz, Inc., 1983,
      Report DM-1-7/23/83.

122. R. Axelsson, E. Mårtensson, and C. Alling, Eur. J. Clin.
      Pharmacol., 1982, 23, 359.

123. F.L.S. Tse and J.I. Williams, Sandoz, Inc., 1981, Report
      DM-1-2/22/81.

124. F.L.S. Tse and J.I. Williams, Sandoz, Inc., 1981, Report
      DM-1-2/25/81.

125. R. Axelsson and E. Mårtensson, Curr. Ther. Res., 1976, 19, 242.

126. R. Bergling, T. Mjorndal, L. Oreland, W. Rapp, and S. Wold, J.
      Clin. Pharmacol., 1975, 15, 178.

127. D.C. Hobbs, W.M. Welch, M.J. Short, W.A. Moody, and C.D. van der
      Velde, Clin. Pharmacol. Ther., 1974, 16, 473.

128. G. Bianchetti, E. Zarifian, M.F. Poirier-Littre, P.L. Morselli,
      and P. Deniker, Int. J. Clin. Pharmacol. Ther. Toxicol., 1980,
      18, 324.

129. J.E.H. Stafford, L.S. Jackson, T.J. Forrest, A. Barrow, and
      R.F. Palmer, J. Pharmacol. Methods, 1981, 6, 261.

130. A. Forsman, E. Mårtensson, G. Nyberg, and R. Öhman, Arch.
      Pharmacol., 1974, 286, 113.

131. W.A. Cressman, J.R. Bianchine, V.B. Slotmick, P.C. Johnson, and
      J. Plostmieks, Eur. J. Clin. Pharmacol., 1974, 7, 99.

132. F.J. Rowell, S.M. Hui, A.F. Fairbairn, and D. Eccleston, Brit.
      J. Clin. Pharmacol., 1981, 11, 377.

133. P.J. Lewi, J.J.P. Heykants, F.T.N. Allewijn, J.G.H. Dony,
      P.A.J. Janssen, Arzneim.-Forsch., 1970, 20, 943.

134. J.J.P. Heykants, P.J. Lewi, and P.A.J. Janssen, Arzneim.-
      Forsch., 1970, 20, 1238.

135. P.J. Lewi, J.J.P. Heykants, and P.A.J. Janssen, Arzneim.-
      Forsch., 1970, 20, 1701.

136. W.A. Cressman, J. Plostneiks, and P.C. Johnson, Anesthesiology,
      1973, 38, 363.

137. W.A. Cressman, N.L. Renzi, and A.C. Bartholomay, J. Pharm. Sci.,
      1972, 61, 1170.

138. F.-A. Wiesel, G. Alfredsson, M. Ehrnebo, and G. Sedvall, Eur.
      J. Clin. Pharmacol., 1980, 17, 385.

139. J.M. Plá-Delfina, J. Moreno, J. Duràn, and A. del Pazo, J.
      Pharmacokin. Biopharm., 1975, 3, 115.

140. R.A. Anderson and W. Sneddon, Med. J. Australia, 1972, No. 1,
      585.

141. V.F. Naggar, M.A. Moustafa, S.A. Khalil, and M.M. Motawi, Canad. J. Pharm. Sci., 1972, 7, 112.

142. S.A. Khalil, M.A. Moustafa, V.F. Naggar, and M.M. Motawi, Canad. J. Pharm. Sci., 1972, 7, 109.

143. E.G. Lovering and D.B. Black, J. Pharm. Sci., 1973, 62, 602.

144. M.F. Sylvestri and C.T. Ueda, Int. J. Clin. Pharmacol. Biopharm., 1979, 17, 492.

145. E. Nelson, J.R. Powell, K. Conrad, K. Likes, J. Byers, S. Baker, and D. Perrier, J. Clin. Pharmacol., 1982, 22, 141.

146. C.T. Viswanathan, H.E. Booker, and P.G. Welling, J. Clin. Pharmacol., 1978, 18, 100.

147. B. Jalling, Devel. Med. Child Neurol., 1974, 16, 781.

148. K. Minagawa, H. Miura, K. Chiba, and T. Ishizaki, Pediat. Pharmacol., 1981, 1, 279.

149. A. Brachet-Liermain, F. Goutieres, and J. Aicardi, J. Pediatr., 1975, 87, 624.

150. B. Jalling, Devel. Med. Child Neurol., 1974, 16, 781.

151. P.J. Neuvonen and E. Elonen, Eur. J. Clin. Pharmacol., 1980, 17, 51.

152. B.B. Coldwell, H.L. Trenholm, B.H. Thomas, and S. Charbonneau, J. Pharm. Pharmacol., 1971, 23, 947.

153. S.J. Enna and L.S. Schanker, Amer. J. Physiol., 1972, 223, 1227.

154. S. Kojima, R.B. Smith, and J.T. Doluisio, J. Pharm. Sci., 1971, 60, 1639.

155. G. Heimann and E. Gladtke, Eur. J. Clin. Pharmacol., 1977, 12, 305.

156. M.J. Painter, C. Pippenger, C. Wasterlain, M. Barmada, W. Pitlick, G. Carter, and S. Abern, Neurology, 1981, 31, 1107.

157. Y.J. Lin, S. Awazu, M. Hanano, and H. Nogami, Chem. Pharm. Bull. (Japan), 1973, 21, 2749.

158. C.T. Viswanathan, H.E. Booker, and P.G. Welling, J. Clin. Pharmacol., 1979, 19, 282.

159. W. Pitlick, M. Painter, and C. Pippenger, Clin. Pharmacol. Ther., 1978, 23, 346.

160. L.O. Boréus, B. Jalling, and N. Kallberg, Acta Paediatr. Scand., 1978, 67, 193.

161. L.O. Boréus, B. Jalling, and A. Wallin, J. Pediatr., 1978, 93, 695.

162. L.N. Rossi, L.M. Nino, and N. Principi, Acta Paediatr. Scand., 1979, 68, 431.

163. I.H. Patel, R.H. Levy, and R.E. Cutler, Clin. Pharmacol. Ther., 1980, 27, 515.

164. A.J. Wilensky, P.N. Friel, R.H. Levy, C.P. Comfort, and S.P. Kaluzny, Eur. J. Clin. Pharmacol., 1982, 23, 87.

165. J.T. Doluisio, R.B. Smith, A.H.C. Chun, and L.W. Dittert, J. Pharm. Sci., 1978, 67, 1586.

166. M. Ehrnebo, J. Pharm. Sci., 1974, 63, 1114.

167. P.J. Howard, S.G. Nair, and M.S. Kennedy, Anaesthesia, 1976, 31, 1032.

168. S.G. Nair, J.W. Dundee, R.S.J. Clarke, and P.J. Howard, Anaesthesia, 1976, 31, 1037.

169. R.B. Smith, L.W. Dittert, W.O. Griffen, and J.T. Doluisio, J. Pharmacokin. Biopharm., 1973, 1, 5.

170. J.O. Brånstad, U. Meresaar, and Å. Agren, Acta Pharm. Suecica, 1972, 9, 129.

171. G. Pagnini, R. Di Carlo, F. Di Carlo, and E. Genazzani, Biochem. Pharmacol., 1971, 20, 3247.

172. M. Ehrnebo and I. Odar-Cederlöf, Eur. J. Clin. Pharmacol., 1977, 11, 37.

173. M. Ehrnebo and I. Odar-Cederlöf, Eur. J. Clin. Pharmacol., 1975, 8, 445.

174. M.M. Ghoneim and H. Pandya, Anesthesiology, 1975, 42, 545.

175. M.M. Reidenberg, I. Odar-Cederlöf, C. von Bahr, O. Borgia, and F. Sjöqvist, New Engl. J. Med., 1971, 285, 264.

176. W.L. Marcus and F. Sperling, Toxicol. Appl. Pharmacol., 1970, 17, 286.

177. M.M. Reidenberg, D.T. Lowenthal, W. Briggs, and M. Gasparo, Clin. Pharmacol. Ther., 1976, 20, 67.

178. L.E. Davis, J.D. Baggot, C.A.N. Davis, and T.E. Powers, Amer. J. Vet. Res., 1973, 34, 231.

179. B.H. Thomas, B.B. Coldwell, G. Solomonraj, W. Zeitz, and H.L. Trenholm, Biochem. Pharmacol., 1972, 21, 2605.

180. G.R. Pearson, J.A. Bogan, and J. Sanford, Brit. J. Anaesthesia, 1973, 45, 586.

181. W.F. Green and J.D. Ireson, Arch. Int. Pharmacodyn. Ther., 1972, 196, 112.

182. S. Kojima, Chem. Pharm. Bull. (Japan), 1973, 21, 2432.

183. K. Balasubramaniam, G.E. Mawer, and P.J. Simons, Brit. J. Pharmacol., 1970, 40, 578P.

184. K. Balasubramaniam, S.B. Lucas, G.E. Mawer, and P.J. Simons, Brit. J. Pharmacol., 1970, 39, 564.

185. D. Kadar, T. Inaba, L. Endrenyi, G.E. Johnson, and W. Kalow, Clin. Pharmacol. Ther., 1973, 14, 552.

186. G.H. Draffan, C.T. Dollery, D.S. Davies, B. Krauer, F.M. Williams, R.A. Clare, B.J. Trudinger, M. Darling, H. Serici, and D.F. Hawkins, Clin. Pharmacol. Ther., 1976, 19, 271.

187. L. Endrenyl, T. Inaba, and W. Kalow, Clin. Pharmacol. Ther., 1977, 20, 701.

188. E.R. Garrett, J. Bres, K. Schnelle, and L.L. Rolf, J. Pharmacokin. Biopharm., 1974, 2, 43.

189. T. Inaba and W. Kalow, Clin. Pharmacol. Ther., 1975, 18, 558.

190. D.D. Breimer, C. Honhoff, W. Zilly, E. Richter, and J.M. van Rossum, J. Pharmacokin. Biopharm., 1975, 3, 1.

191. D.D. Breimer and J.M. van Rossum, Eur. J. Pharmacol., 1974, 26, 321.

192. H.U. Aeschbacher, J. Atkinson, and B. Domahidy, J. Pharmacol. Exp. Ther., 1975, 192, 635.

193. D.D. Breimer and J.M. van Rossum, J. Pharm. Pharmacol., 1973, 25, 762.

194. J.S. McCarthy and R.E. Stitzel, J. Pharmacol. Exp. Ther., 1971, 176, 772.

195. D.D. Breimer, W. Zilly, and E. Richter, Clin. Pharmacol. Ther., 1975, 18, 433.

196. W. Zilly, D.D. Breimer, and E. Richter, Clin Pharmacol. Ther., 1978, 23, 525.

197. S. Mallov and T.J. Baesl, Biochem. Pharmacol., 1972, 21, 1667.

198. J.M. Clifford, J.H. Cookson, and P.E. Wickham, Clin. Pharmacol. Ther., 1974, 16, 376.

199. E.O. Bixler, A. Kales, T.L. Tan, and J.D. Kales, Curr. Ther. Res., 1973, 15, 13.

200. B.O. Hartman and R.E. McKenzie, Aerospace Med., 1966, 37, 1121.

201. R.O. Muhlhauser, W.D. Watkins, R.C. Murphy, and C.A. Chidsey, Drug Metab. Dispos., 1974, 2, 513.

202. S.M. Somani, R.H. McDonald, Jr., and D.P. Schumacher, Arch. Int. Pharmacodyn. Ther., 1975, 215, 301.

203. T.P. Faulkner, J.W. McGinity, J.H. Hayden, D.A. Olson, and E.G. Comstock, J. Clin. Pharmacol., 1979, 19, 605.

204. D.D. Breimer and M.A.C.M. Winten, Eur. J. Clin. Pharmacol., 1976, 9, 443.

205. J.N.T. Gilbert, T. Natunen, J.W. Powell, and L. Saunders, J. Pharm. Pharmacol., 1974, 26, 16P.

206. D.D. Breimer, Eur. J. Clin. Pharmacol., 1976, 10, 263.

207. L.J. Saidman and E.I. Eger, Clin. Pharmacol. Ther., 1973, 14, 12.

208. M. Finster, H.O. Morishima, L.C. Mark, J.M. Perel, P.G. Dayton, and L.S. James, Anesthesiology, 1972, 36, 155.

209. B. Krauer, G.H. Draffan, F.M. Williams, R.A. Clare, C.T. Dollery, and D.F. Hawkins, Clin. Pharmacol. Ther., 1973, 14, 442.

210. J.H. Christensen, F. Andreasen, and J.A. Jansen, Anesthesia, 1982, 37, 398.

211. M.M. Ghoneim, H.B. Pandya, S.E. Kelley, L.J. Fischer, R.J. Corry, Anesthesiology, 1976, 45, 635.

212. R. Dugal, G. Cailé, J. Brodeur, S. Cooper, and J.-G. Besner, L' Union Medicale du Canada, 1973, 102, 1744.

213. K. Korttila and M. Linnoila, Brit. J. Anaesthesia, 1975, 47, 857.

214. H.R. Ochs, H. Otten, D.J. Greenblatt, and H.J. Dengler, Digest Dis. Sci., 1982, 27, 225.

215. F. Moolenaar, S. Bakker, J. Visser, and T. Huizinga, Int. J. Pharmaceut., 1980, 5, 127.

216. S. Dhillon, J. Oxley, and A. Richens, Brit. J. Clin. Pharmacol., 1982, 13, 427.

217. J.H. Gustafson, L. Weissman, R.E. Weinfeld, A.A. Holazo, K.-C. Khoo, and S.A. Kaplan, J. Pharmacokin. Biopharm., 1981, 9, 679.

218. J.A.S. Gamble, J.H. Gaston, S.G. Nair, and J.W. Dundee, Brit. J. Anaesthesia, 1976, 48, 1181.

219. D.W. Sturdee, Brit. J. Anaesthesia, 1976, 48, 1091.

220. D.J. Greenblatt, R.I. Shader, D.R. Weinberger, M.D. Allen, and D.S. MacLaughlin, Psychopharmacology, 1978, 57, 199.

221. U. Laisi, M. Linnoila, T. Seppala, J.-J. Himberg, and M.J. Mattila, Eur. J. Clin. Pharmacol., 1979, 16, 263.

222. D.J. Greenblatt, M.D. Allen, D.S. MacLaughlin, J.S. Harmatz, and R.I. Shader, Clin. Pharmacol. Ther., 1978, 24, 600.

223. A. Langslet, A. Meberg, J.E. Bredesen, and P.K.M. Lunde, Acta Paediatr. Scand., 1978, 67, 699.

224. S.A. Kaplan, M.L. Jack, K. Alexander, and R.E. Weinfeld, J. Pharm. Sci., 1973, 62, 1789.

225. F.B. Eatman, W.A. Colburn, H.G. Boxenbaum, H.N. Posmanter, R.E. Weinfeld, R. Ronfeld, L. Weissman, J.D. Moore, M. Gibaldi, and S.A. Kaplan, J. Pharmacokin. Biopharm., 1977, 5, 482.

226. J.A.S. Gamble, J.W. Dundee and R.C. Gray, Brit. J. Anaesthesia, 1976, 48, 1087.

227. U. Klotz, K.H. Antonin, and P.R. Bieck, Eur. J. Clin. Pharmacol., 1976, 10, 121.

228. J.I. Kanto, V. Lehtinen, and J. Salminen, Psychopharmacologia, 1974, 36, 123.

229. R. Sellman, J. Kanto, E. Raijola, and A. Pekkarinen, Acta Pharmacol. Toxicol., 1975, 37, 345.

230. K. Korttila, M.J. Mattila, and M. Linnoila, Acta Pharmacol. Toxicol., 1975, 36, 90.

231. E. van der Kleijn, J.M. van Rossum, E.T.J.M. Muskens and N.V.M. Rijntjes, Acta Pharmacol. Toxicol., 1971, 29, Suppl. 3, 109.

232. J. Kanto, L. Kanzas, and T. Siirtola, Acta Pharmacol. Toxicol.,
      1975, 36, 328.

233. J. Hendel, Acta Pharmacol. Toxicol., 1975, 37, 17.

234. L.W. Whitehouse, C.J. Paul, B.B. Coldwell, and B.H. Thomas,
      Res. Comm. Chem. Path. Pharmacol., 1975, 12, 221.

235. R. Sellman, A. Pekkarinen, L. Kangas, and E. Raijola, Acta
      Pharmacol. Toxicol., 1975, 36, 25.

236. R. Sellman, J. Kanto, F. Raijola, and A. Pekkarinen, Acta
      Pharmacol. Toxicol., 1975, 36, 33.

237. E.S. Baird and D.M. Hailey, J. Anaesthesiol., 1972, 44, 803.

238. M. Linnoila, K. Korttila, and M.J. Mattila, Acta Pharmacol.
      Toxicol., 1975, 36, 181.

239. D.M. Rutherford, A. Okoko, and P.J. Tyrer, Brit. J. Clin.
      Pharmacol., 1978, 6, 69.

240. D.J. Greenblatt, J.S. Harmatz, and R.I. Shader, Int. J. Clin.
      Pharmacol., 1978, 16, 177.

241. M.M. Reidenberg, M. Levy, H. Warner, C.B. Coutinho, M.A.
      Schwartz, G. Yu, and J. Cheripko, Clin. Pharmacol. Ther., 1978,
      23, 371.

242. S.M. MacLeod, H.G. Giles, B. Bengert, F.F. Liu, and E.M.
      Sellers, J. Clin. Pharmacol., 1979, 19, 15.

243. U. Klotz and C. Lücke, Brit. J. Clin. Pharmacol., 1978, 5, 349.

244. M.D. Allen and D.J. Greenblatt, J. Clin. Pharmacol., 1981, 21,
      219.

245. G.J. DiGregorio, A.J. Piraino, and E. Ruch, Clin. Pharmacol.
      Ther., 1978, 24, 720.

246. H.G. Giles, D.H. Zilm, R.C. Frecker, S.M. Macleod, and E.M.
      Sellers, Brit. J. Clin. Pharmacol., 1977, 4, 711.

247. E. Tsutsumi, T. Inaba, W.A. Mahon, and W. Kalow, Biochem.
      Pharmacol., 1975, 24, 1361.

248. J. Thiessen, E.M. Sellers, P. Denbeigh, and L. Dolman, J. Clin.
      Pharmacol., 1976, 16, 345.

249. C.A. Naranjo, E.M. Sellers, H.G. Giles, and J.G. Abel, Brit. J.
      Clin. Pharmacol., 1980, 9, 265.

250. P.A. Routledge, W.W. Stargel, B.B. Kitchell, A. Barchowsky, and
      D.G. Shand, Brit. J. Clin. Pharmacol., 1981, 11, 245.

251. P.V. Desmond, R.K. Roberts, A.J.J. Wood, G.D. Dunn, G.R.
      Wilkinson, and S. Schenker, Brit. J. Clin. Pharmacol., 1980, 9,
      171.

252. H.R. Ochs, D.J. Greenblatt, H.J. Kaschell, U. Klehr, M. Divoll,
      and D.R. Abernethy, Brit. J. Clin. Pharmacol., 1981, 12, 829.

253. A. Kober, I. Sjöholm, O. Borga, and I. Odar-Cederlöf, Biochem.
      Pharmacol., 1979, 28, 1037.

254. S.H. Grossman, D. Davis, B.B. Kitchell, D.G. Shand, and P.A. Routledge, Clin. Pharmacol. Ther., 1982, **31**, 350.

255. O.M. Bakke and K. Haram, Clin. Pharmacokin., 1982, **7**, 353.

256. J.A.S. Gamble, J. Moore, H. Lamki, and P.J. Howard, Brit. J. Obst. Gynaecol., 1977, **84**, 588.

257. R. Erkkola, L. Kangas, and A. Pekkarinen, Acta Obstet. Gynecol. Scand., 1973, **52**, 167.

258. M. Mandelli, P.L. Morselli, S. Nordio, G. Pardi, N. Principi, F. Sereni, and G. Tognoni, Clin. Pharmacol. Ther., 1975, **17**, 564.

259. J. Kanto, R. Erkkola, and R. Sellman, Ann. Clin. Res., 1973, **5**, 375.

260. M. Guerre-Millo, E. Rey, J.-C. Challier, J.-M. Turquais, Ph. d'Athis, and G. Olive, Eur. J. Clin. Pharmacol., 1979, **15**, 171.

261. K. Haram, O.M. Bakke, K.H. Johannessen, and T. Lund, Clin. Pharmacol. Ther., 1978, **24**, 590.

262. G.T. McCarthy, B. O'Connell, and A.E. Robinson, J. Obstet. Gynaecol. Brit. Commonwealth, 1973, **80**, 349.

263. M.J. Patrick, W.J. Tilstone, and P. Reavey, Lancet, 1972, **i**, 542.

264. R. Erkkola and J. Kanto, Lancet, 1972, **i**, 1235.

265. R. Brandt, Arzneim.-Forsch., 1976, **26**, 454.

266. R.G. Moore and W.G. McBride, Eur. J. Clin. Pharmacol., 1978, **13**, 275.

267. M. Mandelli, G. Tognoni, and S. Garattini, Clin. Pharmacokin., 1978, **3**, 72.

268. H. Dasberg, Pharmako-psychiatrie Neuro-Psychopharmakol., 1975, **8**, 162.

269. H.M. Dasberg, E. van der Kleijn, P.J.R. Guelen, and H.M. van Praag, Clin. Pharmacol. Ther., 1974, **15**, 473.

270. G.N. Bianchi, M.R. Fennessy, J. Phillips, and B.S. Everitt, Psychopharmacologia, 1974, **35**, 113.

271. L. Hilestad, T. Hansen, H. Melsom, and A. Drivenes, Clin. Pharmacol. Ther., 1974, **16**, 479.

272. L. Hillestad, T. Hansen, and H. Melsom, Clin. Pharmacol. Ther., 1974, **16**, 485.

273. D.J. Greenblatt and J. Koch-Weser, Eur. J. Clin. Pharmacol., 1974, **7**, 259.

274. A. Bliding, Eur. J. Clin. Pharmacol., 1974, **7**, 201.

275. H.E. Booker and G.G. Celesia, Arch. Neurol., 1973, **29**, 191.

276. H.G. Giles, E.M. Sellers, C.A. Naranjo, R.C. Frecker, and D.J. Greenblatt, Eur. J. Clin. Pharmacol., 1981, **20**, 207.

277. D.J. Greenblatt, M.D. Allen, J.S. Harmatz, and R.I. Shader, Clin. Pharmacol. Ther., 1980, 27, 301.

278. U. Klotz and I. Reimann, Eur. J. Clin. Pharmacol., 1981, 21, 161.

279. D.R. Abernethy and D.J. Greenblatt, Clin. Pharmacol. Ther., 1981, 29, 757.

280. U. Klotz and I. Reimann, Clin. Pharmacol. Ther., 1981, 30, 513.

281. U. Klotz and I. Reimann, New Engl. J. Med., 1980, 302, 1012.

282. E.M. Sellers, C.A. Naranjo, H.G. Giles, R.C. Frecker, and M. Beeching, Clin. Pharmacol. Ther., 1980, 28, 638.

283. S. Dhillon and A. Richens, Brit. J. Clin. Pharmacol., 1981, 12, 841.

284. W. Löscher and H.-H. Frey, Arch. Int. Pharmacodyn. Ther., 1981, 254, 180.

285. P.B. Andrasen, J. Hendel, G. Greisen, and E.F. Hvidberg, Eur. J. Clin. Pharmacol., 1976, 10, 115.

286. U. Klotz, K.H. Antonin, H. Brugel, and P.R. Bieck, Clin. Pharmacol. Ther., 1976, 21, 430.

287. P.L. Morselli, M. Mandelli, G. Tognoni, N. Principi, G. Pardi, and F. Sereni, in 'Drug Interactions', ed. P.L. Morselli, S. Garattini, and S.N. Cohen, Raven Press, New York, 1974, 259.

288. H. Fukazawa, H. Iwase, H. Ichishita, T. Takizawa, and H. Shimizu, Drug Metab. Dispos., 1975, 3, 235.

289. W.A. Mahon, T. Inaba, T. Umeda, E. Tsutsumi, and R. Stone, Clin. Pharmacol. Ther., 1976, 19, 443.

290. K. Kortilla, M.J. Mattila, and M. Linnoila, Brit. J. Anaesthesia, 1976, 48, 333.

291. D.J. Greenblatt, R.I. Shader, and J. Koch-Weser, Dis. Nervous System, 1975, 36, 6.

292. J. Vessman, G. Freij, and S. Strømberg, Acta Pharm. Suecica, 1972, 9, 447.

293. J.A. Knowles and H.W. Ruelius, Arzneim.-Forsch., 1972, 22, 687.

294. E. Mussini, F. Marcucci, R. Fanelli, A. Guaitani, and S. Garattini, Biochem. Pharmacol., 1972, 21, 127.

295. D.J. Greenblatt, Clin. Pharmacokin., 1981, 6, 89.

296. T.G. Murray, S.T. Chiang, H.H. Koepke, and B.R. Walker, Clin. Pharmacol. Ther., 1981, 30, 805.

297. U. Busch, M. Molzahn, G. Bozler, and F.W. Koss, Arzneim.-Forsch., 1981, 31, 1507.

298. H.J. Shull, G.R. Wilkinson, R. Johnson, and S. Schenker, Ann. Intern. Med., 1976, 84, 420.

299. G. Tomson, N.-O. Lunell, A. Sundwall, and A. Rane, Clin. Pharmacol. Ther., 1979, 25, 74.

300. D.J. Greenblatt, R.I. Shader, K. Franke, D.S. MacLaughlin, J.S.
     Harmatz, M.D. Allen, A. Werner, and E. Woo, J. Pharm. Sci.,
     1979, 68, 57.

301. D.J. Greenblatt, W.H. Comer, H.W. Elliott, R.1. Shader, J.A.
     Knowles, and H.W. Ruelius, J. Clin. Pharmacol., 1977, 17, 490.

302. D.J. Greenblatt, R.T. Schillings, A.A. Kyriakopoulos, R.I.
     Shader, S.F. Sisenwine, J.A. Knowles, and H.W. Ruelius, Clin.
     Pharmacol. Ther., 1976, 20, 329.

303. D.J. Greenblatt, J.A. Knowles, W.H. Comer, R.I. Shader, J.S.
     Harmatz, and H.W. Ruelius, J. Clin. Pharmacol., 1977, 17, 495.

304. L. Aaltonen, J. Kanto, and M. Salo, Acta Pharmacol. Toxicol.,
     1980, 46,]56.

305. H.R. Ochs, J. Busse, D.J. Greenblatt, and M.D. Allen, Brit. J.
     Clin. Pharmacol., 1980, 10, 405.

306. D.J. Greenblatt, M.D. Allen, D.S. MacLaughlin, D.H. Huffman,
     J.S. Harmatz, and R.I. Shader, J. Pharmacokin. Biopharm., 1979,
     7, 159.

307. D.J. Greenblatt, M.D. Allen, A. Locniskar, J.S. Harmatz, and
     R.I. Shader, Clin. Pharmacol. Ther., 1979, 26, 103.

308. J.W. Kraus, P.V. Desmond, J.P. Marshall, R.F. Johnson, S.
     Schenker, and G.R. Wilkinson, Clin. Pharmacol. Ther., 1978, 24,
     411.

309. R. Verbeeck, T.B. Tjandramaga, R. Verberckmoes, and P.J. De
     Schepper, Brit. J. Clin. Pharmacol., 1976, 3, 1033.

310. R.K. Verbeeck, T.B. Tjandramaga, P.J. De Schepper, and R.
     Verberckmoes, Brit. J. Clin. Pharmacol., 1981, 12, 749.

311. J. Rieder, Arzneim.-Forsch., 1973, 23, 212.

312. L. Kangas and D.D. Breimer, Clin. Pharmacokin., 1981, 6, 346.

313. L. Kangas, H. Allonen, R. Lammintausta, M. Salonen, and A.
     Pekkarinen, Acta Pharmacol. Toxicol., 1979, 45, 20.

314. D.D. Breimer, H. Bracht, and A.G. De Boer, Brit. J. Clin.
     Pharmacol., 1977, 4, 709.

315. L. Kangas, E. Iisalo, J. Kanto, V. Lehtinen, S. Pynnonen, I.
     Ruikka, J. Salminen, M. Silanpaa, and E. Syvalahti, Eur. J.
     Clin. Pharmacol., 1979, 15, 163.

316. L. Kangas, J. Kanto, and R. Erkkola, Eur. J. Clin. Pharmacol.,
     1977, 12, 355.

317. L. Kangas, J. Kanto, and A. Pakkanen, Int. J. Clin. Pharmacol.
     Ther. Toxicol., 1982, 20, 585.

318. J. Kanto, L. Kangas, L. Aaltonen, and H. Hilke, Int. J. Clin.
     Pharmacol. Ther. Toxicol., 1981, 19, 400.

319. E. Wickstrøm, R. Amrein, P. Haefelfinger, and D. Hartmann, Eur.
     J. Clin. Pharmacol., 1980, 17, 189.

320. M.A. Schwartz and E. Postma, J. Pharm. Sci., 1970, 59, 1800.

321. S.A. Kaplan, J.A.F. de Silva, M.L. Jack, K. Alexander, N. Strojny, R.E. Weinfeld, C.V. Puglisi, and L. Weissman, J. Pharm. Sci., 1973, 62, 1932.

322. D.J. Greenblatt, M. Divoll, J.S. Harmatz, D.S. MacLaughlin, and R.I. Shader, Clin. Pharmacol. Ther., 1981, 30, 475.

323. M.D. Allen, D.J. Greenblatt, J.S. Harmatz, and R.I. Shader, J. Clin. Pharmacol., 1979, 19, 445.

324. M.T. Smith, I.E.J. Evans, M.J. Eadie, and J.H. Tyrer, Eur. J. Clin. Pharmacol., 1979, 16, 141.

325. R.R. Brodie, L.F. Chasseaud, and T. Taylor, Biopharm. Drug Dispos., 1981, 2, 59.

326. M.D. Allen, D.J. Greenblatt, J.S. Harmatz, and R.I. Shader, Clin. Pharmacol. Ther., 1980, 28, 196.

327. E.S. Vesell, G.T. Passananti, J.-P. Viau, J.E. Epps, and F.J. Di Carlo, Pharmacology, 1972, 7, 197.

328. L.M. Fuccella, G. Tosolini, E. Moro, and V. Tamassia, Int. J. Clin. Pharmacol., 1972, 6, 303.

329. L.M. Fucella, Brit. J. Clin. Pharmacol., 1979, 8, 31S.

330. P. Bittencourt, A. Richens, P.A. Toseland, J.F.C. Wicks, and A.N. Latham, Brit. J. Clin. Pharmacol., 1979, 8, 37S.

331. L.M. Fuccella, G. Bolcioni, V. Tamassia, L. Ferrario, and G. Tognoni, Eur. J. Clin. Pharmacol., 1977, 12, 383.

332. H.J. Schwarz, Brit. J. Clin. Pharmacol., 1979, 8, 23S.

333. S.A.M. Salem, C.D. Kinney, and D.G. McDevitt, Brit. J. Pharmacol., 1981, 73, 412P.

334. H.R. Ochs, D.J. Greenblatt, and H. Heuer, J. Clin. Pharmacol., 1984, 24, 58.

335. M. Divoll, D.J. Greenblatt, J.S. Harmatz, and R.I. Shader, J. Pharm. Sci., 1981, 70, 1104.

336. D.J. Greenblatt, R.I. Shader, M. Divoll, and J.S. Harmatz, Brit. J. Clin. Pharmacol., 1981, 11, 11S.

337. D.J. Hoffman and A.H.C. Chun, J. Pharm. Sci., 1975, 64, 1668.

338. P.J. Carrigan, G.C. Chao, W.M. Barker, D.J. Hoffman, and A.H.C. Chun, J. Clin. Pharmacol., 1977, 17, 18.

339. H.R. Ochs, E. Steinhaus, A. Locniskar, M. Knuchel, and D.J. Greenblatt, Klin. Wochenschr., 1982, 60, 411.

340. R.I. Shader, A. Georgotas, D.J. Greenblatt, J.S. Harmatz, and M.D. Allen, Clin. Pharmacol. Ther., 1978, 24, 308.

341. C.W. Abruzzo, T. Macasieb, R. Weinfeld, J.A. Rider, and S.A. Kaplan, J. Pharmacokin. Biopharm., 1977, 5, 377.

342. C.W. Abruzzo, M.A. Brooks, S. Cotler, and S.A. Kaplan, J. Pharmacokin. Biopharm., 1976, 4, 29.

343. A.H.C. Chun, P.J. Carrigan, D.J. Hoffman, R.P. Kershner, and J.D. Stuart, Clin. Pharmacol. Ther., 1977, 22, 329.

344. R.I. Shader, D.A. Ciraulo, D.J. Greenblatt, and J.S. Harmatz, Clin. Pharmacol. Ther., 1982, 31, 180.

345. H.R. Ochs, D.J. Greenblatt, M.D. Allen, J.S. Harmatz, R.I. Shader, and G. Bodem, Clin. Pharmacol. Ther., 1979, 26, 449.

346. D.R. Abernethy, D.J. Greenblatt, M. Divoll, and R.I. Shader, J. Pharm. Sci., 1982, 71, 942.

347. T.R. Norman, A. Fulton, G.D. Burrows, and K.P. Maguire, Eur. J. Clin. Pharmacol., 1981, 21, 229.

348. E. Rey, Ph. d'Athis, P. Giraux, D. de Lauture, J.M. Turquais, J. Chavinie, and G. Olive, Eur. J. Clin. Pharmacol., 1979, 15, 175.

349. E. Rey, P. Giraux, Ph. d'Athis, J.M. Turquais, J. Chavinie, and G. Olive, Eur. J. Clin. Pharmacol., 1979, 15, 181.

350. L.A. Gottschalk, R. Biener, and E.C. Dinovo, Res. Comm. Chem. Path. Pharmacol., 1974, 8, 697.

351. D.J. Greenblatt, R.I. Shader, and J. Koch-Weser, New Engl. J. Med., 1974, 291, 1116.

352. P.J. Perry, D.C. Wilding, R.C. Fowler, C.D. Hepler, and J.F. Caputo, Clin. Pharmacol. Ther., 1978, 23, 535.

353. D.J. Greenblatt, R.I. Shader, S.M. MacLeod, E.M. Sellers, K. Franke, and H.G. Giles, Eur. J. Clin. Pharmacol., 1978, 13, 267.

354. D.J. Greenblatt, R.I. Shader, J.S. Harmatz, K. Franke, and J. Koch-Weser, Amer. J. Psychiat., 1977, 134, 559.

355. R.I. Shader, A. DiMascio, and J.S. Harmatz, Amer. J. Psychiat., 1972, 128, 1576.

356. D.J. Greenblatt, R.I. Shader, and J. Koch-Weser, Amer. J. Psychiat., 1974, 131, 1395.

357. E.M. Sellers, D.J. Greenblatt, D.H. Zilm, and N. Degani, Brit. J. Clin. Pharmacol., 1978, 6, 370.

358. D.J. Greenblatt R.I. Shader, S.M. MacLeod, and E.M. Sellers, Clin. Pharamcokin., 1978, 3, 381.

359. H.G. Boxenbaum, K.A. Geitner, M.L. Jack, W.R. Dixon, H.E. Spiegel, J. Symington, R. Christian, J.D. Moore, L. Weissman, and S.A. Kaplan, J. Pharmacokin. Biopharm., 1977, 5, 3.

360. D.J. Greenblatt, R.I. Shader, K. Franke, D.S. MacLaughlin, B.J. Ransil, ad J. Koch-Weser, Clin. Pharmacol. Ther., 1977, 22, 893.

361. H.G. Boxenbaum, K.A. Geitner, M.L. Jack, W.R. Dixon, and S.A. Kaplan, J. Pharmacokin. Biopharm., 1977, 5, 25.

362. D.J. Greenblatt, J.S. Harmatz, D.R. Stanski, R.I. Shader, K. Franke, and J. Koch-Weser, Psychopharmacology, 1977, 54, 277.

363. S.A. Kaplan, M. Lewis, M.A. Schwartz, E. Postma, S. Cotler, C.W. Abruzzo, T.L. Lee, and R.E. Weinfeld, J. Pharm. Sci., 1970, 59, 1569.

364. M.A. Schwartz, E. Postma, and S.J. Kolis, J. Pharm. Sci., 1971, 60, 438.

365. M.A. Schwartz, E. Postma, and Z. Gaut, J. Pharm. Sci., 1971, 60, 1500.

366. R.K. Roberts, P.V. Desmond, G.R. Wilkinson, and S. Schenker, Clin. Pharmacol. Ther., 1979, 25, 826.

367. B. Whiting, J.R, Lawrence, G.G. Skellern, and J. Meier, Brit. J. Clin. Pharmacol., 1979, 7, 95.

368. A.M. Hoyumpa, Southern Med. J., 1978, 71, 23.

369. P.V. Desmond, R.V. Patwardhan, S. Schenker, and A.M. Hoyumpa, Eur. J. Clin. Pharmacol., 1980, 18, 275.

370. D.D. Morgan, J.D. Robinson, and C.L. Mendenhall, Eur. J. Clin. Pharmacol., 1981, 19, 279.

371. J.D. Christensen, Acta Pharmacol. Toxicol., 1973, 33, 262.

372. G.M. Stirrat, P.T. Edington, and D.J. Berry, Brit. Med. J., 1974, ii, 729.

373. J.J. Vallner, J.A. Kotzan, J.T. Stewart, I.L. Honigberg, T.E. Needham, and W.J. Brown, J. Clin. Pharmacol., 1980, 20, 444.

374. M. Divoll, D.J. Greenblatt, D.A. Ciraulo, S.K. Puri, I. Ho, and R.I. Shader, J. Clin. Pharmacol., 1982, 22, 69.

375. S.A Kaplan, M.L. Jack, R.E. Weinfeld, W. Glover, L. Weissman, and S. Cotler, J. Pharmacokin. Biopharm., 1976, 4, 1.

376. I. Bekersky, A.C. Maggio, V. Mattaliano, Jr., H.G. Boxenbaum, D.E. Maynard, P.D. Cohn, and S.A. Kaplan, J. Pharmacokin. Biopharm., 1977, 5, 508.

377. F.S. Eberts, Jr., Y. Philopoulos, L.M. Reineke, and R.W. Vliek, Clin. Pharmacol. Ther., 1981, 29, 81.

378. P.J. Pentikäinen, P.J. Neuvonen, and K.-G. Jostell, Eur. J. Clin. Pharmacol., 1980, 17, 275.

379. D.D. Breimer, Brit. J. Anaesthesia, 1976, 48, 643.

380. R.L. Nation, B. Learoyd, J. Barber, and E.J. Triggs, Eur. J. Clin. Pharmacol., 1976, 10, 407.

381. D.D. Breimer, Clin. Pharmacokin., 1977, 2, 93.

382. K. Chang and W.L. Chiou, Res. Comm. Chem. Path. Pharmacol., 1976, 13, 357.

383. M.E. Williams, M.J. Kendall, M. Mitchard, S.S. Davis, and R. Poxon, Brit. J. Clin. Pharmacol., 1974, 1, 99.

384. C. White, E. Doyle, L.F. Chasseaud, and T. Taylor, Eur. J. Clin. Pharmacol., 1976, 10, 343.

385. G. Alván, Ö. Ericsson, S. Levander, and J.-E. Lindgren, Eur. J. Clin. Pharmacol., 1974, 7, 449.

386. R.K. Nayak, R.D. Smyth, J.H. Chamberlain, A. Polk, A.F. DeLong, T. Herczeg, P.B. Cnemburkar, R.S. Joslin, and N.H. Reavey-Cantwell, J. Pharmacokin. Biopharm., 1974, 2, 107.

387. J.M. Christensen and S. Holfort, J. Pharm. Pharmacol., 1975, 27, 538.

388. L.M. Cummins, Y.C. Martin, and E.E. Scherfling, J. Pharm. Sci.,
      1971, 60, 261.

389. M. Simpson and E.L. Parrott, J. Pharm. Sci., 1980, 69, 227.

390. E.M. Sellers, M. Lang, J. Koch-Weser, E. LeBlanc, and H. Kalant,
      Clin. Pharmacol. Ther., 1972, 13, 37.

391. E.M. Sellers, G. Carr, J.G. Bernstein, S. Sellers, and J. Koch-
      Weser, Clin. Pharmacol. Ther., 1972, 13, 50.

392. P.K. Gessner, Arch. Int. Pharmacodyn. Ther., 1973, 202, 392.

393. E.R. Garrett and H. J. Lambert, J. Pharm. Sci., 1973, 62, 550.

394. H. Meinardi, E. van der Kleijn, J.W.A. Meijer, and H. van Rees,
      Epilepsia, 1975, 16, 353.

395. A.J. Glazko, Epilepsia, 1975, 16, 367

396. H. Kutt, Clin. Pharmacol. Ther., 1974, 16, 243.

397. E.F. Hvidberg and M. Dam, Clin. Pharmacokin., 1976, 1, 161.

398. H. Kutt, Epilepsia, 1975, 16, 393

399. H. Kutt and J.K. Penry, Arch. Neurol., 1974, 31, 283.

400. H. Kutt, Pediatrics, 1974, 53, 557.

401. A. Windorfer, R. Gadeke, and M. Sauer, Z. Kinderheilkunde, 1975,
      119, 15.

402. A. Windorfer, R. Gadeke, and M. Sauer, Z. Kinderheilkunde, 1975,
      119, 25.

403. M.J. Eadie, Clin. Pharmacokin., 1976, 1, 52.

404. S. Livingston, W. Berman, and L.L. Pauli, J. Amer. Med. Assoc.,
      1975, 232, 60.

405. P.J. Neuvonen, Clin. Pharmacokin., 1979, 4, 91.

406. J.I. Manson, S.M. Beal, A. Magarey, A.C. Pollard, W.J. O'Reilly,
      and L.N. Sansom, Med. J. Austral., 1975, 2, 590.

407. S.I. Borst and C.H. Lockwood, Int. J. Clin. Pharmacol.
      Biopharm., 1975, 12, 309.

408. A.P. Melikian, A.B. Straughn, G.W.A. Slywka, P.L. Whyatt, and
      M.C. Meyer, J. Pharmacokin. Biopharm., 1977, 5, 133.

409. P.J. Neuvonen, P.J. Pentikainen, and S.M. Elfving, Int. J.
      Clin. Pharmacol., 1977, 15, 84.

410. L.N. Sansom, W.J. O'Reilly, C.W. Wiseman, L.M. Stern, and J.
      Derham, Med. J. Austral., 1975, 2, 593.

411. B. Rambeck, H.E. Boenigk, and E. Stenzel, Eur. J. Clin.
      Pharmacol., 1977, 12, 285.

412. L. Lund, Eur. J. Clin. Pharmacol., 1974, 7, 119.

413. R. Gugler, C.V. Manion, and D.L. Azarnoff, Clin. Pharmacol.
      Ther., 1976, 19, 135.

414. K.S. Albert, E. Sakmar, M.R. Hallmark, D.J. Weidler, and J.G. Wagner, Clin. Pharmacol. Ther., 1974, 16, 727.

415. T.C. Smith and A. Kinkel, Clin. Pharmacol. Ther., 1977, 20, 738.

416. E. Zylber-Katz, L. Granit, and M. Levy, Isr. J. Med. Sci., 1978, 14, 489.

417. S. Sved, R.D. Hossie, I.J. McGilveray, N. Beaudoin, and R. Brein, Canad. J. Pharm. Sci., 1979, 14, 67.

418. S.S. Chen, J. Allen, J. Oxley, and A. Richens, Epilepsia, 1982, 23, 149.

419. D. Jung, J.R. Powell, P. Walson, and D. Perrier, Clin. Pharmacol. Ther., 1980, 28, 479.

420. V.K. Kulshresthsa, M. Thomas, J. Wadsworth, and A. Richens, Brit. J. Clin. Pharmacol., 1978, 6, 177.

421. A. Melander, G. Brante, O. Johansson, T. Lindberg, and E. Wahlin-Boll, Eur. J. Clin. Pharmacol., 1979, 15, 269.

422. H.B. Kostenbauder, R.P. Rapp, J.P. McGovern, T.S. Foster, D.G. Perrier, H.M. Blacker, W.C. Hulon, and A.W. Kinkel, Clin. Pharmacol. Ther., 1975, 18, 449.

423. M.J. Painter, C. Pippenger, H. MacDonald, and W. Pitlick, J. Pediatr., 1978, 92, 315.

424. J.C. McElnay, P.F. D'Arcy, and O. Throne, Int. J. Pharmaceut., 1980, 7, 83.

425. H. Van Rees and E.L. Noach, Arch. Int. Pharmacodyn. Ther., 1973, 206, 76.

426. J.D. Robinson, B.A. Morris, G.W. Aherne, and V. Marks, Brit. J. Clin. Pharmacol., 1975, 2, 345.

427. L. Lund, G. Alván, A. Berlin, and B. Alexanderson, Eur. J. Clin. Pharmacol., 1974, 7, 81.

428. W.J. Jusko, J.R. Koup, and G. Alván, J. Pharmacokin. Biopharm., 1976, 4, 327.

429. E. Martin, T.N. Tozer, L.B. Sheiner, and S. Riegelman, J. Pharmacokin. Biopharm., 1977, 5, 579.

430. R.G. Feldman and C.E. Pippenger, J. Clin. Pharmacol., 1976, 16, 51.

431. D.G. Lambie, R.N. Nanda, R.H. Johnson, and J.A. Shakir, Lancet, 1976, ii, 386.

432. G.W. Houghton, A. Richens, P.A. Toseland, S. Davidson, and M.A. Falconer, Eur. J. Clin. Pharmacol., 1975, 9, 73.

433. A.S. Troupin and P. Friel, Epilepsia, 1975, 16, 223.

434. F. Vajda, F.M. Williams, S. Davidson, M.A. Falconer, and A. Breckenridge, Clin. Pharmacol. Ther., 1974, 15, 597.

435. D.G. Ferry, D. Ferry, and E.G. McQueen, New Zealand Med. J., 1975, 81, 3.

436. E.H. Reynolds, Proc. Roy. Soc. Med., 1975, 68, 102.

437. E.H. Reynolds and R.D. .Travers, Brit. J. Psychiat., 1974, 124, 440.

438. L. Lund, Arch. Neurol., 1974, 31, 289.

439. G.R. Matzke, J.C. Cloyd, and R.J. Sawchuk, J. Clin. Pharmacol., 1981, 21, 92.

440. T.M. Ludden, J.P. Allen, W.A. Valutsky, A.V. Vicuna, J.M. Nappi, S.F. Hoffman, J.E. Wallace, D. Lalka, and J.L. McNay, Clin. Pharmacol. Ther., 1977, 21, 287.

441. S. Vozeh, K.T. Muir, L.B. Sheiner, and F. Follath, J. Pharmacokin. Biopharm., 1981, 9, 131.

442. A. Richens and A. Dunlop, Lancet, 1975, ii, 247.

443. B. Rambeck, H.E. Boenigk, A. Dunlop, P.W. Mullen, J. Wadsworth, and A. Richens, Ther. Drug. Monit., 1979, 1, 325.

444. W.E. Dodson, Clin. Pharmacol. Ther., 1980, 27, 704.

445. J.G. Wagner, J. Pharmacokin. Biopharm., 1978, 6, 209.

446. M. Patterson, R. Heazelwood, B. Smithurst, and M.J. Eadie, Brit. J. Clin. Pharmacol., 1982, 13, 423.

447. D.T. Casto, T.M. Ludden, J.M. Bertoni, L.C. Littlefield, R.A. Sagraves, and R.W. Mackey, Clin. Pharmacol. Ther., 1982, 32, 628.

448. M. Ehrnebo and I. Odar-Cederlöf, Eur. J. Clin. Pharmacol., 1975, 8, 445.

449. I. Odar-Cederlöf and O. Borga, Clin. Pharmacol. Ther., 1976, 20, 36.

450. D.G. Fraser, T.M. Ludden, R.P. Evens, and E.W. Sutherland, III, Clin. Pharmacol. Ther., 1980, 27, 165.

451. M.A. Goldberg and T. Todoroff, J. Pharmacol. Exp. Ther., 1976, 196, 579.

452. J.W. Paxton, Clin. Pharmacol. Ther., 1980, 27, 170.

453. R.F. Leonard, P.J. Knott, G.O. Rankin, D.S. Robinson, and D.E. Melnick, Clin. Pharmacol. Ther., 1981, 29, 56.

454. E.A. De Leacy, C.D. McLeay, M.J. Eadie, and J.H. Tyrer, Brit. J. Clin. Pharmacol., 1979, 8, 33.

455. M. Furianut, P. Benetello A. Avogaro, and R. Dainese, Clin. Pharmacol. Ther., 1978, 24, 294.

456. A. Monks and A. Richens, Clin. Pharmacol. Ther., 1980, 27, 89.

457. G.M. Frigo, S. Lecchini, G. Gatti, E. Perucca, and A. Crema, Brit. J. Clin. Pharmacol., 1979, 8, 553.

458. J.Q. Rose, S.A. Barron, and W.J. Jusko, Int. J. Clin. Pharmacol., 1978, 16, 547.

459. W. Löscher, J. Pharmacol. Exp. Ther., 1979, 208, 429.

460. H.E. Booker and B. Darcey, *Epilepsia*, 1973, *14*, 177.

461. The Boston Collaborative Drug Surveillance Program, *Clin. Pharmacol. Ther.*, 1973, *14*, 529.

462. L. Lund, A. Berlin, and P.K.M. Lunde, *Clin. Pharmacol. Ther.*, 1972, *13*, 196.

463. M.R. Blum and S. Riegelman, *New Engl. J. Med.*, 1972, *286*, 109.

464. T.F. Blaschke, P.J. Meffin, K.L. Melmon, and M. Rowland, *Clin. Pharmacol. Ther.*, 1975, *17*, 685.

465. I. Odar-Cederlöf and O. Borga, *Eur. J. Clin. Pharmacol.*, 1974, *7*, 31.

466. W.H. Steele, J.R. Lawrence, H.L. Elliott, and B. Whiting, *Eur. J. Clin. Pharmacol.*, 1979, *15*, 69.

467. O.B. Paulson, A. Györy, and M.M. Hertz, *Clin. Pharmacol. Ther.*, 1982, *32*, 466.

468. H. Vapaatalo and L. Lehtinen, *Eur. Neurol.*, 1975, *5*, 303.

469. D.B. Appleton, M.J. Eadie, W.D. Hooper, B. Lucas, J.M. Sutherland, and J.H. Tyrer, *Med. J. Austral.*, 1972, *1*, 410.

470. L.G. Borofsky, S. Louis, H. Kutt, and M. Roginsky, *J. Pediatr.*, 1972, *81*, 995.

471. N. Barth G. Alván, O. Borga, and F. Sjöqvist, *Clin. Pharmacokin.*, 1976, *1*, 444.

472. F. Reynolds, N.F. Jones, P.N. Ziroyanis, and S.E. Smith, *Lancet*, 1976, *ii*, 384.

473. J.C. Mucklow, M.R. Bending, G.C. Kahn, and C.T. Dollery, *Clin. Pharmacol. Ther.*, 1978, *24*, 563.

474. S.N. Anavekar, R.H. Saunders, W.M. Wardell, I. Shoulson, F.G. Emmings, C.E. Cook, and A.J. Gringeri, *Clin. Pharmacol. Ther.*, 1978, *24*, 629.

475. G.J. Ayers and D. Burnett, *Lancet*, 1977, *i*, 656.

476. G.J. Conrad, C.O. Haavik, and K.F. Finger, *J. Pharm. Sci.*, 1971, *60*, 1642.

477. C.M. Lander, V.E. Edwards, M.J. Eadie, and J.H. Tyrer, *Neurology*, 1977, *27*, 128.

478. S.-S. Chen, E. Perucca, J.-N. Lee, and A. Richens, *Brit. J. Clin. Pharmacol.*, 1982, *13*, 547.

479. K.I. Mygind, M. Dam, and C. Christiansen, *Acta Neurol. Scand.*, 1976, *54*, 160.

480. B.L. Mirkin, *J. Pediatr.*, 1971, *78*, 329.

481. T. Ishizaki, K. Yokochi, K. Chiba, T. Tabuchi, and T. Wagatsuma, *Pediat. Pharmacol.*, 1981, *1*, 291.

482. A. Rane, M. Garle, O. Borga, and F. Sjöqvist, *Clin. Pharmacol. Ther.*, 1974, *15*, 39.

483. K. Arnold and N. Gerber, Clin. Pharmacol. Ther., 1970, 11, 121.

484. A. Richens, Clin. Pharmacokin., 1979, 4, 153.

485. A. Vicuna, D. Lalka, P. duSouich, N. Vicuna, T.M. Ludden, and A.J. McLean, Res. Comm. Chem. Path. Pharmacol., 1980, 28, 3.

486. L.K. Garrettson and W.J. Jusko, Clin. Pharmacol. Ther., 1975, 17, 481.

487. R. Holcomb, R. Lynn, B. Harvey, B.J. Sweetman, and N. Gerber, J. Pediatr., 1972, 80, 627.

488. N. Gerber, R. Lynn, and J. Oates, Ann. Intern. Med., 1972, 77, 765.

489. W.E. Dodson, Neurology, 1982, 32, 42.

490. P.G. Blain, J.C. Mucklow, C.J. Bacon, and M.D. Rawlins, Brit. J. Clin. Pharmacol., 1981, 12, 659.

491. L.A. Bauer, and R.A. Blouin, Clin. Pharmacol. Ther., 1982, 31, 301.

492. B. Bach, J.M. Hansen, J.P. Kampmann, S.N. Rasmussen, and L. Skovsted, Clin. Pharmacokin., 1981, 6, 389.

493. P.M. Loughnan, A. Greenwald, W.W. Purton, J.V. Aranda, G. Watters, and A.H. Neims, Arch. Dis. Child, 1977, 52, 302.

494. R.G. Curless, P.D. Walson, and D.E. Carter, Neurology, 1976, 26, 715.

495. P.W. Mullen, Clin. Pharmacol. Ther., 1978, 23, 228.

496. T.M. Ludden, J.P. Allen, L.W. Schneider, and S.A. Stavchansky, J. Pharmacokin. Biopharm., 1978, 6, 399.

497. J.P. Allen, T.M. Ludden, S.R. Burrow, W.A. Clementi, and S.A. Stavchansky, Clin. Pharmacol. Ther., 1979, 26, 445.

498. P.W. Mullen and R.W. Foster, J. Pharm. Pharmacol., 1979, 31, 100.

499. E. Perucca, K. Makki, and A. Richens, Clin. Pharmacol. Ther., 1978, 24, 46.

500. O. Borga, C. Hoppel, I. Odar-Cederlöf, and M. Garle, Clin. Pharmacol. Ther., 1979, 26, 306.

501. F. Bochner, W.D. Hooper, J.M. Sutherland, M.J. Eadie, and J.H. Tyrer, Clin. Pharmacol. Ther., 1973, 14, 791.

502. J.M. Letteri, H. Mellk, S. Louis, H. Kutt, P. Durante, and A.J. Glazko, New Engl. J. Med., 1971, 285, 648.

503. G. Levy and J.J. Ashley, J. Pharm. Sci., 1973, 62, 161.

504. D.S. Adler, E. Martin, J.G. Gambertoglio, T.N. Tozer, and J.P. Spire, Clin. Pharmacol. Ther., 1975, 18, 65.

505. E. Perucca and A. Richens, Drugs, 1981, 21, 120.

506. E. Perucca, Clin. Pharmacokin., 1982, 7, 57.

507.   P.J. Neuvonen, R.A. Tokola, and M. Kaste, Eur. J. Clin. Pharmacol., 1981, 21, 215.

508.   P. Sandor, E.M. Sellers, M. Dumbrell, and V. Khouw, Clin. Pharmacol. Ther., 1981, 30, 390.

509.   T. Lysbo Svendsen, M.B. Kristensen, J.M. Hansen, and L. Skovsted, Eur. J. Clin. Pharmacol., 1976, 9, 439.

510.   R.D. Haribson and B.A. Becker, Toxicol. Appl. Pharmacol., 1971, 20, 573.

511.   I.E. Leppik, V. Ramani, R.J. Sawchuk, and R.J. Gumnit, New Engl. J. Med., 1979, 300, 481.

512.   M. Dam, J. Christiansen, O. Munck, and K.I. Mygind, Clin. Pharmacokin., 1979, 4, 53.

513.   A. Küpfer, R.K. Roberts, S. Schenker, and R.A. Branch, J. Pharmacol. Exp. Ther., 1981, 218, 193.

514.   R.A. Buchanan, A.W. Kinkel, and T.C. Smith, Int. J. Clin. Pharmacol., 1973, 7, 213.

515.   J.W. Warren, Jr., J.D. Benmaman, B.B. Wannamaker, and R.H. Levy, Clin. Pharmacol. Ther., 1980, 28, 646.

516.   D. Battino, C. Cusi, S. Franceschetti, A. Moise, S. Spina, and G. Avanzini, Clin. Pharmacokin., 1982, 7, 176.

517.   I.H. Patel, R.H. Levy, and J.S. Lockard, J. Pharm. Sci., 1977, 66, 650.

518.   M.A. el Sayed, W. Löscher, and H.H. Frey, Arch. Int. Pharmacodyn. Ther., 1978, 234, 180.

519.   G.A. Smith, L. McKauge, D. Dubetz, J.H. Tyrer, and M.J. Eadie, Clin. Pharmacokin., 1979, 4, 38.

520.   N. Gerber and J.G. Wagner, Clin. Pharmacokin., 1972, 3, 455.

521.   J.R. Koup, J.Q. Rose, and M.E. Cohen, Epilepsia, 1978, 19, 535.

522.   P.J. Nicholls and T.C. Orton, Brit. J. Pharmacol., 1972, 45, 48.

523.   S.B. Karch, J. Amer. Med. Assoc., 1973, 223, 1463.

524.   M.R. Dobrinska and P.G. Welling, J. Pharm. Sci., 1977, 66, 688.

525.   R.H. Levy, W.H. Pitlick, A.S. Troupin, J.R. Green, and J.M. Neal, Clin. Pharmacol. Ther., 1975, 17, 657.

526.   M. Anttila, P. Kahela, M. Panelius, T. Yrjäna, R. Tikkanen, and R. Aaltonen, Eur. J. Clin. Pharmacol., 1979, 15, 421.

527.   J.A. Wada, A.S. Troupin, P. Friel, R. Remick, K. Leal, and J. Pearmain, Epilepsia, 1978, 19, 251.

528.   K. Richter and B. Terhaag, Int. J. Clin. Pharmacol., 1978, 16, 377.

529.   L.M. Cotter, M.J. Eadie, W.D. Hooper, C.M. Lander, G.A. Smith, and J.H. Tyrer, Eur. J. Clin. Pharmacol., 1977, 12, 451.

530. M. Dam, J. Christiansen, C.B. Kristensen, Aa. Helles, A. Jaegerskou, and M. Schmiegelow, Eur. J. Clin. Pharmacol., 1981, 20, 59.

531. M. Eichelbaum, K. Ekbom, L. Bertilsson, V.A. Ringberger, and A. Rane, Eur. J. Clin. Pharmacol., 1975, 8, 337.

532. M.D. Rawlins, P. Collste, L. Bertilsson, and L. Palmer, Eur. J. Clin. Pharmacol., 1975, 8, 91.

533. I.H. Patel and R.H. Levy, Epilepsia, 1980, 21, 103.

534. M. Eichelbaum, L. Bertilsson, L. Lund, L. Palmer, and F. Sjöqvist, Eur. J. Clin. Pharmacol., 1976, 9, 417.

535. S.I. Johannessen, M. Gerna, J. Bakke, R.E. Strandjord, and P.L. Morselli, Brit. J. Clin. Pharmacol., 1976, 3, 575.

536. M.L. Friis, J. Christiansen, and E.F. Hvidberg, Eur. J. Clin. Pharmacol., 1978, 14, 47.

537. J.W. Faigle, K.F. Feldmann, and V. Balzer, 'Antiepileptic Drug Monitoring', Pitman, Kent, England, 1977, pp. 104-110.

538. E. Rey, Ph. d'Athis, D. de Lauture, O. Dulac, J. Aicardi, and G. Olive, Int. J. Clin. Pharmacol. Biopharm., 1979, 17, 90.

539. A. Rane, B. Höjer, and J.T. Wilson, Clin. Pharmacol. Ther., 1976, 19, 276.

540. J.W. Paxton and R.A. Donald, Clin. Pharmacol. Ther., 1980, 28, 695.

541. J.J. MacKichan, P.K. Duffner, and M.E. Cohen, Brit. J. Clin. Pharmacol., 1981, 12, 31.

542. H.G.M. Westenberg, E. van der Kleijn, T.T. Oei, and R.A. de Zeeuw, Clin. Pharmacol. Ther., 1978, 23, 320.

543. B. Terhaag, K. Richter, and H. Diettrich, Int. J. Clin. Pharmacol., 1978, 16, 607.

544. S. Pynnönen, Acta Pharmacol. Toxicol., 1977, 41, 465.

545. S. Pynnönen, J. Kanto, M. Sillanpää, and R. Erkkola, Acta Pharmacol. Toxicol., 1977, 41, 244.

546. A.P. Gerardin, F.V. Abadie, J.A. Campestrini, and W. Theobald, J. Pharmacokin. Biopharm., 1976, 4, 521.

547. L.M. Cotter, M.J. Eadie, W.D. Hooper, C.M. Lander, G.A. Smith, and J.H. Tyrer, Eur. J. Clin. Pharmacol., 1977, 12, 451.

548. W.H. Pitlick, R.H. Levy, A.S. Troupin, and J.R. Green, J. Pharm. Sci., 1976, 65, 462.

549. P.J. MacNamara, W.A. Colburn, and M. Gibaldi, J. Pharmacokin. Biopharm., 1979, 7, 63.

550. M. Eichelbaum, K.W. Köthe, F. Hoffman, and G.E. von Unruh, Clin. Pharmacol. Ther., 1979, 26, 366.

551. I.H. Patel, R.H. Levy, and W.F. Trager, J. Pharmacol. Exp. Ther., 1978, 206, 607.

552. S. Pynnönen, H. Frey, and M. Sillanpää, Int. J. Clin. Pharmacol. Ther. Toxicol., 1980, 18, 247.

553. L. Bertilsson, B. Höjer, G. Tybring, J. Osterloh, and A. Rane, Clin. Pharmacol. Ther., 1980, 27, 83.

554. A. Rane, L. Bertilsson, and L. Palmer, Eur. J. Clin. Pharmacol., 1975, 8, 283.

555. J.S. Lockard, R.H. Levy, V. Uhlir, and J. Farquhar, Epilepsia, 1974, 15, 351.

556. R.A. Ronfeld and L.Z. Benet, Res. Comm. Chem. Path. Pharmacol., 1975, 10, 303.

557. F. Hassan, B.M. Assael, L. Bossi, S. Garattini, M. Gerna, R. Gomeni, and P.L. Morselli, Arch. Int. Pharmacodyn. Ther., 1976, 220, 125.

558. A.A. Lai and R.H. Levy, J. Pharm. Sci., 1979, 68, 416.

559. A.A. Lai, R.H. Levy, and R.E. Cutler, Clin. Pharmacol. Ther., 1978, 24, 316.

560. M. Theisohn and G. Heimann, Eur. J. Clin. Pharmacol., 1982, 22, 545.

561. R. Gugler, and G.E. von Unruh, Clin. Pharmacokin., 1980, 5, 67.

562. A.H.C. Chun, D.J. Hoffman, N. Friedmann, and P.J. Carrigan, J. Clin. Pharmacol., 1980, 20, 30.

563. W. Oelkers, G. Stoffels, H. Schafer, and H. Reith, Arzneim.-Forsch., 1977, 27, 1088.

564. U. Klotz and K.H. Antonin, Clin. Pharmacol. Ther., 1977, 21, 736.

565. V. Nitsche and H. Mascher, Epilepsia, 1982, 23, 153.

566. U. Klotz, Int. J. Clin. Pharmacol. Ther. Toxicol., 1982, 20, 24.

567. P. Loiseau, A. Brachet, and P. Henry, Epilepsia, 1975, 16, 609.

568. J.C. Cloyd and R.L. Kriel, Neurology, 1981, 31, 1348.

569. F. Moolenaar, W.J. Greving, and T. Huizinga, Eur. J. Clin. Pharmacol., 1980, 17, 309.

570. J. Bruni, B.J. Wilder, L.J. Willmore, R.J. Perchalski, and H.J. Villarreal, Clin. Pharmacol. Ther., 1978, 24, 324.

571. W. Löscher, J. Pharmacol. Exp. Ther., 1978, 204, 255.

572. D. Brewster and N.C. Muir, Clin. Pharmacol. Ther., 1980, 27, 76.

573. J.M. Orr, F.S. Abbott, K. Farrell, S. Ferguson, I. Sheppard, and W. Godolphin, Clin. Pharmacol. Ther., 1982, 31, 642.

574. S. Dhillon and A. Richens, Brit. J. Clin. Pharmacol., 1982, 13, 553.

575. F. Pisani, G. Oteri, and R. Di Perri, Brit. J. Clin. Pharmacol., 1981, 12, 81.

576. W. Löscher and H. Esenwein, <u>Arzeim.-Forsch.</u>, 1978, <u>28</u>, 782.

577. S.I. Johannessen, <u>Arzneim.-Forsch.</u>, 1977, <u>27</u>, 1083.

578. R.G. Dickinson, C.H. Lawyer, S.N. Kaufman, R.K. Lynn, N. Gerber, M.J. Novy, and M.J. Cook, <u>Pediat. Pharmacol.</u>, 1980, <u>1</u>, 71.

579. T.A. Bowdle, I.H. Patel, R.H. Levy, and A.J. Wilensky, <u>Clin. Pharmacol. Ther.</u>, 1980, <u>28</u>, 486.

580. R.H. Levy, J.S. Lockard, I.H. Patel, and W.C. Congdon, <u>J. Pharm. Sci.</u>, 1977, <u>66</u>, 1154.

581. J.S. Lockard, R.H. Levy, L.L. DuCharme, W.C. Congdon, and I.H. Patel, <u>Epilepsia</u>, 1977, <u>18</u>, 183.

582. J.S. Lockard, R.H. Levy, W.C. Congdon, L.L. DuCharme, and I.H. Patel, <u>Epilepsia</u>, 1977, <u>18</u>, 205.

583. R.H. Levy, C.T. Viswanathan, and J.S. Lockard, <u>J. Pharm. Sci.</u>, 1982, <u>71</u>, 723.

584. G.W. Mihaly, F.J. Vajda, J.L. Miles, and W.J. Louis, <u>Eur. J. Clin. Pharmacol.</u>, 1979, <u>16</u>, 23.

585. M.I. Reunanen, P. Luoma, V.V. Myllylä, and E. Hokkanen, <u>Curr. Ther. Res.</u>, 1980, <u>28</u>, 456.

586. G.J. Schapel, R.G. Beran, C.J. Doecke, W.J. O'Reilly, P.A. Reece, R.H.C. Rischbieth, L.N. Sansom, and P.E. Stanley, <u>Eur. J. Clin. Pharmacol.</u>, 1980, <u>17</u>, 71.

587. U. Klotz, T. Rapp, and W.A. Müller, <u>Eur. J. Clin. Pharmacol.</u>, 1978, <u>13</u>, 55.

588. F. Pisana, A.A. D'Agostino, A. Fazio, G. Oteri, G. Primerano, and R. Di Perri, <u>Epilepsia</u>, 1982, <u>23</u>, 115.

589. W.A. Colburn, I. Bekersky, B.H. Min, B.J. Hodshon, and W.A. Garland, <u>Res. Comm. Chem. Path. Pharmacol.</u>, 1980, <u>27</u>, 73.

590. F.E. Dreifuss, J.K. Penry, S.W. Rose, H.J. Kupferberg, P. Dyken, and S. Sato, <u>Neurology</u>, 1975, <u>25</u>, 255.

591. K.-C. Khoo, J. Mendels, M. Rothbart, W.A. Garland, W.A. Colburn, B.H. Min, R. Lucek, J.J. Carbone, H.G. Boxenbaum, and S.A. Kaplan, <u>Clin. Pharmacol. Ther.</u>, 1980, <u>28</u>, 368.

592. O. Sjö, E.F. Hvidberg, J. Naestoft, and M. Lund, <u>Eur. J. Clin. Pharmacol.</u>, 1975, <u>8</u>, 249.

593. M.E. Miller, W.A. Garland, B.H. Min, B.T. Ludwick, R.H. Ballard, and R.H. Levy, <u>Clin. Pharmacol. Ther.</u>, 1981, <u>30</u>, 343.

594. H.-H. Frey, W. Göbel, and W. Löscher, <u>Arch. Int. Pharmacodyn. Ther.</u>, 1979, <u>242</u>, 14.

595. B.B. Gallagher, I.P. Baumel, and R.H. Mattson, <u>Neurology</u>, 1972, <u>22</u>, 1186.

596. R.E. Kauffman, R. Habersang, and L. Lansky, <u>Clin. Pharmacol. Ther.</u>, 1977, <u>22</u>, 200.

597. C.-S. C. Lee, T.C. Marbury, R.T. Perchalski, and B.J. Wilder, <u>J. Clin. Pharmacol.</u>, 1982, <u>22</u>, 301.

598. J.C. Cloyd, K.W. Miller, and I.E. Leppik, <u>Clin. Pharmacol. Ther.</u>, 1981, <u>29</u>, 402.

599. P.R. Cottrell, J.M. Streete, D.J. Berry, H. Schäfer, F. Pisani, E. Perucca, and A. Richens, <u>Epilepsia</u>, 1982, <u>23</u>, 307.

3 Antimicrobial Agents

Penicillins

Introduction

Although the penicillins as a drug class rank among the oldest of
the antimicrobial agents, new derivatives of this class continue to be
reported. Improved efficacy of the newer penicillins is often based
on bioavailability and pharmacokinetic characteristics. Investigation
of these concepts, together with continued interest in the disposition
of established compounds, has generated a considerable literature on
the pharmacokinetics of the penicillins, often comparing old and new
forms.

For example, Dittert et al.[1] studied the distribution of
ampicillin, methicillin, penicillin G, oxacillin, and dicloxacillin in
man and showed that, despite considerable differences in binding to
serum proteins, all compounds except dicloxacillin had similar overall
volumes of distribution of 20 - 30 l. Blood levels of all penicillins
fitted the two-compartment open model and similar fractions of each
drug reached the peripheral compartment. Higher p.o. absorption rates
and higher blood levels of the monobasic penicillins, nafcillin,
dicloxacillin, and penicillin G were obtained in female dogs than in
male dogs.[2] Studies have shown that beagle dogs can be used to predict bioavailability characteristics of penicillins in man,[3] differences in peak serum levels, peak times, and absorption efficiencies
from various formulations being accurately reflected in human subjects. A study of the salivary secretion of phenoxymethylpenicillin,
ampicillin, cloxacillin, and cephalexin in man showed that only trace
amounts of these antibiotics appeared in either mixed or parotid

saliva when therapeutic levels were present in serum.[4] It is suggested that these antibiotics would be of limited use in salivary
gland infections.

Penicillin V

The bioavailability characteristics of penicillin V[5] and the
pharmacokinetics of some penicillins in man[6] have been reviewed.
Different absorption rates and plasma levels of penicillin V have been
observed from different p.o. dosed tablets, liquid formulations, and
powders.[7,8] Peak serum levels of penicillin varied as much as
sixfold between some treatments. Similar bioavailability characteristics were demonstrated from two commercial penicillin V-K formulations in volunteers, and with both preparations a significant linear
correlation was obtained between areas under serum drug profiles and
dose over a wide dosage range.[9] Higher serum penicillin levels were
obtained in children from p.o. K^+ penicillin V than from Ca^{2+} and
benzathine salts of penicillin, all doses being given as suspensions.[10] Interestingly, higher serum levels were also obtained from
the K^+ salt administered as a dilute solution compared with a concentrated solution. Coeliac disease in children caused a marked decrease
in the absorption of Ca^{2+} penicillin V, and a smaller decrease for
the K^+ salt. Relatively poor absorption has also been reported for
the Ca^{2+} and benzathine salts of phenoxymethylpenicillin in man
compared with the K^+ salt. Poorer bioavailability of Ca^{2+} salt
tablets was associated with longer _in vitro_ dissolution times.

Oral doses of penicillin V were most efficiently absorbed when
administered on an empty stomach.[12] Reducing the fasting period from
2 to 0 h before dosing resulted in decreased plasma concentrations of
the antibiotic. Administration of penicillin V in a small volume of
oily suspension also yielded a lower peak concentration than in a
larger volume of aqueous solution. Based on total recovery of penicillin in urine, the bioavailability of a 1 g tablet of penicillin V

was doubled after jejunoileal bypass, probably due to reduced metabolism in the gut wall.[12] A more profound effect of the surgery was observed on the serum drug concentrations, which averaged 6.7 and 164 units ml^{-1} before and after bypass, respectively.

Penicillin V and some other antibiotics entered pericardial fluid rapidly following i.m. administration to man and dogs.[14] In both species, drug levels in pericardial fluid equalled or exceeded plasma levels within 2 - 3 h of dosing. Drug penetration into pericardial fluid tended to increase in pericardial infection. Uptake of penicillin and cephalothin by dog-kidney tissue was markedly impaired by probenecid.[15] However, accumulation of drug in kidney occurred with time, owing to inhibition of tubular secretion of penicillin by probenecid. Probenecid increases c.s.f. levels of penicillin G and of other penicillins and cephalosporins by inhibiting their secretion from c.s.f. into plasma.[16] In patients undergoing tonsillectomy who received multiple doses of penicillin V, drug concentrations in tonsillar tissue reached a level approximately 25% of those in serum.[17]

Penicillin G

Oral doses of 500 mg potassium penicillin G to human subjects result in urinary concentrations of <u>ca.</u> 600 µg ml^{-1} for 2 h and 300 µg ml^{-1} for 4 h after dosing.[18] Although the relative importance of serum and urine levels of antibiotic in the treatment of pyelonephritis is problematical, these data suggest that p.o. penicillin G therapy may be suitable for some types of urinary tract infections. Experiments in animals show that duration of serum penicillin levels, and also persistence of antibiotic in bone tissue, may be markedly influenced by both the formulation and the dosage regimen.[19,20]

Serum penicillin levels in newborn infants are higher and more prolonged than in children and adults after equivalent doses.[21] This effect is seen only in the first 4 or 5 d of life, and renal clearance of antibiotic increases after this time with rapid maturation of kidney tubular function.

Slow placental transfer of penicillin G in the goat gives rise to maternal:foetal serum concentration ratios of <u>ca</u>. 9.0 during infusion into the mother and from 3×10^{-3} to 6×10^{-4} during infusion into the foetus.[22] Inefficient placental transfer is consistent with the low lipid solubility and low ionization constant of penicillin G, and there is no evidence of active placental transport.

<u>Ampicillin</u>

Numerous reports have discussed the absorption of ampicillin from different formulations, physical forms, and prodrugs. Many of the reports are conflicting. Whyatt et al.[23] failed to find any significant differences in serum levels, peak serum levels, times of peak levels, and area profiles among 17 different brands of ampicillin capsules. Another study, however, reported differences in bioavailability from commercial ampicillin formulations, one product producing areas under serum level curves <u>ca</u>. 30% higher than two competitive brands.[24] No differences could be detected between different lots of the more bioavailable product. In a more recent study absorption efficiency of a 500 mg dose of ampicillin in capsule was reported to be <u>ca</u>. 40%.[25] Ampicillin absorption appeared to be independent of age, but was significantly reduced by food.[26] In a comparative study mean peak serum ampicillin levels and areas under serum ampicillin curves were reduced from 6.5 µg ml^{-1} and 19.4 µg ml^{-1} h, respectively, in fasted individuals, to 2.9 µg ml^{-1} and 9.6 µg ml^{-1} h following a 500 mg p.o. dose after a meal.[27] Equivalent values for amoxicillin were 12.6 µg ml^{-1} and 39.4 µg ml^{-1} h in fasted individuals and 5.4 µg ml^{-1} and 21.7 µg ml^{-1} h after a meal.

Newborn children behave similarly to adults in that they absorb the anhydrous form of ampicillin more efficiently than the trihydrate.[28-31] Serum levels of antibiotic in the newborn are further elevated owing to the underdeveloped excretory capacity of the neonatal kidney (Figure 3.1). It has been proposed that p.o. dosed

anhydrous ampicillin may be a suitable alternative to parenteral doses
in the newborn.[32]

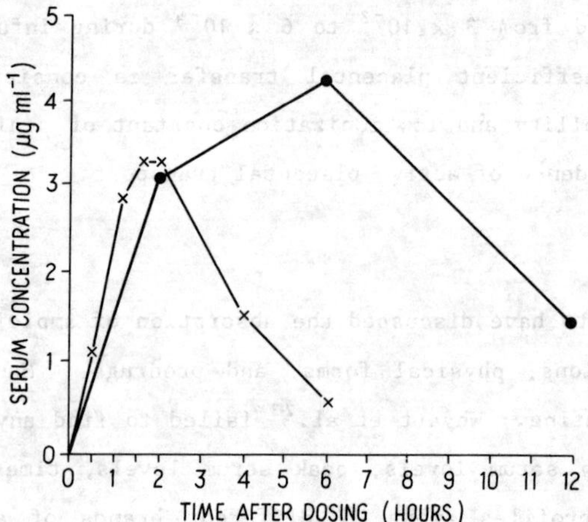

Figure 3.1   Mean serum levels of anhydrous ampicillin
in newborn infants (●——●) (24 - 48 h, 10 mg kg^{-1})
and adults x——x (500 mg).   Reproduced by permission
from *Pediatrics*, 1973, **51**, 578.

The absorption efficiency, and the rate of elimination of
ampicillin and nalidixic acid, are both decreased in patients with
shigellosis.[33]   Poor absorption was generally observed in younger
patients with marked diarrhoea but there was no ready explanation for
the delayed excretion. The absorption of antibiotic from i.m. injections of ampicillin trihydrate suspension and a dicloxacillin solution
was slower than from an ampicillin sodium solution in man.[34]   Blood
levels from dicloxacillin and ampicillin solutions were fitted to the
two-compartment model with first-order absorption, whereas those resulting from the ampicillin suspension required two successive first-
order absorption steps to obtain a good fit of actual to theoretical
blood level versus time curves.

Experiments in animals[35] and man[36] have shown rapid penetration
of ampicillin into both subcutaneous tissue and blister fluid after a
single i.v. dose. Distribution into tissues and extravascular fluids
was enhanced by administration of bacampicillin, a prodrug of ampicil-

lin, apparently due to improved p.o. absorption.[37] In healthy mongrel dogs, i.v. administration of 100 and 200 mg ampicillin resulted in subtherapeutic antibiotic concentrations in pancreatic fluid, mean C_{max} values being 0.4 and 2.7 µg ml^{-1}.[38] After inducing pancreatitis in the same animals, a significant increase in ampicillin excretion in pancreatic juice was observed; peak concentrations were 19 and 38.5 µg ml^{-1}, respectively, from the 100 and 200 mg doses. However, serum drug levels appeared to be unaffected by pancreatitis.

Both ampicillin and flucloxacillin penetrate bone tissue to reach levels that inhibit <u>Staph. aureus</u> and <u>E. coli</u>.[39] However the doses employed, 2 g ampicillin and 2 g flucloxacillin, were ineffective against some Gram-negative anaerobes in bone marrow.

The mean biological $t_{0.5}$ of ampicillin in neonates is 1.1 h, which is similar to the value in adults.[40] However, the elimination $t_{0.5}$ varies sixfold from 0.67 to 4.0 h in neonates, and is closely correlated with postmenstrual age.

Studies in rats demonstrated marked differences in tissue distribution characteristics of ampicillin, doxycycline, and cephalothin.[41] Doxycycline penetrated most tissues to a greater extent than ampicillin, while values for cephalothin were variable. However, greater tissue retention occurred with ampicillin compared to doxycycline as tissue levels of the former, but not the latter, declined at a slower rate than serum levels.

Plasma levels of ampicillin after both p.o. and i.v. doses were lower in pregnant women, using the same subjects in nonpregnant conditions as controls.[42] Decreased plasma levels were accompanied by increased apparent body distribution volumes, decreased elimination $t_{0.5}$, and increased plasma clearances. These data suggest that usual ampicillin doses may be too low in pregnant women, and this may apply also to other drugs used in pregnancy.

After continuous i.v. infusion, the ratio of steady-state levels of ampicillin in c.s.f. and plasma was 0.025 in patients without

meningitis.[43] In patients with meningitis the blood-c.s.f. barrier
was partially abolished and the c.s.f.:plasma ampicillin ratio increased to 0.061. Coadministration of probenecid increased the elimination $t_{0.5}$ of ampicillin from 60 to 100 min in man,[44] such that
serum levels obtained from 2 g of ampicillin with probenecid generally
exceeded those from 3 g of amoxicillin alone.

After a 500 mg i.v. dose of sodium ampicillin, average clearance
of the drug was 0.18 l h^{-1} kg^{-1} in young adults (22 - 36 yr) but
decreased to 0.08 l h^{-1} kg^{-1} in the elderly (67 - 84 yr).[25] The
respective $t_{0.5}$ values were 1.7 and 6.7 h, which were similar to
those observed after p.o. administration of ampicillin trihydrate to
the same subjects. Marked retention of ampicillin in plasma has been
noted in patients with renal failure.[45] As ampicillin obeys two-
compartment kinetics in the body, dose adjustment in renal failure
should be based on the magnitude of the rate constant for elimination
of drug from the central compartment, or total body clearance, rather
than the terminal plasma $t_{0.5}$.[45]

Biliary excretion accounted for 65 - 75% of ^{35}S after ^{35}S-
ampicillin, ^{35}S-azidocillin, and ^{35}S-benzylpenicillin were injected
i.v. into rats.[46] However, the proportion of excreted radioactivity
due to biologically active material was higher for ampicillin than for
the other compounds. Biliary excretion accounted for only 0.1% of
p.o. or i.v. dosed ampicillin in patients with T-tube drainage.[47]
However, concentrations of antibiotic in bile exceeded MIC values for
susceptible organisms.

Ampicillin Prodrugs and Derivatives

Superior absorption and distribution qualities have been demonstrated for a number of ampicillin precursors. GI absorption of
bacampicillin was both more rapid and more complete compared to
ampicillin in healthy subjects, yielding a 30 - 40% increase in drug
bioavailability,[50] while penetration of ampicillin into prostatic

fluid and spinal fluid was superior after i.v. doses of a methoxy-methyl ester of hetacillin in dogs compared with equivalent doses of ampicillin.

In other studies p.o. doses of bacampicillin yielded similar serum levels of antibiotic compared to equivalent doses of parenteral ampicillin in healthy individuals[52] and, together with pivampicillin, gave rise to serum levels twice as high as those obtained from equivalent doses of ampicillin.[53] On the other hand, no increase was observed in antibiotic levels in bronchial mucosa tissue after bacampicillin compared with ampicillin.[54] Repeated p.o. 500 mg doses of combined bacampicillin and mecillinam gave rise to mean peak tissue levels of 2.1 μg ml^{-1} ampicillin and 1.5 μg ml^{-1} mecillinam, these values being approximately one-half of those in serum.[55] Although the overall AUC values of both compounds in lymph were less than in serum, penetration into lymph, which may represent levels in unmanipulated tissues, was considered satisfactory. In 2 - 9 m infants, a bacampicillin dose of 10 mg kg^{-1} produced mean peak drug levels in serum of 7.2 μg ml^{-1}.[56] Although this value is less than peak levels obtained from an equivalent dose of bacampicillin in adults,[57] it is nonetheless greater than levels obtained from pivampicillin in children.

Serum and tissue levels of ampicillin are increased when the antibiotic is administered as pivampicillin[58-61] and may be increased still further by concurrent treatment with pivampicillin and metoclopramide.[62] However absorption of pivampicillin may be reduced at high doses.[60] The bioavailability of pivampicillin is superior to that of ampicillin from suspension dosage forms in children[63] and the systemic availability of pivampicillin is similar from different commercial formulations.[64] Esters of ampicillin are absorbed from different regions of the gut compared to parent drug.[65] Some 90% of radioactive label was absorbed proximal to the upper jejunum from p.o. dosed solutions of ^{35}S-pivampicillin and ^{35}S-carampicillin in healthy volunteers; after p.o. ^{35}S-ampicillin the corresponding value was 24 - 45%. The ampicillin esters may be hydrolysed in the blood, the lumen, the gut wall, and also by first-pass metabolism. However major hydrolysis occurs in intestinal tissue, as pivampicillin constitutes less than 1% of total drug in both the portal and peripheral circulations after p.o. doses.[66] Direct measurement of blood and bile levels in this study demonstrated the ability of the liver to excrete ampicillin against a concentration gradient.

Pivampicillin is absorbed more efficiently than ampicillin in pregnant women, but plasma levels of antibiotic from both compounds are lower than in nonpregnant women.[67] This trend persists after both single and repeated doses. GI absorption of pivampicillin was reduced and varied in patients in the postabsorptive phase following urological surgery.[68]

Unlike pivampicillin, the derivative metampicillin gives rise to lower circulating levels of ampicillin after p.o. doses.[69] After i.m. doses both the derivative and ampicillin appear in serum, although only ampicillin is detectable in urine.

Epicillin is poorly absorbed compared with ampicillin after p.o. dosing.[70] Only 27% of an epicillin p.o. dose was recovered in 24 h urine compared with 50% for ampicillin and 57% for amoxicillin. A serial effect was postulated in this study in that ampicillin serum levels were higher if epicillin had been dosed the previous week than when ampicillin was taken first. Tissue distribution of epicillin was superior to that of ampicillin in rabbits.[71] Blood levels of both compounds declined biexponentially after 50 mg kg^{-1} and 100 mg kg^{-1} doses but declined triexponentially after 200 mg kg^{-1} doses. Also, the apparent distribution of epicillin was dose-independent, while ampicillin appeared to distribute less efficiently at higher doses.

After equivalent p.o. doses to man, hetacillin was absorbed more slowly and produced more persistent serum levels than ampicillin.[72]

Increased serum levels of ampicillin, reported after parenterally dosed hetacillin[73] may be due partially to a technical artifact, caused by the assay of biologically inactive hetacillin as ampicillin.[74] Studies using specific assays for both compounds have nonetheless shown that GI absorption of ampicillin is somewhat improved when the antibiotic is administered as the hetacillin derivative.[75]

<u>Amoxicillin</u>

Amoxicillin is rapidly absorbed from the GI tract. Following a single 500 mg p.o. dose to 9 healthy subjects, peak serum concentrations of 6.0 - 15 μg ml^{-1} were reached between 1.25 and 2 h.[76] The absolute bioavailability of p.o. amoxicillin in the study averaged 77% while the serum clearance, measured after giving the same dose intravenously, was 13.3 l h^{-1}. Amoxicillin absorption from p.o. and i.m. doses was independent of dose size in the 250 - 1000 mg range.[77] Equimolar p.o. doses of amoxicillin (290 mg) and bacampicillin (400 mg) yielded comparable bioavailability of antibiotic in man, although the latter appeared to be absorbed more rapidly.[78] In patients who had undergone vagotomy and pyloroplasty, the absorption of amoxicillin was delayed, with serum T_{max} ranging from 2 to 3 h.[79]

There have been variable reports on the influence of food on amoxicillin absorption. Results of one study indicated no effect by food in adults.[80] Although this study indicated no effect on the extent of amoxicillin absorption, the mean absorption lag time was increased from 0.56 to 1.2 h, and the T_{max} increased from 1.9 to 2.4 h in the presence of food. Other studies have demonstrated reduced amoxicillin absorption due to ingested food.[81]

A study in children showed a reduced mean peak serum level of amoxicillin from 5.4 μg ml^{-1} in fasting children to 3.2 μg ml^{-1} in nonfasting children following a 15 mg kg^{-1} dose.[82] This reduction in peak levels due to food is similar to a previous observation in adults.[81] The effect of food in children was attenuated somewhat at a dose level of 25 mg kg^{-1}, mean peak amoxicillin levels being 8.9 and 7.9 µg ml^{-1} in fasting and nonfasting infants, respectively, and AUC values were unaffected by food. The relative serum levels obtained following fasting and nonfasting doses of 25 mg kg^{-1} ampicillin and 15 mg kg^{-1} amoxicillin in this population are illustrated in Figure 3.2.

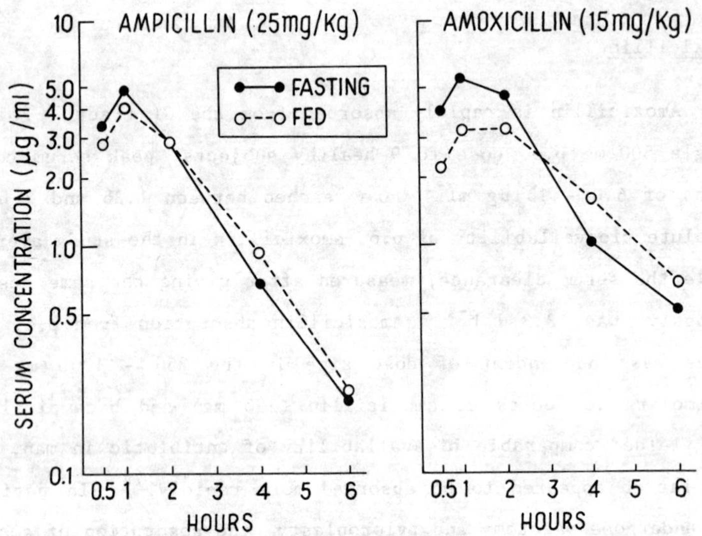

Figure 3.2   Serum concentration time curves for ampicillin (25 mg kg^{-1}) and amoxicillin (15 mg kg^{-1}) in infants and children. Reproduced by permission from *Pediatrics*, 1979, **64**, 627.

Combining clavulanic acid with amoxicillin extends the antibacterial activity of amoxicillin to include β-lactamase producing strains, although it does not influence the absorption or disposition of either drug.[83,84]   In 17 infants and children who received a liquid suspension of amoxicillin and potassium clavulanate (6.6 and 1.7 mg kg^{-1}, respectively), peak plasma concentrations of 2.8 and 0.8 µg ml^{-1}, respectively, were reached in <u>ca</u>. 1 h.[85] Doubling the dose in a second group of 17 children doubled the peak antibiotic concentrations but had no effect on elimination $t_{0.5}$ values, 1.3 - 1.5 h for amoxicillin and 1.1 - 1.2 h for clavulanic acid. The bioavailability of amoxicillin and clavulanic acid from a combination tablet (250 mg amoxicillin as the trihydrate and 125 mg clavulanic acid as the potassium salt) was unaffected when taken with food; serum concentration profiles of both compounds were virtually identical under fasting and nonfasting conditions.[86]

After rapid i.v. injection to man, amoxicillin serum levels obeyed two-compartment model kinetics, and the drug had an overall distribution volume $(V_{d,ss})$ 29% larger than that of ampicillin.[87] Although both ampicillin and amoxicillin obey two-compartment model kinetics after i.v. doses to adults, studies in neonates obtained almost identical values for the central and overall drug distribution volumes for ampicillin, indicating single-compartment kinetic behavior.[88] Following i.v. injection to infants and children, serum levels of amoxicillin were related to dose size over the dosage range 14.8 - 41.5 mg kg^{-1} and the biological $t_{0.5}$ was independent of dose.[89]

Following a 1 g i.m. dose in man, amoxicillin concentrations in bile, lung, liver, and gallbladder were approximately twice the respective values after an equal dose of ampicillin.[90] Clinically effective levels of amoxicillin were found also in bronchial secretion after 50 - 100 mg kg^{-1} p.o. doses.[91]

Amoxicillin is capable of entering the c.s.f. but at low levels relative to those in plasma.[92] In 21 patients without meningeal inflammation, a single p.o. dose of 250 mg clavulanic acid yielded little or no detectable drug in the c.s.f.[93] Tissue distribution studies in the rat showed that the highest concentrations of amoxicillin and clavulanic acid were found in the excretory organs, i.e. kidney and liver.[94] In the mouse, rat, and dog, serum $t_{0.5}$ values of clavulanic acid were 0.3, 0.5, and 0.7 h, respectively, approximately one-half those for amoxicillin (0.7, 1, and 1.4 h, respectively).[94] In contrast, the elimination rate of the two compounds was similar in the squirrel monkey and man.

Renal excretion of amoxicillin, which amounts to 68% of an i.v. dose in normal kidney function, is reduced in renal failure and the elimination rate constant, β, is related to corrected creatinine clearance, Cl_{CR}, by equation 3.1.[95]

$$\beta = 0.0055\ (Cl_{CR}) + 0.043 \tag{3.1}$$

The observed $t_{0.5}$ of amoxicillin in 8 patients with Cl_{CR} values less than 7 ml min^{-1} was 7.5 - 21 h, but this value fell to 3 h during haemodialysis,[96] and 6.6 - 7 h during peritoneal dialysis.[96] Amoxicillin is not concentrated in bile, and biliary levels of antibiotic are normally one-half of those in serum. Unlike the aminoglycosides and tetracyclines, amoxicillin is removed from bile at the same rate as from serum.[97]

Nafcillin

The systemic availability of nafcillin is erratic and is reduced in the presence of food.[98] Single p.o. doses of 500 mg nafcillin to fasted volunteers yielded a mean peak serum level of 3.2 µg ml^{-1} at 1 h, which was reduced to 1.7 µg ml^{-1} and delayed to 1.5 h when dosed postprandially. Single 1 g doses gave peak serum levels of drug approximately double those from 500 mg doses, and they occurred at about the same time.

Inflammation enhances penetration of nafcillin into ventricular fluid.[99] Following 100 - 200 mg kg^{-1} nafcillin per day in divided i.v. doses, serum antibiotic $t_{0.5}$ was <u>ca</u>. 3 h in infants under 3 wk of age but decreased to 1.5 h in those older than 1 m.[99,100] In adult male volunteers who received an i.v. dose of 500 mg sodium nafcillin, the mean $t_{0.5}$ and total clearance were 42 min and 6.9 ml min^{-1} kg^{-1}, respectively.[101] Coadministration of probenecid with nafcillin in the same subjects prolonged nafcillin $t_{0.5}$ to 59 min while reducing the clearance to 3.3 ml min^{-1} kg^{-1}. The kidney is a minor route for nafcillin elimination in man since only 17% and 30%

of the dose administered with and without probenecid, respectively, was recovered in urine. Two studies have shown that neither the elimination kinetics nor the distribution of nafcillin are changed in moderate or severe renal failure.[102,103] The rate of nafcillin elimination is unaffected by haemodialysis.

Piperacillin

The pharmacokinetics of piperacillin have been examined in healthy volunteers after single i.v.[104,105] and i.m.[106] doses. Serum levels of drug are dose-related. The drug is 20% bound to plasma proteins and distributes into an apparent volume of 20 - 24 l 1.73 m^{-2}. The $t_{0.5}$ and also peak serum levels of piperacillin are increased by 30% in the presence of probenecid, and $V_{d\beta}$ is increased by 20%.

A single 5 g i.v. dose of piperacillin achieved therapeutic levels in gallbladder wall, intraabdominal skeletal muscle, and adipose tissue in 14 patients undergoing biliary tract surgery.[107] Piperacillin also penetrated into c.s.f. of patients with meningitis, achieving an average c.s.f.:serum concentration ratio of 0.32.[108]

In healthy subjects, 67.5% of a 2 g i.v. dose of piperacillin was recovered in 0 - 8 h urine.[109] The serum $t_{0.5}$ and clearance of the drug were 0.9 h and 20 l h^{-1} 1.73 m^{-2}, respectively, similar to those observed for ticarcillin and carbenicillin. In paediatric patients (3 -14 yr), the serum $t_{0.5}$ of piperacillin averaged 37 min, somewhat shorter than in adults.[110] The ratio of renal clearance to total clearance was approximately 0.6, suggesting significant nonrenal elimination. In a study in patients undergoing cholecystectomy, Giron et al.[111] reported excretion of piperacillin via the bile. Piperacillin elimination is only moderately affected during renal impairment.[112-114] In 7 patients with creatinine clearance values less than 7 ml min^{-1} who were undergoing chronic, intermittent haemodialysis, piperacillin $t_{0.5}$ while off dialysis was 1 - 3 h.[115] The mean $t_{0.5}$ during dialysis was 1.3 h and clearance was 0.09 l h^{-1} kg^{-1}. Although 40 - 70% of dosed piperacillin is cleared unchanged in urine,[104,109] extrarenal pathways appear to compensate for renal excretion mechanisms in renal failure, so that dosage adjustment in these patients is probably unnecessary.

Methicillin

The pharmacokinetics of methicillin in neonates have been shown to be similar to those of other penicillins in this age group.[116] Following 25 and 50 mg kg^{-1} i.m. doses, peak antibiotic concentrations of 58 and 80 µg ml^{-1} in serum were obtained at 1 h. The average serum $t_{0.5}$ ranged from 1 to 3 h, and this value declined while plasma clearance and drug distribution volume tended to increase, with increasing gestational and chronological age.

After i.v. infusion of methicillin (5 - 125 mg kg^{-1} h^{-1}) to rabbits with staphylococcal meningitis, the c.s.f.:serum antibiotic concentration ratio ranged from 0.04 to 0.06.[117] This ratio was lower than that of vancomycin (0.08 - 0.12) but was slightly higher than those for oxacillin, nafcillin, and cephalothin (0.01 - 0.03). Methicillin concentration was also higher in fibrin-scarred heart valves than in normal heart of the rabbit.[118] Serum protein binding averaged 17% over a wide concentration range of 11.5 - 125 µg ml^{-1}. Mean total body clearance of methicillin in this animal model was 0.86 l h^{-1} kg^{-1}, and excretion occurred predominantly via the kidneys.

Gradnik and Fleischmann[119] presented evidence that renal enzymes in the rat, but not hepatic enzymes, are capable of hydrolyzing the $-N=CH_2$ group of methicillin, and they suggest that methicillin circulates unchanged in the body until excreted by the kidneys.

Cyclacillin and Propicillin

The pharmacokinetics of cyclacillin and amoxicillin after 15 mg kg^{-1} p.o. doses were compared in 12 children who received both drugs in crossover fashion.[120]   Cyclacillin was absorbed more rapidly and reached higher serum concentrations, with T_{max} and C_{max} values of 30 min and 15.6 µg ml^{-1}, respectively, compared with 60 min and 7.3 µg ml^{-1} for amoxicillin.   The C_{max} of cyclacillin increased proportionately to ca. 26 µg ml^{-1} after 25 mg kg^{-1} doses, and bioavailability was unaffected by feeding status.   However, in situ perfusion studies using rat small intestine showed that cyclacillin absorption at relatively low concentrations (< 1 mg ml^{-1}) may follow Michaelis-Menten kinetics.[121]   The average elimination $t_{0.5}$ of cyclacillin in children was approximately 0.7 h, about one-half that of amoxicillin.[120]

Elderly patients appear to absorb and eliminate propicillin as efficiently as young adults.[122] However, serum levels from equal doses are twice as high in geriatric patients, owing to reduced tissue uptake and a smaller drug distribution volume of 19.9 l compared with 28.7 l.

Carbenicillin and Ticarcillin

Carbenicillin and ticarcillin are not absorbed from p.o. doses. The indanyl ester of carbenicillin is rapidly absorbed from a solution after p.o. dosing to man, yielding peak serum levels at 1 - 2 h.[123] Absorption from capsules is poor, but tablet formulations with glycerine or citrate provide rapid and efficient absorption with peak serum levels occurring at 1 h. Efficient but more variable absorption of indanyl carbenicillin from sodium glycinate and citrate tablets has been demonstrated in dogs.[124]

Penetration of carbenicillin into renal parenchymal tissue was severely impaired in the hydropoenic state in dogs and also in severe renal disease in man.[125]   In diseased renal tissue, carbenicillin levels were 4 - 14 times less than in normal renal tissue. Although carbenicillin has been claimed to interfere with renal excretion of gentamicin, no interactions were observed between these compounds in rats with normal or one-fifth normal renal parenchyma.[126] Elimination rate constants of both carbenicillin and gentamicin were reduced only to one-half normal values in rats with one-fifth parenchyma, indicating high excretion by residual nephrons.

Renal elimination of carbenicillin is increased in children with early diabetes mellitus, resulting in a reduction in serum carbenicillin $t_{0.5}$ from 50 to 34 min.[127] Increased carbenicillin clearance is accompanied by increased GFR, which may in turn be related to increased kidney size. Increased clearance in early-stage diabetic children was demonstrated previously for penicillin G.[128] The pharmacokinetics of two carbenicillin esters, carfecillin and carindacillin, were found to be similar in man.[129] After 1 g p.o. doses, peak serum levels of antibiotic averaging 15.6 - 17.0 μg ml^{-1} were obtained at 1 h. Both drugs had $t_{0.5}$ values of < 1 h, and 24-h urinary recovery accounted for 42 - 44% of the dose.

Although carbenicillin is excreted by both glomerular filtration and kidney tubular secretion in man, serum $t_{0.5}$ values, and also urinary carbenicillin excretion, correlate well with creatinine clearance.[130-133] Serum $t_{0.5}$ values of 1 h in normal adults are prolonged to 2.7 h in newborn infants, and to 4 h in babies of low birth weight.[131]

The pharmacokinetics of carbenicillin and ticarcillin have been compared in humans.[134] Ticarcillin had a biological $t_{0.5}$ of 72 min which was significantly, but probably not clinically, different from the value of 65 min for carbenicillin. The distribution of ticarcillin (15.7 1) was also larger than that of carbenicillin (12.3 1) and it was less bound to plasma proteins (50% versus 60%).

After a single 5 g i.v. dose of ticarcillin to patients undergoing abdominal surgery, the drug distributed rapidly into muscle and fat.[135] Tissue:serum concentration ratios averaging 0.1 - 0.3 were observed during 1 - 9 h postdose. In 12 healthy volunteers, the mean $t_{0.5}$ values from i.v. and i.m. doses of ticarcillin were similar,

0.9 and 1.3 h, respectively, while the serum clearance was 192 ml min^{-1} 1.73 m^{-2} for the i.v. dose.[136] Intramuscular dosage preparations of ticarcillin in aqueous solution and in 3% benzyl alcohol yielded similar rates and extents of systemic bioavailability; urinary recoveries from these formulations over 12 h were 83 and 76%, respectively, compared with 86% after an i.v. dose.

Predosing with probenecid increased ticarcillin $t_{0.5}$, from a mean control value of 1.3 h to 2.1 h.[137] Data from a single patient showed that the pharmacokinetics of ticarcillin were unaffected by concurrent administration of the cancer chemotherapeutic agent cisplatin.[138]

The elimination $t_{0.5}$ of ticarcillin is markedly dependent on renal function, increasing from <u>ca</u>. 1 h in normal renal function to 15 - 20 h in severe renal impairment.[139-142] However, therapeutic levels of antibiotic are obtained at all levels of renal function, and the elimination $t_{0.5}$ of ticarcillin is reduced to 3 - 4 h during haemodialysis, and to 9 h during peritoneal dialysis.[141-142]

<u>Oxacillin, Cloxacillin, Dicloxacillin, Flucloxacillin</u>

This group of penicillinase-resistant penicillins is characterized by their p.o. activity and extensive binding to plasma proteins in man. Oxacillin is extensively metabolized in man. Approximately 27% of a 500 mg p.o. dose was recovered intact in the 0 - 10 h urine whereas the metabolites penicilloic acid, 5-hydroxymethyl derivative, and pencilloic acid of the 5-hydroxymethyl derivative accounted for 16, 22, and 22% of the dose, respectively.[143]

High protein binding of oxacillin, cloxacillin, dicloxacillin, and nafcillin in dogs caused less efficient penetration of these compounds into ascitic fluid compared to some other penicillins, although the binding effect was reduced after repeated doses.[144] Total concentrations of antibiotic in ascitic fluid could be predicted with some accuracy from relative binding to serum and ascitic fluid proteins. While both oxacillin and methicillin penetrate into bone to some extent, superior penetration was obtained with cephalothin in patients, despite lower serum levels of the cephalosporin.[145]

Serum levels of oxacillin, and other penicillins and cephalosporins, may be predicted with some accuracy when binding to both serum and tissue proteins is taken into account. By incorporating the binding characteristics to various tissues, Peterson et al.[146] obtained high correlations between predicted and actual β-point (extrapolated β-phase) serum levels for 5 of 6 antibiotics. The values obtained are given in Table 3.1.

Table 3.1 Predicted and actual peak equilibrium serum antibiotic concentration (β-point) for 30 mg kg^{-1} rapid i.v. dose. Predicted values are based on observed binding of antibiotics to serum and tissue proteins.

Antibiotic	Predicted β point (mg 100 ml^{-1})	Actual β point (mg 100 ml^{-1})
Methicillin	5.1	5.1
Cefazolin	6.9	6.7
Cefamandole	7.5	7.2
Penicillin G	10.6	11.8
Oxacillin	6.5	5.6
Nafcillin	16.5	2.2

Reproduced by permission from *J. Antimicrob. Chemother.*, 1979, *5*, 219.

Oral doses of sodium cloxacillin give rise to similar serum antibiotic levels to equivalent i.m. doses of sodium oxacillin.[147] In another study, the availability of dicloxacillin and cloxacillin from 2 g p.o. doses to volunteers was calculated to be 49 and 37%, respectively, from area analysis, but higher estimates of 74 and 49% were obtained from urinary excretion data.[148] Absorption of cloxacillin was somewhat lower and was more variable than that of dicloxacillin. Some evidence was presented for dose-dependent elimination kinetics of dicloxacillin, with elimination rates decreasing at higher doses, presumably due to saturation of renal tubular secretion. Intra-ocular penetration of cloxacillin is extremely poor, and the antibiotic was not detected in aqueous humour following 1 - 4 g doses to patients undergoing cataract surgery.[149] Even with subconjunctival injections, a dose of 250 mg was required to obtain therapeutically effective cloxacillin levels in aqueous humour.[150]

Probenecid significantly reduced tissue distribution of ampicillin, benzylpenicillin and cloxacillin in lactating ewes.[151] Reduced excretion of antibiotics in milk due to probenecid was rationalized by identifying milk with a pharmacokinetic tissue compartment, as no changes in drug partitioning or protein binding due to probenecid were observed. Probenecid had no effect on the distribution kinetics of cloxacillin in man in the absence of kidney function.[152] Thus, evidence has been presented that reported changes in drug disposition due to probenecid are due to kinetic rather than distribution factors. On the other hand, probenecid has been shown to increase the penetration of oxacillin into fibrin clots *in vitro*.[153] The mechanism for this is not known, but it appears to be unrelated to changes in drug-protein interactions.

Subtherapeutic levels of dicloxacillin were reported in a neonate, even after daily doses of 175 mg kg^{-1} d^{-1}.[151] The cause of inadequate levels is obscure, but enhanced renal secretion, due possibly to induction by dicloxacillin itself or by coadministered phenobarbital, may have been responsible.

Following single i.v. doses of 10, 20, and 40 mg kg^{-1} in the rabbit, dicloxacillin rapidly distributed into muscle tissue.[154] Elimination $t_{0.5}$ values in serum and muscle were similar, about 40 to 60 min, and were independent of dose (Figure 3.3). In man, administration of dicloxacillin (250 mg i.v.) in the presence of sulfaethidole, a protein binding displacer, resulted in significantly elevated serum concentrations of the penicillin.[155] The mean $t_{0.5}$ of dicloxacillin also increased from 0.96 h to 1.43 h, apparently due to sulfaethidole-induced changes in its extravascular distribution.

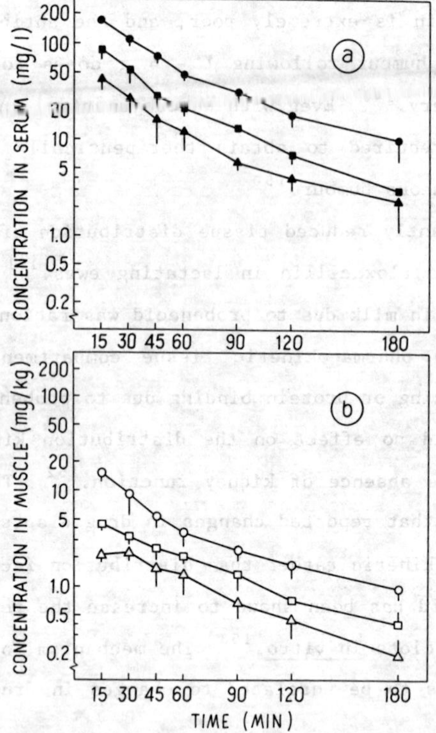

Figure 3.3   Concentrations of dicloxacillin in rabbit
serum (a; filled symbols) and muscle pieces (b; open
symbols) after intravenous injection at the following
dose levels: 10 mg kg^{-1} (▲,△); 20 mg kg^{-1} (■ , □);
and 40 mg kg^{-1} (●,o). Reproduced by permission from
<u>J. Antimicrob. Chemother</u>., 1982, <u>9</u>, 201.

After p.o. dosing to man flucloxacillin gives generally higher
serum levels of total and free drug compared to oxacillin, cloxacillin, and dicloxacillin.[156]   Absorption of flucloxacillin was delayed
in unfasted subjects and serum levels were <u>ca</u>. one-half those in
fasting subjects.

Plasma protein binding of cloxacillin and flucloxacillin was
examined in 7 newborn infants and their mothers and in 7 healthy non-
pregnant women serving as controls.[157]   As shown in Figures 3.4 and
3.5, binding of these drugs in the mothers increased during the first
postnatal week while that in the infants decreased. The decrease in

binding in the infants correlated with an increase in bilirubin levels. In the controls, both cloxacillin and flucloxacillin were greater than 90% bound. The maternal:foetal ratio of blood or plasma concentration was <u>ca</u>. 1 for cloxacillin and 0.8 for flucloxacillin. Flucloxacillin was rapidly distributed into human heart and lung tissues, reaching concentrations as much as 22 and 36%, respectively, of the serum antibiotic level following an i.m. dose.[158] In contrast, practically no flucloxacillin was found in pericardial fluid.

After p.o. (0.75 - 1 g) or i.v. (0.5 g) doses of flucloxacillin to patients with normal kidney function, the plasma $t_{0.5}$ and renal clearance values were 49 min and 69 ml min^{-1}, respectively, for parent compound and 56 min and 144 ml min^{-1} for the active metabolite hydroxyflucloxacillin.[159] In patients with severe renal insuf-

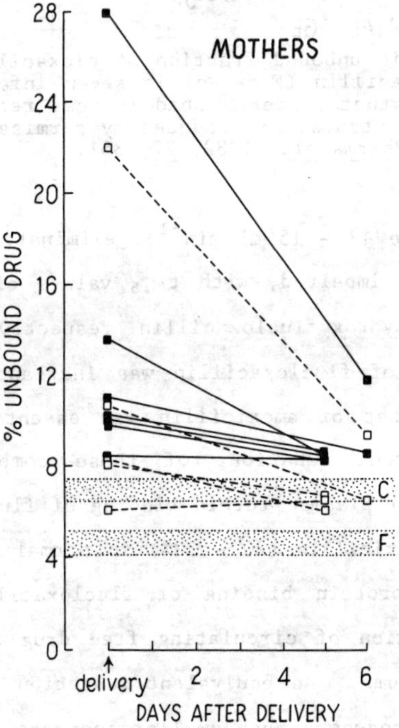

Figure 3.4   Change in unbound fraction of cloxacillin (C, ▪——▪) and flucloxacillin (F, ▫--▫) in seven mothers during the first postnatal week. Shaded areas represent range of controls. Reproduced by permission from <u>Eur. J. Clin. Pharmacol</u>., 1982, <u>22</u>, 351.

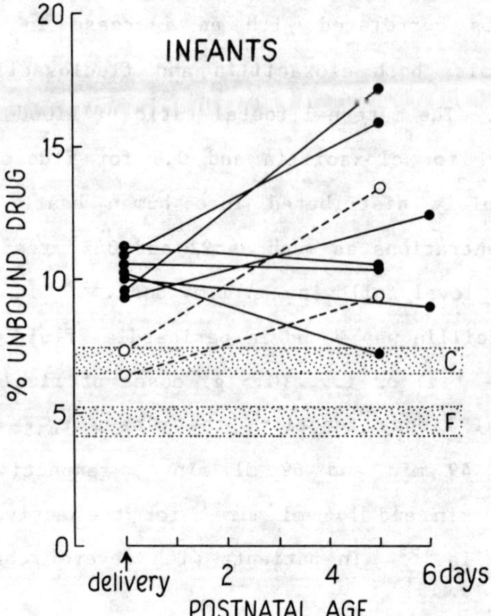

Figure 3.5 Change in unbound fraction of cloxacillin (C,●-●) and flucloxacillin (F,o---o) in seven infants during the first postnatal week. Shaded areas represent range of the controls. Reproduced by permission from Eur. J. Clin. Pharmacol., 1982, 22, 351.

ficiency (creatinine clearance 13 - 15 ml min^{-1}), elimination of the antibiotics was significantly impaired, with $t_{0.5}$ values of 2.6 and 4.9 h for flucloxacillin and hydroxyflucloxacillin, respectively.

The distribution volume of flucloxacillin was increased in the uraemic condition, whereas that of amoxicillin was essentially unchanged.[160,161] The different behaviour of these compounds is probably due to the high (90%) plasma protein binding of flucloxacillin compared with that of amoxicillin (20 - 30%) in normal subjects. Thus a small reduction in protein binding of flucloxacillin will markedly increase the proportion of circulating free drug and hence the apparent distribution volume. An equivalent reduction in amoxicillin protein binding will produce a much smaller increase in circulating free drug and consequently only a small increase in apparent distribution volume. The high protein binding of flucloxacillin, even in severe uraemia, is reflected in the low plasma clearance of this compound during haemodialysis.[162,163]

Azlocillin, Azidocillin, Mezlocillin

Azlocillin is well absorbed after p.o. doses to children, resulting in serum levels of total drug considerably higher than those obtained with p.o. dosed ampicillin.[164] Rapid absorption of azidocillin has been demonstrated also in dogs and rats.[165] Azidocillin is less bound to serum proteins than ampicillin and has a biological $t_{0.5}$ of $\underline{ca}$. 30 min.

Penetration of azlocillin and mezlocillin into c.s.f. was studied in the rabbit.[166] As shown in Figure 3.6, antibiotic concentrations in c.s.f. were negligible after parenteral doses in normal rabbits, but increased considerably in rabbits with meningitis. Concentrations in c.s.f. and serum were directly related to administered dose. For both compounds, the ratio of mean peak c.s.f. to serum concentration ranged from 0.05 after i.m. dosing to greater than 0.1 following i.v. administration. Similarly, in 9 patients with acute meningitis who received 5 g i.v. mezlocillin, c.s.f.:serum concentration ratios of 0 - 0.11 were observed.[167] Other investigators have described the distribution of azlocillin, mezlocillin, and oxacillin into the bone, tissues, and peritoneal and pleural cavities.[168-171]

In healthy subjects who received 1 g i.v. mezlocillin the mean elimination $t_{0.5}$ and total body clearance were $\underline{ca}$. 50 min and 400 ml min^{-1} 1.73 m^{-2}, respectively.[172] Similar $t_{0.5}$ value was reported after i.m. doses of mezlocillin, and this was not affected by probenecid, although the latter significantly reduced renal and non-renal clearances of mezlocillin. Approximately 50% of an i.v. dose of mezlocillin was recovered unchanged in the urine, indicating that 50% of the dose is cleared by extrarenal routes. Following 2 g i.v. doses of mezlocillin[173] and azlocillin[174] to patients with T-tube drainage, biliary excretion averaged 22.1% and 5.3% of the respective doses in patients with normal liver function, but decreased to 3.2 and 0.4%, respectively, in those with impaired liver function. Brogard et al.[175] administered 1 g i.m. mezlocillin to cholecystectomized patients with T-tubes and reported a 12 h biliary excretion of 2.6% of

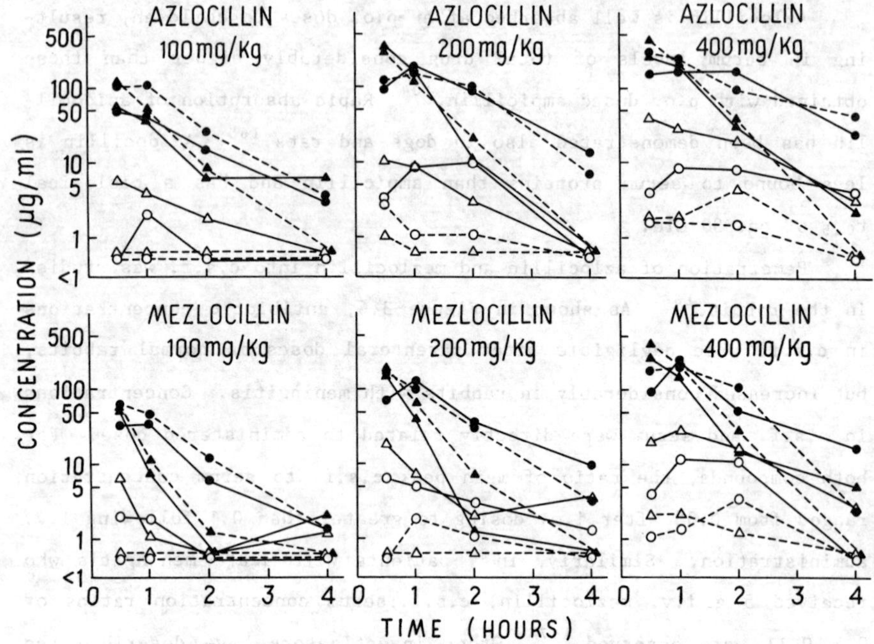

Figure 3.6   Mean serum concentrations (solid symbols) and cerebrospinal fluid concentrations (open symbols) of azlocillin and mezlocillin after i.m. (circles) or i.v. (triangles) administration to normal rabbits (broken lines) and rabbits with experimentally induced *P. aeruginosa* meningitis (solid lines). Reproduced by permission from *Antimicrob. Ag. Chemother.*, 1982, *22*, 909.

the dose. In these studies, $t_{0.5}$ of mezlocillin was 80 – 90 min, shorter than that of azlocillin, 110 min. Azlocillin also appeared in bronchial secretions, observed drug concentrations being 30 – 240 µg g^{-1} after a 75 mg kg^{-1} i.v. dose to children.[176]

The elimination kinetics of azlocillin and mezlocillin in newborn infants appear to be independent of the state of maturity at birth,[177,178] but are determined by age.[178]   After 75 – 100 mg i.v. or i.m. doses, the $t_{0.5}$ of mezlocillin averaged 2.6 h in infants over 7 d of age and 4.3 h in those 7 d or younger.[179]

Azlocillin pharmacokinetics were shown to be dose-dependent, with saturation of both renal and nonrenal elimination pathways at elevated dose levels.[180,181] After i.v. doses of 1, 2, and 5 g azlocillin to 10 healthy volunteers in a crossover study, respective serum $t_{0.5}$ values were 0.9, 1.0, and 1.5 h.[181] In addition to a disproportionate increase in serum AUC, cumulative urinary recovery of unchanged azlocillin also increased from 59% of the 1 g dose to 75% of the 5 g dose. Renal clearances for the 1, 2, and 5 g doses were 7.1, 6.5, and 4.8 l h^{-1}, respectively, while the nonrenal clearances were 5.1, 2.9, and 1.8 l h^{-1}. After a 30 min i.v. infusion of 80 mg kg^{-1} to subjects with chronic renal impairment, azlocillin $t_{0.5}$ values were 2.0, 4.0, and 5.7 h in patients with creatinine clearances of 30 - 50, 10 - 30, and < 10 ml min^{-1} 1.73 m^{-2}, respectively.[182] The $t_{0.5}$ was reduced by <u>ca.</u> 50% during haemodialysis.[182-184]

The disposition kinetics of mezlocillin are similarly influenced by both dose size and renal function over the 1 - 5 g dosage range.[185] After administering 1, 3, and 5 g mezlocillin as single i.v. doses at 1 week intervals to 6 normal subjects and 6 anuric patients, dose-dependent kinetics were observed only in the latter.[186] The respective clearance values, which reflected nonrenal excretion, were 194, 97, and 68 ml min^{-1} while the corresponding $t_{0.5}$ values were 1.7, 2.2, and 2.3 h with increasing dose. Reduced clearance from high mezlocillin doses appears to be related primarily to saturable non-renal elimination, either metabolism or biliary excretion. The elimination $t_{0.5}$ of mezlocillin is 30% shorter than that of carbenicillin after equivalent doses to healthy individuals.[187]

Other investigators have reported mezlocillin $t_{0.5}$ values varying from <u>ca.</u> 1 h in patients with creatinine clearances over 60 ml min^{-1} to 1.6 - 3.6 h in those with creatinine clearances below 10 ml min^{-1}.[188-191] As shown in Figure 3.7, cumulative urinary recovery of mezlocillin progressively decreased with declining renal function.[192] However, since extrarenal pathways also play an important role in mezlocillin elimination, the overall clearance of this drug is only moderately impaired in renal insufficiency.

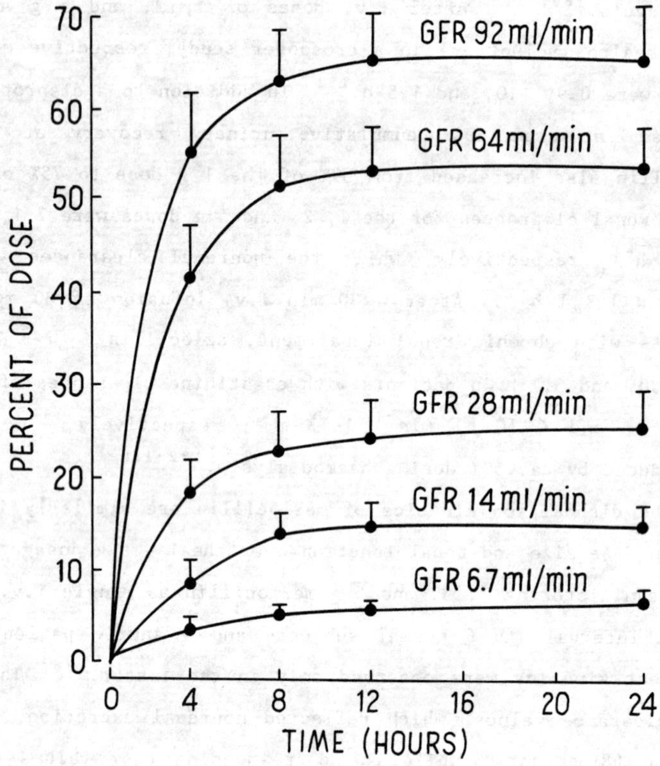

Figure 3.7 Cumulative urinary recovery of mezlocillin (as percentage of dose administered) for various degrees of renal insufficiency (GFR). Bars represent mean ± standard error, n = 40. Reproduced by permission from <u>Antimicrob. Ag. Chemother</u>., 1980, <u>18</u>, 81.

Dosage adjustment of mezlocillin is thus necessary only in severe renal impairment.[189,192,193] Haemodialysis is somewhat more effective than peritoneal dialysis in clearing mezlocillin, although both contribute to only a minor degree to mezlocillin elimination.[192,194,195]

Other Penicillin Derivatives

Sultamicillin is hydrolyzed during enteral absorption to form ampicillin and sulbactam, a β-lactamase inhibitor. Multiple dosing studies in 6 healthy male subjects showed that serum ampicillin levels from sultamicillin were approximately 2-fold higher than those following an equivalent dose of ampicillin.[196] Urinary recovery data also suggested greater bioavailability of ampicillin from sultamicillin. The $t_{0.5}$ values of both ampicillin and sulbactam were <u>ca</u>. 1 h, thus causing no accumulation of drug during a t.i.d. regimen.

After i.v. dosing, the mean serum $t_{0.5}$ of sulbenicillin was 27 min in control subjects, 1.5 h in patients with GFR values between 14 and 45 ml min^{-1}, and 4.6 h when GFR was 8 - 10 ml min^{-1}.[197] The sulbenicillin dose was completely recovered in urine within 12 h except in patients with GFR values less than 10 ml min^{-1}.

Temocillin penetrated readily into blister fluids, reaching concentrations <u>ca</u>. 50% of those in serum at 2 - 3 h after an i.v. dose.[198] The mean elimination $t_{0.5}$ of temocillin in serum was 4.5 h, similar to that in blister fluid, while plasma and renal clearances were 25 and 20 ml min^{-1}, respectively.

Intravenous doses of 200 mg mecillinam produced initial serum levels of 6.9 μg ml^{-1} in healthy volunteers.[199] Thereafter, drug levels declined biexponentially with a mean terminal $t_{0.5}$ of 0.8 h. The systemic availability of mecillinam from p.o. dosed pivmecillinam in tablets is 65 - 70%, and a 400 mg dose of pivmecillinam produced peak serum levels of 2.0 μg ml^{-1} at 1 - 1.5 h postdose.

The bioavailability of mecillinam after a p.o. dose of bacmecillinam appeared to be greater than that from pivmecillinam. In 12 healthy fasting subjects who received 400 mg tablets of the two drugs as the respective hydrochloride salts peak plasma mecillinam concentrations were 4.6 μg ml^{-1} from bacmecillinam and 2.4 μg ml^{-1} from pivmecillinam.[200] Absorption efficiency of mecillinam is identical from i.m. and i.v. doses, while serum AUC values are proportional to dose size for 200, 400, and 800 mg doses.[201]

The mean $t_{0.5}$ of mecillinam was 51 min following a 10 mg kg^{-1} i.v. infusion, while the plasma and renal clearances averaged 3.5 and 2.5 ml min^{-1} kg^{-1}.[202] Approximately 70% of the dose was recovered unchanged in 24 h urine. Therapeutic concentrations of mecillinam were obtained in bile at 1 - 3 h following a single 800 mg i.m. dose, averaging 40 mg l^{-1} in the functioning gallbladder and 49 mg l^{-1} in the common bile duct.[203]

The serum mecillinam $t_{0.5}$ is increased to approximately 1.5 h, and serum levels of drug are increased, by probenecid.[204] Resting subjects experienced a reduced rate of drug clearance compared to moderately active individuals, but peak serum drug levels were also reduced, suggesting a larger drug distribution volume in resting individuals.[205] The elimination of mecillinam is less efficient in elderly (> 65 yr) patients than in younger individuals, and the bio-logical $t_{0.5}$ is increased from a normal value of 0.9 h to 4.0 h.[206] Reduced elimination in elderly patients occurs despite renal function being normal for that age group, and is associated with reduced drug recovery in urine.

The pharmacokinetics of azthreonam were examined following a 1 g i.v. dose to 6 healthy male subjects.[207] The decline in serum drug levels was rapid and biexponential, showing an apparent distribution volume, V_β, of 17.2 l and a terminal $t_{0.5}$ of 1.9 h. Total clearance of azthreonam was 89 ml min^{-1}, and 74% of the dose was recovered in 24 h urine. Drug penetrated into blister fluid, reaching a maximum level of 25.4 µg ml^{-1} at 1.8 h postdose and subsequently was eliminated at a rate similar to serum azthreonam.

In rabbits with meningitis, 25 mg kg^{-1} i.v. doses of N-formimi-doyl thienamycin yielded a mean peak c.s.f. concentration of 2.5 µg ml^{-1} at 45 min.[208] The c.s.f.:serum AUC ratio was 0.31, and the $t_{0.5}$ of the antibiotic was similar in serum and in c.s.f., *ca.* 1.5 h. In contrast, negligible levels of N-formimidoyl thienamycin were found in animals without meningeal inflammation (Figure 3.8).

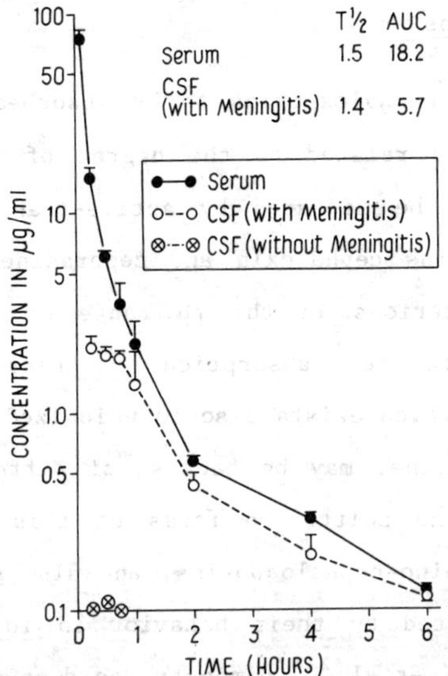

Figure 3.8   Serum and c.s.f. concentrations of N-formimidoyl thienamycin after a 25 mg kg^{-1} dose given intravenously to rabbits with (or without) experimental E. coli Kl meningitis. $t_{0.5}$ values are in hours and AUC values are in microgram hours per milliliter. Reproduced by permission from <u>Antimicrob. Ag. Chemother.</u>, 1982, <u>21</u>, 390.

Cephalosporins and Cephamycins

The cephalosporins became established as a major class of semi-synthetic broad spectrum antibiotics during the review period and new derivatives have continued to be generated, giving rise to first, second, and third generation compounds. A considerable number of reviews have been published on the pharmacology, pharmacokinetics, clinical pharmacokinetics, and pharmacodynamics of both new and established cephalosporins.[209-213] Despite the large number of compounds that have been developed only a small number have been shown to be orally active, the majority requiring parenteral administration. In this review, attention will focus first on the orally active cephalosporins and subsequently on the first, second, and third and later generation parenteral compounds.

The Orally Active Cephalosporins

The ability of the amino-cephalosporins to be absorbed systemically after p.o. doses may be related to the degree of ionization within the GI tract, and may be mediated by active-transport processes. The oral cephalosporins cephalexin and cephradine exist as uncharged molecules and zwitterions in the pH range of the small intestine, and this may promote their absorption.[214] Less efficient absorption of cephaloglycine, which exists also in unionized forms and zwitterion forms in the intestine, may be because of different proportions of unionized forms and zwitterion forms of this compound. Saturable absorption of the amino-cephalosporins, and also some other compounds, is strongly suggested by their behavior in _in situ_ rat intestinal preparations. Tsuji et al.[215] demonstrated dose-dependency in the disappearance of cephalexin and cephradine from intestinal loops, the proportion of drug absorbed decreasing with increasing dose, and proposed that absorption occurs by combined first-order and Michaelis-Menten kinetics as shown in equation 3.2. In this equation,

$$\frac{dC}{dt} = - \frac{V_{max}C}{K_m + C} - (k_1 + k_2)C \qquad (3.2)$$

C is drug concentration in the intestine and k_1 and k_2 are first-order absorption and degradation constants. Saturable cephalosporin absorption has not been demonstrated in man.

Cephalexin, Cephradine, Cefaclor, Cefadroxil, Cefroxadine, Cefatrizine

Studies carried out over a limited therapeutic dose range have failed to demonstrate dose dependency in the absorption of cephalexin and cephradine from commercial dosage forms.[216,217] Their absorption characteristics are almost identical at the same dose level.[218] The reliability of cephalexin absorption is demonstrated by the very small effect that different formulations[219] or acute illness[220] have on serum profiles of this antibiotic.

Absorption of cephalexin and cephradine is more rapid under fasting compared to nonfasting conditions.[221] Peak serum concentrations of cephalexin are related to the magnitude of p.o. doses, but not to the size of i.m. injections. This may be due to deposition and subsequent slow release of drug from the injection site.[222] Depot formation may also explain the relatively low serum levels and long $t_{0.5}$ values of cephalexin after i.m. administration, but it does not explain almost quantitative urinary recovery of antibiotic from this route compared with 50% of i.v. and p.o. doses.[223] Both the absorption and excretion of cephalexin are impaired in newborn infants, in which the 24 h urinary recovery of antibiotic accounted for 5 - 66% of a daily p.o. dose.[224]

In contrast to sodium cephalexin,[225] the l-lysine salt of cephalexin was efficiently absorbed following deep i.m. injection in man.[226] Intramuscular injection of 1 g lysine cephalexin yielded mean peak serum cephalexin levels of 24 $\mu g\ ml^{-1}$ after 30 min compared with 27 $\mu g\ ml^{-1}$ at 60 min following an equivalent dose of cephalexin monohydrate. These levels were considerably higher than those obtained from i.m. sodium cephalexin and are probably due to better solubility and buffering capacity of the lysine salt.

Penetration of cephalexin into human sinus mucosal tissue and secretions was extremely variable following p.o. doses.[227] Although mucosal drug levels were considerably higher than those found in secretions, cephalexin would not be expected to be readily effective against <u>Haemophilis influenzae</u> at these sites. Cephalexin also penetrated poorly into human prostatic tissue and semen, with drug levels at these sites constantly falling below the MIC values of organisms associated with chronic bacterial prostatitis.[228]

Comparison of antibiotic concentrations in sputum and serum in patients with acute respiratory infections suggested that cephalexin enters bronchial mucus by a passive process.[229] High sputum levels in some patients may be due to loss of integrity of the blood-bronchus barrier during inflammation. Cephalexin rapidly crosses the human placenta, and peak maternal and cord-serum levels both occur at about 1.5 - 2 h after p.o. dosing to the mother.[230]

Cephalexin, cephalothin, and cephaloridine were shown, unlike the tetracyclines, to penetrate into bone to a very limited extent after s.c. or p.o. doses to rats.[231] Ratios of bone to serum concentrations averaged 1:4 for cephalothin, 1:7 for cephaloridine, and 1:9 for cephalexin during 0.25 - 4 h after dosing. Despite the differences in concentrations, the $t_{0.5}$ values in bone and serum were similar. Greene et al.[232] suggest that evaluation of cephalexin pharmacokinetics in terms of a simple one-compartment model can give incorrect estimates of drug elimination and distribution. The discussion is based principally on the observation by Wagner[233] that the two-compartment model collapses to a one-compartment model, provided that the ratio in equation 3.3, where A and B are intercepts of the fast (α) and slow (β) drug elimination slopes, k_{21} is a distribution rate constant, and

$$\frac{B}{A + B} = \frac{(k_{21} - \beta)}{(\alpha - \beta)} = \frac{V_1}{V_{d(extrap)}} \tag{3.3}$$

V_1 and $V_{d(extrap)}$ are the central and extrapolated distribution volumes, is equal to or greater than 0.9. Greene et al.[232] obtained a mean value for B/(A + B) of 0.44 indicating the requirement of two-compartment model interpretation for cephalexin. However one-compartment model interpretation may be sufficiently accurate for most clinical purposes.

The pharmacokinetics of cephalexin were studied using a temporal curve-displacement method based on normalized times for peak serum concentrations.[234] Dose-independent kinetics were observed in man over the dose range 250 - 1000 mg. Drug accumulation occurred during five 1000 mg doses at 6 h intervals, but not with 500 mg doses.

Cephalexin is normally rapidly eliminated and has a plasma $t_{0.5}$ of $\underline{ca}$. 1 h.   In patients with renal failure the $t_{0.5}$ of cephalexin may increase up to $\underline{ca}$. 18 h depending on the severity of the condition.   The $t_{0.5}$ is only partially reduced by haemodialysis.[235] Cephalexin is excreted in human bile, although biliary concentrations are considerably lower than in serum, and peak concentrations do not occur until 2 - 3 h after dosing.   Biliary excretion is decreased in obstructive biliary disease but may be increased by probenecid administration.[236,237]

The oral cephalosporin cefaclor yields somewhat lower serum levels compared with cephradine, cephalexin, and cefadroxil in human volunteers.[238,239]   Cefaclor also has a somewhat shorter biological $t_{0.5}$ of 0.6 h compared with the value of 1 h commonly reported for the other oral cephalosporins, and this is probably related to the relative chemical instability of cefaclor.[239]   Typical serum profiles from 500 mg doses of the four oral cephalosporins are shown in Figure 3.9.   Although peak serum levels of cefaclor are reduced by

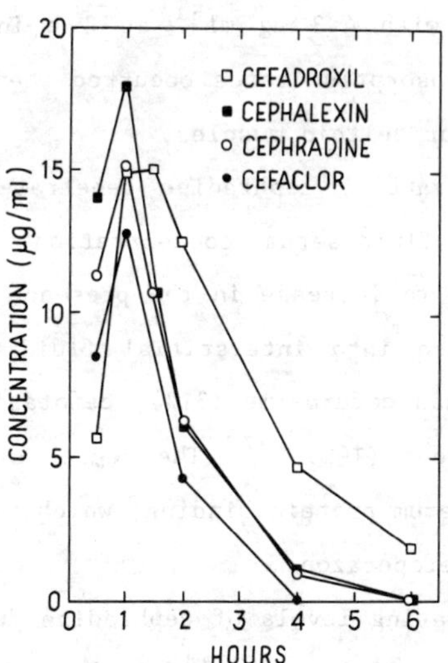

Figure 3.9   Serum concentrations of cefadroxil, cephradine, and cefaclor after single oral doses of 500 mg of each drug.   Reproduced by permission from J. Clin. Pharmacol., 1978, 18, 174.

concomitant milk in children, the overall availability of drug is unaffected.[240]

Cephradine is efficiently absorbed after p.o., i.v., and s.c. doses to mice, rats, and dogs, while absorption was poor following rectal doses.[241] The antibiotic is extensively distributed in the rat, with concentrations in kidneys and liver exceeding plasma levels eightfold and threefold, respectively. The drug $t_{0.5}$ value in both dogs and rats was about 1 h. The absorption of p.o. dosed cephradine in man was delayed in nonfasted subjects, and serum antibiotic levels were considerably reduced.[242] However, the overall absorption efficiency, estimated from areas under serum level curves, was similar in fasted and nonfasted subjects. Cephradine has been shown to be equally bioavailable from i.v. and i.m. injections, and from p.o. dosed capsules and suspensions.[243]

Sex differences have been noted in the absorption rates of cephradine from the gluteus maximus muscle in humans.[244] Drug absorption was faster in males, producing peak plasma levels of 11 µg ml^{-1} at 0.6 h compared with 4.3 µg ml^{-1} at 2 h in females. No sex-related differences in absorption rates occurred when drug was injected into vastus lateralis or deltoid muscles.

After i.m. doses to the rabbit, cephradine penetrated rapidly into pleural fluid.[245] The fluid:serum concentration ratio was approximately 0.6, and appeared to increase in the presence of infection.[246] Cephradine penetration into interstitial fluid in humans averaged 47%, more efficient than cefuroxime (31%), cefotaxime (27%), cefoxitine (25%), and cefoperazone (10%).[247] The degree of penetration was inversely related to serum protein binding, which ranged from 10% for cephradine to 90% for cefoperazone.

Marked increases in circulating levels of cephradine due to probenecid treatment have been reported in mice.[248] Probenecid inhibits renal tubular secretion of cephradine but has little effect on its distribution characteristics.[249] Cephradine serum clearance and

$t_{0.5}$ were 17.2 ml min^{-1} and 0.8 h, respectively, after a 500-mg i.v. dose alone compared with 9.4 ml min^{-1} and 1.5 h in the presence of probenecid.

Renal elimination of cephradine, which contains both a carboxylic acid group and an amino group, is reduced in alkaline urine but is not altered in acidic urine.[250] This is consistent with the pKa values of the functional groups. However, the area under the serum level-time curve is also reduced in prealkalinized subjects, and speculated causes for this include hydrolysis of cephradine in the gut lumen or gut wall, and base trapping in the kidney tubules.[251]

The bioavailability of p.o. cefaclor appears to be dose-independent within the therapeutic range. Peak serum concentrations averaged 9 µg ml^{-1} following a 250 mg dose[252] and 35 µg ml^{-1} following a 1000 mg dose,[253] both attained at <u>ca</u>. 1 h. In normal subjects, mean cefaclor $t_{0.5}$ was 0.5 h, and 67% of a single dose was excreted unchanged in 24 h urine.[254]

Circulating levels of cefaclor are increased by probenecid, as are the elimination $t_{0.5}$ and corrected AUC values of cefaclor and cephradine.[255] This study provides another example of a possible interaction by probenecid directly influencing drug distribution. The concept of a specific interaction with probenecid is supported by the observation that peak serum levels of cefaclor in patients with mild renal impairment are similar to those in normal renal function despite an increased elimination $t_{0.5}$ of 1.4 - 2.7 h in uraemic patients.[256]

Although cefaclor is cleared largely by renal excretion, drug clearance is not markedly influenced in renal failure.[257] The drug $t_{0.5}$ was 40 - 60 min in normal individuals, and this value increased to 3 h in essentially anephric patients. Analysis of the data suggests either that 25% of the drug is normally cleared via extrarenal routes, or that these routes come into play when renal function is compromised. In another study, cefaclor $t_{0.5}$ averaged 2.2 h in patients with creatinine clearances of 5 - 15 ml min^{-1} 1.73 m^{-2}.

Less than 9% of the dose was recovered in urine during 0 - 24 h.
Haemodialysis removed <u>ca</u>. 34% of the cefaclor dose and reduced its
$t_{0.5}$ to 1.4 h.[254]   In cholecystectomized patients with inserted
T-tubes, the cumulative biliary excretion of cefaclor amounted to only
0.05% of a 1 g p.o. dose.[258]

The bioavailability of cefadroxil was similar from single 500 mg
p.o. doses given as a solution, suspension, and capsule, approximately
80 - 90% of an i.v. reference dose.[259] Plasma peak concentrations and
AUC values were proportional to dose in the 250 - 1500 mg range
(Figure 3.10), and 80 - 90% of each single dose was recovered in 24 h
urine.[260,261]   Administration of 2.5 g of probenecid with 500 mg
cefadroxil prolonged the mean cefadroxil serum $t_{0.5}$ from 1.1 to 1.6

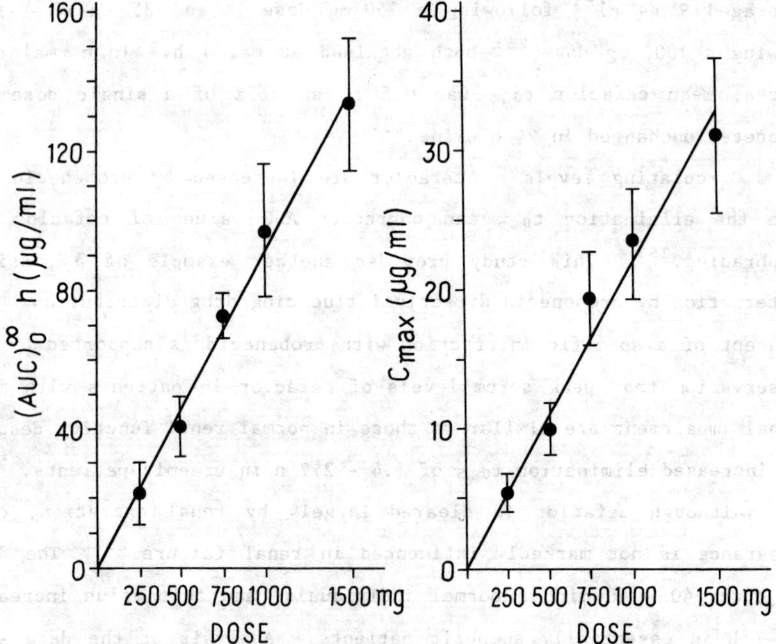

Figure 3.10   Linear relationship between $(AUC)_0^\infty$ and
C_{max} for cefadroxil, and dose.   Reproduced by permission from <u>Eur. J. Clin. Pharmacol</u>., 1980, <u>18</u>, 505.

h while having no significant effect on its distribution volume.[262]
The cefadroxil $t_{0.5}$ in children (1 - 11 yr) appeared to be similar

to that in adults,[263,264] but it was considerably longer in infants (4 - 10 months), averaging _ca_. 2.3 h following a 25 mg kg^{-1} p.o. dose.[264]

During multiple p.o. doses of 1000 mg cefadroxil t.i.d. in 8 healthy volunteers, mean peak serum concentrations increased from 27.5 µg ml^{-1} on day 1 to 35.5 µg ml^{-1} on day 8, suggesting some accumulation of the antibiotic.[265] The plasma $t_{0.5}$ of cefadroxil increased from 1.4 - 1.6 h in normal subjects to 20 - 25 h in patients with severe renal impairment.[266-270] During haemodialysis, the elimination $t_{0.5}$ was reduced to 3.4 h.[268] Renal impairment does not significantly modify the distribution of cefadroxil.

Oral doses of cefroxadine were rapidly and almost completely absorbed; peak serum drug levels were reached at 0.5 - 1.5 h[271,272] and concentrations were dose-proportional (Figure 3.11).

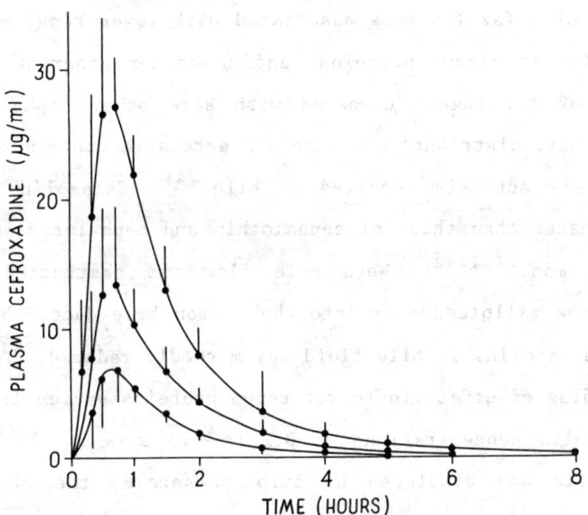

Figure 3.11 Cefroxadine concentrations in plasma after administration of 212, 424, and 847 mg (mean of six subjects ± SD). Reproduced by permission from _J. Pharmacokin. Biopharm._, 1982, _10_, 15.

Cefroxadine elimination kinetics also were linear, with a mean terminal $t_{0.5}$ of 1 h and cumulative urinary excretion of _ca_. 95%

after p.o. and i.v. doses. Although systemic availability of cefatrizine from p.o. doses is only one-half that from i.m. doses,[273] serum and urine levels obtained from a 500 mg p.o. dose exceeded the minimum inhibitory concentrations of susceptible organisms.

Cefazolin, Cephalothin, Cephaloridine, Cephapirin

Intravenous doses of cefazolin yielded higher and more prolonged serum levels than cephaloridine, cephradine, cefazaflur, cephalothin, cephacetril, and cephapirin,[274,275] while i.v. cefamandole yielded 50% higher drug levels in serum than cephapirin and cephalothin.[276] Cefazolin is rapidly absorbed after i.m. injections yielding serum levels twice as high as an equivalent dose of cephalothin.[277] Dose-related peak cefazolin levels were reached 1 h following a single i.m. injection and declined with a plasma $t_{0.5}$ of 2-3 h.[278-280] Higher serum levels of cefazolin were associated with lower renal clearance, greater binding to plasma proteins, and a smaller apparent distribution volume of this agent compared with some other cephalosporins. Despite the small distribution volume and extensive protein binding of cefazolin it is actively secreted in bile.[281] Cefazolin levels in bile were greater than those of cephalothin and cephaloridine both in rats and in man.[281,282] When bile flow was obstructed in man, either into the gallbladder or into the common bile duct, the appearance of cephalosporins in bile fluid was markedly reduced.[283,284]

The binding of cefazolin to rat serum proteins varied from 81% to 59% at cefazolin concentrations of 0.2 to 1.0 mmol l^{-1}.[285] Protein bound cefazolin was displaced by sulphaphenazole, the displacement effect being dependent on sulphaphenazole concentration. Binding of cefazolin to serum albumin is reduced in uraemic patients, although serum albumin levels are unchanged and the reduced binding is reflected in greater distribution volumes for cefazolin in renal insufficiency. In the dog, cefazolin readily permeates into normal and osteomyelitic bone.[286] In man, serum concentrations of cefazolin resulting from a 10 mg kg^{-1} i.v. infusion of cefazolin were similar when drug was administered alone or together with an equal dose of moxalactam.[287] Elimination $t_{0.5}$ values were 2.0 and 2.2 h for cefazolin and moxalactam, respectively.

Although cefazolin is 80% bound to plasma proteins, compared with 10% for cephaloridine, levels of cefazolin in dog interstitial fluid were higher than those of cephaloridine after i.v. injection.[288] Cefazolin also yielded higher levels in interstitial fluid than cephaloridine in rabbits, while cefamandole yielded lower interstitial fluid levels than the other 2 drugs given i.m.[289] Cephaloridine, however, penetrated into interstitial tissue more rapidly than either cefazolin or cefamandole and yielded the highest levels during 4 h postdose. The longer $t_{0.5}$ of cefazolin compared with the other cephalosporins led to greater accumulation of this drug in interstitial fluid after repeated doses. The degree of accumulation observed for the three compounds is shown in Figure 3.12.

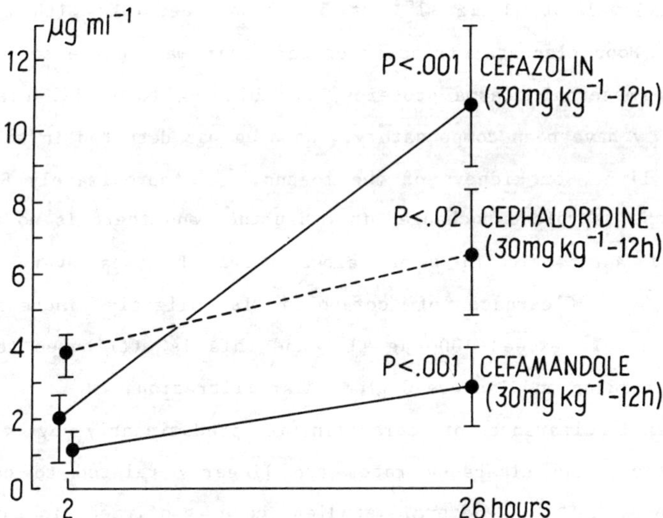

Figure 3.12 Cumulative effect of 3 i.m. injections (30 mg kg^{-1} every 12 h). Comparison of the interstitial concentrations (± 1 SEM) obtained 2 h after the first injection (2 h) and 2 h after the third injection (26 h) of cefazolin, cephaloridine, and cefamandole in rabbits. Reproduced by permission from *Antimicrob. Ag. Chemother.*, 1977, **11**, 594.

Despite their relatively easy entry into interstitial fluid, neither cefazolin nor cephaloridine penetrate the blood brain barrier.[290] Cephalosporin levels in c.s.f. were below the limits of detection in 7 patients receiving 1 g of cephaloridine i.v. and in 5 patients receiving 1 g of cefazolin i.v. Cefazolin crosses inflammed synovial membranes, yielding synovial fluid antibiotic concentrations greater than those in serum within 2 h of an i.m. dose.[291] Both cefazolin and cephaloridine penetrate effectively into wound fluids, achieving levels significantly higher than those in serum.[292] Penetration of cefazolin into human milk is poor, however, and although levels in milk are measurable they are approximately 50-fold lower than simultaneous levels in serum.[293] Cefazolin crosses the placenta inefficiently.[294,295] Following single 14 mg kg^{-1} i.m. doses to healthy pregnant women, maternal serum levels of drug reached peak values of 48 µg ml^{-1} at about 1 h and then declined with a $t_{0.5}$ of 1.5 h. Compared with these values, drug levels in cord serum reached a peak level of 11 µg ml^{-1} at 5.5 h and declined with a $t_{0.5}$ of 5.4 h. Poor placental transfer of cefazolin may be due to binding of drug to maternal plasma proteins, but binding to foetal plasma proteins may have been compensatory. No drug was detected in the c.n.s., lungs, liver, or kidneys of the foetus.[290] Approximately 80% of an i.m. dose is voided unchanged in 6 h urine, and there is no accumulation of antibiotic in serum after repeated doses every 6 or 12 h.[296,297] Clearance of cefazolin is slightly increased when plasma levels exceed 1000 µg ml^{-1} and this is attributed to reduced plasma binding and increased glomerular filtration.

Renal clearance of cefazolin is predominantly by glomerular filtration, and clearance rates are linearly related to creatinine clearance.[298,299] Several studies have confirmed inhibition of cefazolin elimination in impaired renal function.[300,301] In severe uraemia, cefazolin $t_{0.5}$ was reduced from 30 – 40 h to about 4 h during haemodialysis, although peritoneal dialysis had little influence on cefazolin clearance. The apparent distribution volume of cefazolin was significantly increased at creatinine clearance values below 25 ml min^{-1}, presumably resulting from decreased drug binding to plasma proteins.[302]

Reports on the dialysability of cefazolin in uraemic patients are conflicting and appear to depend upon the type of condition, azotaemic or nonazotaemic, the degree of protein binding, and the type of dialyser used.[303,304] Craig et al.[305] found that haemodialysis reduced the drug $t_{0.5}$ from 22.5 h to 2.7 h, and from 21.3 h to 5.0 h in anephric and oliguric patients, respectively, using a Gambro dialyser with cuprophane membranes. Persistence of circulating drug levels, despite dialysis, may be explained in part by back-diffusion of antibiotic from dialysate into blood.

Cefazolin clearance may be reduced to a greater extent in elderly patients than might be predicted from standard renal function indicators.[306] Otaya and Hayashi[307] described an expression for i.v. infusion of rapidly eliminated drugs, with particular reference to cephalothin. The expression includes terms for drug binding to plasma proteins and the fraction of plasma water in blood. Results from this study suggest that cephalothin is rapidly deactivated in plasma water in the absence of, but not in the presence of, protein; assayed drug levels were approximately five times greater in the presence of than in the absence of protein. The stabilizing mechanism of plasma proteins was not elucidated.

Cephalothin penetrates bone less efficiently than lincomycin in rabbits, and bone penetration by both compounds is increased in osteomyelitic bones.[308] Bone antibiotic levels peak at the same time, and concentration-time profiles are similar to those in serum. Cephalothin enters aqueous humour after subconjunctival injections yielding peak levels _ca._ 1 - 2 h after dosing. The ratio of aqueous humour : serum antibiotic levels ranges from 4.0 to 67.0 during 5 h after dosing, and loss of antibiotic from aqueous humour occurs by a biphasic process.[309]

There have been conflicting reports on the effect of cardiopulmonary surgery on cephalothin levels. One study reports that serum antibiotic levels are considerably reduced, and that in children undergoing this treatment conventional cephalothin doses fail to provide therapeutic levels.[310] Another study reports that elimination of cephalothin is reduced during cardiopulmonary by-pass, and this is attributed not only to extra-corporeal circulation but also to reduced hepatic clearance under the surgical conditions.[311]

Early microbiological assays indicated that cephalothin activity had a biological $t_{0.5}$ of 30 - 50 min. However, later HPLC assays showed that unchanged cephalothin has a $t_{0.5}$ of <u>ca</u>. 11 - 15 min in adults and <u>ca</u>. 19 min in children.[312,313] The major desacetylcephalothin metabolite, which has 25% of the antimicrobial activity of the parent drug, has a $t_{0.5}$ of 18 min.

Serum $t_{0.5}$ values of cephalothin were increased in renal failure, and linear relationships have been established between antibiotic $t_{0.5}$ values and serum creatinine and also chrom-EDTA-clearance values.[314] Although furosemide and mercaptomerin interfere with renal secretory mechanisms,[315,316] these diuretic agents had no effect on the rate of cephalothin elimination in man.[317] The osmotic diuretic mannitol was also without effect on cephalothin clearance.

Although the use of cephaloridine in patients with renal insufficiency is generally deprecated in favour of cephalothin, observed relationships between the clearance rate of cephaloridine and creatinine clearance made it practicable to retain cephaloridine therapy for uraemic patients. Bechtol[318] described a nomogram (Figure 3.13) relating cephaloridine maintenance dose to creatinine clearance. In difficult cases, however, it would be desirable to monitor serum cephaloridine concentrations. A method has been described that permits calculation of the time course of cephaloridine concentrations in wound tissue and the best means of obtaining optimal antibiotic concentrations at these sites.[319]

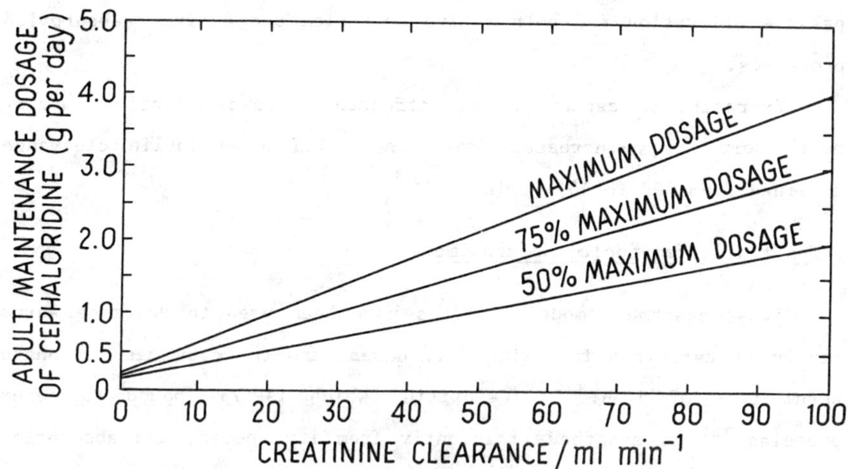

Figure 3.13   Calculated equivalent daily maintenance doses of cephaloridine as a function of endogenous creatinine clearance. Reproduced by permission from Curr. Ther. Res., 1972, 14, 790.

Comparative drug disposition studies in mice, rats, dogs, and humans indicate that cephapirin is metabolized to desacetylcephapirin in these species. Pharmacokinetic analyses of the concentrations of cephapirin and desacetylcephapirin in plasma and urine reveal that the rate and extent of deacetylation decrease from rodents to dogs to humans. The kinetic analyses suggest also that the kidney performs a role not only in the excretion but also in the metabolism of cephapirin to desacetylcephapirin.[320]

Peak serum levels of 73 μg ml^{-1} and 24 μg ml^{-1} were observed 15 min and 30 min, respectively, following single 1 g i.v. and i.m. doses of cephapirin. During the first 6 h after injection, 72% and 53% of the i.v. and i.m. doses, respectively, were recovered in urine.[321]   Saturable reabsorption of cephapirin, and to a lesser extent of cephaloridine, is suggested by a study in healthy male volunteers in which renal clearances declined when plasma levels were reduced.[322] Thus, renal elimination of these compounds may include passive filtration and both active secretion and active reabsorption processes.

Excretion of cephapirin was affected by renal function impairment; serum $t_{0.5}$ increased from 0.9 to 2.7 h as inulin clearance declined from 100 to 10 ml min^{-1}.[323]

Cefoxitin, Cefamandole, Cefuroxime

Two-compartment model kinetics have been used to describe serum levels of cefoxitin following i.v. doses, and the drug has a β-phase serum $t_{0.5}$ of 1 h.[324] Cefoxitin, which is 73% bound to serum proteins,[325] is absorbed efficiently from i.m. doses, and absorption efficiency is unaffected by the presence of lidocaine.[326] Despite its high protein binding, tissue levels of cefoxitin are generally higher than those of cephalothin after equivalent doses.[327] Cefoxitin penetrates efficiently into dermabrasion tissue fluid,[328] achieving levels comparable to those in plasma.

Following 50 mg kg^{-1} i.m. doses of cefoxitin to the rat, interstitial fluid:blood AUC ratios averaged 0.77.[329] The decline of cefoxitin concentration in interstitial fluid was slower than that in blood, respective $t_{0.5}$ values being 75 and 25 min. In patients the penetration efficiency of cefoxitin into muscle tissue and fat, measured by tissue:serum concentration ratios, reached 100% and 60%, respectively.[330] Cefoxitin also penetrated rapidly into the peritoneal fluid, reaching peak fluid concentrations within 20 min of an i.v. dose.[331] The mean peritoneal fluid concentration was 86% of the simultaneous serum level, and penetration appeared to be unaffected by acute peritonitis. In cirrhotic patients with ascites, a 30 mg kg^{-1} i.v. dose of cefoxitin yielded a peak antibiotic concentration in ascitic fluid of 32.8 µg ml^{-1} at 2 h.[332] Two grams of cefoxitin administered i.v. to patients undergoing open heart surgery maintained adequate concentrations in the right atrial appendage (60 µg g^{-1})

and pericardial fluid (19 μg ml^{-1}) to protect against possible Staphylococcal infections.[333] Cefoxitin penetrates efficiently into the c.s.f. of experimental animals and man,[334,335] and particularly into c.s.f. of patients with bacterial meningitis.[336,337] During a multiple dosing regimen of 2 g every 4 h by i.v. infusion, the mean c.s.f. cefoxitin concentration at steady state averaged 3 - 5 μg ml^{-1}, compared with a simultaneous serum level of 8 - 9 μg ml^{-1}.[338] Effective antimicrobial concentrations were found in the uterine tissue following i.m. administration of 2 g cefoxitin in 31 premenopausal women immediately before vaginal hysterectomy.[339] In patients scheduled for cholecystectomy, i.v. doses of 2 g cefoxitin resulted in concentrations in gallbladder bile greater than 10 μg ml^{-1}.[340] Cefoxitin also diffuses rapidly into the human foetus.[341] In 35 pregnant women who received 1 g cefoxitin i.m. 15 to 180 min before delivery, peak serum concentrations in maternal and foetal blood were 25 and 15 μg ml^{-1}, respectively, both achieved at 30 - 45 min postinjection. In contrast, no cefoxitin was detected in the milk of nursing mothers. Serum levels of cefoxitin were higher and more prolonged after i.v. dosage than equivalent doses of cephalothin,[342] as renal clearance of cephalothin exceeded that of cefoxitin.[343] Only 0.1 - 6% of dosed cefoxitin was metabolized to the descarbamyl derivative, compared with > 35% deacetylation of cephalothin.

Cefoxitin is eliminated primarily by glomerular filtration and tubular secretion. Probenecid competes with cefoxitin for tubular sites of secretion, thus retarding excretion of the latter.[344] Renal clearance and serum $t_{0.5}$ of cefoxitin were 231 ml min^{-1} and 0.8 h, respectively, when 2 g of cefoxitin are administered i.v. alone and 91 ml min^{-1} and 1.6 h when given concomitantly or 1 h after 1 g of probenecid.[345] However, cumulative urinary excretion during 24 h, _ca._ 84% of dose, was unaffected by probenecid. Cefoxitin $t_{0.5}$ in infants and children (3 - 151 m)[346] was similar to that in young adults (15 - 55 yr),[347] approximately 40 min. In geriatric patients (66 - 94 yr), the $t_{0.5}$ averaged 1.1 h.[347] The elderly also exhibited a decrease in cefoxitin binding to plasma proteins, <u>ca</u>. 69% compared with 79% in the young subjects. Cefoxitin clearance is impaired in renal failure, and is not increased by peritoneal dialysis.[348] Its mean $t_{0.5}$ increased from 40 min in healthy subjects to 22 - 24 h in severe renal impairment, with a corresponding decrease in total body clearance from 340 to 13 ml min^{-1} 1.73 m^{-2}.[349-352] After a single 40 mg kg^{-1} i.m. dose to rabbits with varying degrees of renal impairment induced by uranyl nitrate, cefoxitin $t_{0.5}$ varied from 1 to 16 h, compared with a mean of 0.37 h in rabbits with normal renal function.[353] Biliary excretion of cefoxitin increased considerably in renal impairment; average recovery ranged from 0.47% of the dose in normal rabbits to 9.09% in those with severe renal impairment.

The pharmacokinetics of cefamandole have been reviewed in relation to other cephalosporins.[354] Cefamandole obeys two-compartment kinetics following i.v. doses, and has a reported β-phase $t_{0.5}$ of 1 - 1.5 h. However, studies using a specific liquid chromatographic assay have suggested that a three-compartment open model with $t_{0.5}$ values of 5, 24, and 74 min may more accurately describe cefamandole kinetics.[355] Most of the drug is eliminated in urine, and its renal and serum clearances are similar. Cefamandole is 70% bound to serum proteins, and penetrates poorly into c.s.f.[356] In rabbits the concentration of antibiotic in c.s.f. exceeded the MIC for <u>Haemophilus influenzae</u> only after a 150 mg kg^{-1} dose. On the other hand, cefamandole penetrates effectively into pulmonary and s.c. tissue and is recommended as a drug suitable for perioperative prophylaxis.[357]

The penetration of cefamandole into pancreatic fluid, as measured by the fluid:serum AUC ratio following a 25 mg kg^{-1} i.v. dose, was 0.23 in dogs with a normal pancreas but increased to 0.44 after induction of pancreatitis.[358] This change was associated with a decrease in serum albumin concentration during acute pancreatitis, resulting in increased free drug concentration. On the other hand, clearance of cefamandole was 290 ml min^{-1} both before and after induction of pancreatitis.

As may be predicted from its high renal clearance, the biological $t_{0.5}$ of cefamandole is prolonged in renal failure, increasing to 14 - 18 h in patients with severe renal impairment.[359,360] The $t_{0.5}$ is reduced to _ca_. 4 h by haemodialysis[361] while peritoneal dialysis is less effective.[362] Dosage schedules have been described that allow for variable elimination characteristics of cefamandole in dialysis patients.[363]

Following single 1 g i.v. doses, cefuroxime penetrated readily into peritoneal and pleural fluids with concentrations exceeding 15 μg ml^{-1} and 5 - 10 μg ml^{-1}, respectively.[364-366] The drug also achieved a bone:serum concentration ratio of 0.1 - 0.2, and was considered to be suitable for prophylactic use in patients undergoing hip replacement surgery.[367] While some investigators reported limited penetration of cefuroxime into the c.s.f.,[368] others have observed penetrations of 6 and 10% after i.v. doses of 50 and 75 mg kg^{-1}, respectively, and found the antibiotic satisfactory for the treatment of bacterial meningitis.[369]

The site of i.m. injection may influence circulating levels of cefuroxime.[370] Although similar serum profiles were obtained following thigh and buttock injections in male volunteers, absorption of antibiotic was slower, and peak drug levels in serum were reduced from the buttock injection site compared with the thigh site in females. Overall drug availability was similar from the two injection sites in both sexes.

The disposition of cefuroxime after i.m. injections of the sodium and lysine salts were similar.[371] The drug was excreted almost exclusively by the kidneys, and its clearance tended to decrease in the elderly (71 - 92 yr), apparently due to declining renal function in this patient population.[372,373] Serum levels of cefuroxime declined with a terminal $t_{0.5}$ of 70 min after bolus i.v. doses to volunteers.[374]   The cefuroxime:creatinine clearance ratio indicated that 40 - 50% of the drug was secreted into the renal tubules and this was confirmed by a 40% reduction in cefuroxime clearance, with simultaneous probenecid administration. The pharmacokinetics of cefuroxime are similar in hospitalised patients, with a reported $t_{0.5}$ of 1.4 h, and urinary excretion accounting for greater than 80% of parenteral doses as active compound within 8 h.[375] Analysis of serum cefuroxime levels in terms of the two-compartment model yielded mean central compartment and total distribution volumes of 5.3 and 11.7 1 1.73 m^{-2}, respectively, after a single 500 mg dose.[376] The drug is 33% bound to plasma proteins at therapeutic levels.

After a single 750 mg i.v. dose of cefuroxime to 3 groups of male volunteers with creatinine clearances of 60 - 120, 20 - 59, and < 20 ml min^{-1} 1.73 m^{-2}, mean serum $t_{0.5}$ values for cefuroxime were 1.7, 2.4, and 17.6 h, respectively (Figure 3.14).[377] The correspond-

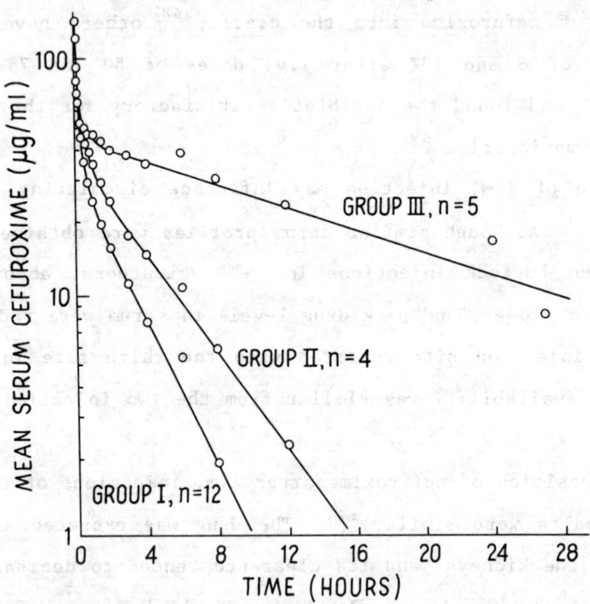

Figure 3.14   Mean serum levels of cefuroxime as measured by HPLC assay in Groups 1 (Cl$_{CR}$ = 60 to 120 ml min^{-1} 1.73 m^{-2}), 2 (Cl$_{CR}$ =120 - 59 ml min^{-1} 1.73 m^{-2}), and 3 (Cl$_{CR}$ < 20 ml min^{-1} 1.73 m^{-2}). Each subject received 750 mg of cefuroxime during 2 min i.v. Reproduced by permission from Antimicrob. Ag. Chemother., 1981, 19, 443.

ing serum clearances were 123, 79, and 13 ml min^{-1} 1.73 m^{-2}, while the volume of distribution appeared to be independent of renal function. Cumulative excretion of cefuroxime in 24 h urine was essentially complete in normal and moderately impaired renal function, but accounted for only 40% of the dose in uraemic patients with creatinine clearances < 20 ml min^{-1} 1.73 m^{-2}, indicating the need for dose reduction in this group. Urine antibiotic levels in all patients exceeded the MIC for susceptible organisms for more than 12 h.

Cefotaxime, Cephacetrile, Ceforanide, Ceftezole

The pharmacokinetics of cefotaxime have been described after i.m. and i.v. doses to healthy volunteers.[378] This cephalosporin has kinetic properties similar to other cephalosporins, as characterized by a $t_{0.5}$ of 1 - 1.5 h and a distribution volume of 22 1 1.73 m^{-2}. Cefotaxime, like cephalothin and cephapirin, is converted to a less active 0-deacetyl metabolite, and urinary recovery of unchanged drug is only 33 - 66%.

The extravascular concentration of cefotaxime following a 1 g i.m. injection appeared to be greater than the MIC for most susceptible organisms.[379] However, the drug penetrated poorly through non-inflammed meninges; concentrations in c.s.f. ranged from 0.01 to 0.7 μg ml^{-1} after a 30 mg kg^{-1} i.v. dose.[380] Similarly, low cefotaxime levels were found in the milk of lactating mothers, the milk:serum concentration ratios being less than 0.17.[381] In pregnant women, cefotaxime readily crosses the placenta, producing bactericidal concentrations in the foetus. Cefotaxime penetrates prostatic and renal tissues, achieving tissue:serum concentration ratios as high as 0.31 and 0.54, respectively.[382] Following a 1 g i.m. dose, cefotaxime is 35 - 45% bound to serum proteins.[383]

Cefotaxime is rapidly eliminated by healthy individuals and approximately 50 - 60% of an i.v. or i.m. dose is excreted in 24 h urine.[383-385] Fifteen percent of the dose is recovered in urine as the desacetyl derivative. Multiple dosing of 1 g cefotaxime every 6 h for 2 wk resulted in no drug accumulation or altered pharmacokinetics.[383,385] Probenecid inhibits renal tubular secretion of cefotaxime, causing a 2-fold reduction in its renal and total body clearances.[383,386] Mean cefotaxime elimination $t_{0.5}$ was 5 - 6 h in premature infants with a low birth weight of 1.1 - 1.2 kg, and decreased to 3.4 h in normal birth weight (2.6 kg) neonates.[387,388] In older infants and children (5 m - 12 yr), cefotaxime disposition kinetics were similar to those in adults.[389]

Renal dysfunction decreases urinary excretion of cefotaxime and desacetylcefotaxime, and the $t_{0.5}$ of parent drug is prolonged to <u>ca</u>. 3 h in patients with creatinine clearances less than 10 ml min^{-1},[390-392] although $t_{0.5}$ values as great as 11 h have been reported in some uraemic patients.[393] Since nonrenal mechanisms of elimination may assume importance when kidney function is compromised, cefotaxime dose adjustment is generally considered necessary only in severe renal insufficiency. Haemodialysis significantly reduces the $t_{0.5}$ of cefotaxime. A 4-6 h haemodialysis session removed approximately 60% of the dose, while peritoneal dialysis was less effective.[392,393]

After i.v. doses to man, cephacetrile obeyed two-compartment model kinetics, each compartment representing about 12% of the total body volume.[394] The drug is completely absorbed from i.m. doses and is cleared from plasma after both i.m. and i.v. doses with a $t_{0.5}$ of <u>ca</u>. 1.4 h. Studies in rats using ^{14}C-cephacetrile show that ^{14}C widely distributes into tissues, with highest levels occurring in the kidneys, plasma, and liver and the lowest levels in the brain. Radioactivity levels in tissues declined at approximately the same rate as those in plasma, and the kinetics of drug in plasma were unaffected by repeated doses.[395]

Elimination of cephacetrile occurs almost entirely via the kidneys, and urinary excretion occurs by both filtration and secretion.[396,397] Tubular secretion has been proposed as a possible reason for low renal lymph concentrations of this antibiotic in comparison with cephaloridine in dogs.

Cephacetrile elimination is markedly affected by renal function and the elimination $t_{0.5}$ may increase from a normal value of <u>ca</u>. 1 h to 20 - 40 h in severe renal impairment.[398-402] The overall relationship between drug elimination rate constant and creatinine clearance is given in equation 3.4. Loading and maintenance dose recom-

$$k_{el} = 0.008 + 0.0061 \ (Cl_{CR}) \tag{3.4}$$

mendations are based on this relationship. Haemodialysis has been reported to decrease the serum $t_{0.5}$ of cephacetrile in severe uraemia to one-fifth and one-eighth its predialysis value.[403] Biliary excretion of cephacetrile is low in humans but increases in renal impairment.[404]

Intramuscular 556 mg and 1132 mg doses of ceforanide were completely bioavailable in man; peak plasma concentrations of 38 and 74 μg ml^{-1} were reached at 1.0 - 1.3 h postdose.[405] The drug is approximately 80% bound to plasma proteins over the concentration range of 27 - 200 μg ml^{-1}. Ceforanide elimination kinetics are dose-independent, with a mean terminal $t_{0.5}$ of 3 h. Plasma and renal clearances averaged 46 and 35 ml min^{-1} 1.73 m^{-2}, respectively, and 85% of the dose is excreted unchanged in 12 h urine. Multiple dosing at 12 h intervals for 10 d results in no drug accumulation. Similar pharmacokinetic data were obtained in cancer patients following i.v. doses of 500 mg or 1 g ceforanide by infusion over 30 min.[406] Approximately 55% of the dose was recovered in urine within 6 h, and ceforanide serum $t_{0.5}$ ranged from 2.2 to 2.9 h. Healthy subjects who received 1 or 2 g i.m. ceforanide either alone or simultaneously with 1 g probenecid showed similar mean antibiotic $t_{0.5}$ values of 3.2 - 3.7 h and plasma clearances of 37 - 42 ml min^{-1} 1.73 m^{-2}.[407] Probenecid had no significant effect on plasma concentration (Figure

3.15) or urinary excretion of ceforanide, suggesting that tubular
secretion plays a minor role in its excretion. Saliva obtained from
the same subjects contained less than 0.5 μg ml^{-1} of ceforanide at
all sampling times. Since ceforanide is eliminated primarily by the
kidneys, its plasma clearance declines with increasing renal impairment. Mean ceforanide $t_{0.5}$ increased from 3 h in normal subjects to
29 h in dialysis patients.[408] Haemodialysis removed <u>ca</u>. 20% of the
ceforanide dose, thus reducing its concentration in plasma but
appeared to have no effect on its $t_{0.5}$. In the rat and the dog,
ceforanide $t_{0.5}$ was approximately 1 h and plasma clearance averaged

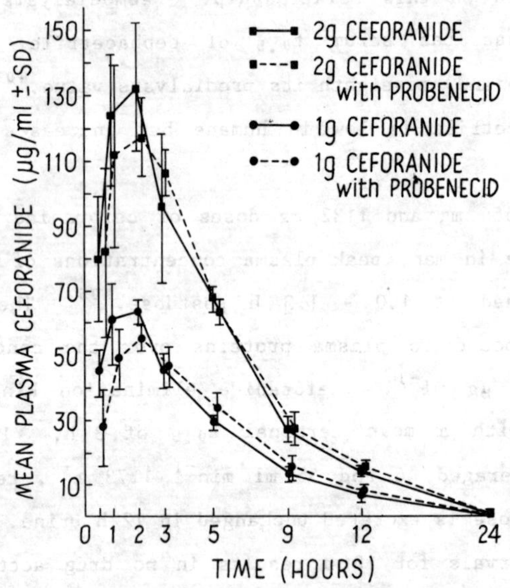

Figure 3.15 Mean plasma concentrations of ceforanide
versus time after administration of 1 and 2 g of
ceforanide with or without probenecid. Reproduced by
permission from <u>Antimicrob. Ag. Chemother.</u>, 1981, <u>20</u>,
530.

5 - 6 ml min^{-1} kg^{-1}.[409,410] Urinary recovery of the antibiotic in these animals was similar to that in humans, 80 - 90% in 24 h.
Ceforanide $t_{0.5}$ in rat tissues was similar to that in plasma. Concomitantly administered ceforanide (100 mg kg^{-1} s.c.) and amikacin
(25 mg kg^{-1} s.c.) resulted in no pharmacokinetic interactions.

Blood levels of ceftezole were lower than those of cefazolin, but higher than those of cephaloridine and cephalothin after single 10 and 20 mg kg^{-1} i.v. doses to rats and rabbits.[411] However, blood levels of ceftezole in dogs were similar to those of cefazolin and cephaloridine. Following a single 500 mg i.m. dose to healthy volunteers, a maximum ceftezole serum level of 23 µg ml^{-1} was obtained at 30 min, but levels were undetectable at 6 h. Greater than 90% of the dose is recovered in urine as unchanged drug. No changes in plasma level or urinary excretion patterns were observed after repeated i.m. injection to rabbits twice daily for 14 d.

Moxalactam, Cefmetazole, Cefoperazone, Cefsulodin

Moxalactam pharmacokinetics are linear over the parenteral (i.v. and i.m.) dose range of 0.25 - 4 g,[412] and are similar after single and multiple doses, with no accumulation of drug following repeated administration.[412,413] The antibiotic is eliminated primarily via the kidneys, and approximately 55 - 75% of the dose is recovered in urine.[412,414-416] Renal excretion occurs almost exclusively by glomerular filtration and is therefore not affected by probenecid.[414] Unchanged moxalactam has been found in faeces after parenteral doses, suggesting biliary excretion and possibly enterohepatic circulation of the antibiotic.[412,416] In patients with indwelling T-tubes who received single i.v. doses of 500 or 2000 mg moxalactam, peak concentrations in bile averaged 34 and 74 µg ml^{-1}, respectively.[417] Reported $t_{0.5}$ values for moxalactam in normal adults are 2 - 3 h, similar to those reported for cefazolin.[412,415,416] In children, Romagnoli et al.[418] found prolonged moxalactam $t_{0.5}$ with decreasing age, averaging 1.6 h at 1 - 24 m, 4.4 h at 1 - 4 wk, and 6.2 h in neonates.

In 19 adult patients scheduled for coronary bypass surgery, higher serum concentrations of cefazolin than moxalactam were observed at all times after simultaneous administration of the two drugs (10 mg kg^{-1}, i.v. or i.m).[419] However, moxalactam and cefazolin concentrations in atrial appendages were similar, <u>ca</u>. 20 µg g^{-1} after i.v. doses and 10 µg g^{-1} after i.m. doses. This is probably due to the moderate degree of serum protein binding of moxalactam relative to cefazolin. Data in the rabbit[420] and man[421] showed efficient penetration of moxalactam into c.s.f. when the meninges were inflamed, reaching maximum c.s.f. concentrations of 5 - 10 µg ml^{-1} following 20 - 25 mg kg^{-1} i.v. infusions. Moxalactam penetration into rabbit c.s.f. was greater than cefotaxime, cefoperazone, and ceftriaxone.[420]

Total body clearance of moxalactam correlates well with creatinine clearance, while nonrenal clearance is unaffected by kidney function.[422-424] In 20 patients with varying degrees of renal impairment, mean moxalactam $t_{0.5}$ increased from 2.2 h in patients with creatinine clearance > 60 ml min^{-1} 1.73 m^{-2} to 22.3 h in those with creatinine clearance < 10 ml min^{-1} 1.73 m^{-2}.[425] No corresponding changes in moxalactam distribution volume were detected.

Haemodialysis in anephric patients reduced the moxalactam $t_{0.5}$ from <u>ca</u>. 20 h to <u>ca</u>. 2.8 h, removing approximately 50% of the dose during a single dialysis.[426-429] In contrast, the amount of moxalactam removed by peritoneal dialysis was insignificant.[429] It was suggested that the normal moxalactam dose of 1 g twice daily should be reduced to 1 g daily for patients with a creatinine clearance of 30 ml min^{-1}, and 1 g on alternate days if creatinine clearance is below 10 ml min^{-1}.

In healthy subjects with normal renal function, the relatively new cephamycin, cefmetazole, was rapidly eliminated; approximately 70% of a 1 g i.v. dose was excreted in the urine within 6 h.[430] The serum $t_{0.5}$ and clearance were 0.8 h and 164 ml min^{-1} 1.73 m^{-2}, respectively. In patients with severe renal insufficiency the $t_{0.5}$ increased to 15 h while serum clearance was reduced to 14 ml min^{-1} 1.73 m^{-2}.

Cefoperazone, and also moxalactam and cefotaxime, penetrated poorly into the c.s.f. of rabbits with normal meninges.[431] The c.s.f.:serum concentration ratios were 1 - 2%, compared with 20% for sulphamethoxazole and 36% for trimethoprim. In rabbits with meningitis, a two- to threefold increase in c.s.f. concentration was observed for all compounds except sulphamethoxazole.

Cefoperazone pharmacokinetics after a 2 - 3 g i.v. dose to normal subjects were described by a linear two-compartment model. The mean terminal $t_{0.5}$ was 2 h while serum clearance ranged from 85 - 96 ml min^{-1}. Urinary recovery of cefoperazone averaged 29%, indicating a minor role of kidney excretion.[432,433] Pharmacokinetic parameters of cefoperazone in anephric patients were almost identical to those in normal subjects.[433] Sekine et al.[434] reported prolonged serum $t_{0.5}$ values of cefoperazone in patients with liver dysfunction suggesting that the drug is excreted mainly via the bile. In 4 patients with cholelithiasis and 1 patient with carcinoma of the head of the pancreas, a 1 g i.v. dose of cefoperazone yielded peak concentrations of 373 - 3100 µg ml^{-1} in the common duct bile, 6.8 - 680 µg ml^{-1} in gallbladder bile, and 16.8 - 48 µg g^{-1} in gallbladder wall.[435] Repeated i.v. administration of cefoperazone, 4 g d^{-1} in divided doses, resulted in no drug accumulation or change in $t_{0.5}$.[436]

The tissue distribution of cefsulodin has been examined in patients undergoing various operations.[437] After a 2 g i.v. bolus dose, adequate antibacterial concentrations were found in the skin, fat, muscle, prostatic tissue, and peritoneal secretion. Cefsulodin concentrations in tissues at 30 min postdose were between 10 and 20 µg g^{-1}, compared with 78 µg ml^{-1} in serum. Others have reported adequate antibacterial concentrations in sputum, bile, bone, and pleural and peritoneal fluids from comparable doses of cefsulodin, although drug penetration through non-inflammed meninges was relatively poor.[438] A study in guinea pigs showed marked penetration of cefsulodin into perilymph and aqueous humour after parenteral doses.[439]

In normal subjects with creatinine clearances > 80 ml min^{-1}, cefsulodin $t_{0.5}$ was 1.9 h and plasma and renal clearances were 2.0 and 1.1 ml min^{-1} kg^{-1}, respectively.[440] The $t_{0.5}$ increased progressively to 13 h in anuric patients, while a linear correlation was established between cefsulodin plasma clearance and GFR. Cumulative excretion in 24 h urine was <u>ca</u>. 55% from patients with normal and mildly impaired kidney function and 37% in those with moderate renal impairment. Haemodialysis was effective in removing cefsulodin, shortening its $t_{0.5}$ to 2.1 h and reducing plasma concentrations by 60%. Cefsulodin $t_{0.5}$ in anuric patients on peritoneal dialysis averaged 8.9 h.[441]

Ceftriaxone, Ceftazidime, Ceftizoxime, Ceftezole, Cefonicid, Cefotiam, Cefmenoxime

In 6 healthy volunteers who received 3 g ceftriaxone i.v., the volume of distribution and total body clearance of unbound drug averaged 168 l and 258 ml min^{-1}, respectively, while the corresponding values for total drug were 12.7 l and 18.5 ml min^{-1}.[442] The mean ceftriaxone $t_{0.5}$ in this study was 7.8 h. Other investigators[443-445] who studied ceftriaxone doses of 150 mg - 2 g i.v. in normal subjects reported similar dose-independent $t_{0.5}$ values of 6 - 8 h, but invariably observed increased clearance and AUC values with increasing dose. The phenomenon was explained in terms of concentration-dependent binding of ceftriaxone to plasma proteins, the average free drug fraction being 0.04 and 0.17 at total plasma concentrations of 0.5 and 300 µg ml^{-1}, respectively.[443] A small discrepency was observed in the reported urinary recovery of unchanged ceftriaxone, <u>ca</u>. 65% in some studies[442,443] and <u>ca</u>. 40% in others.[444,445] Following a 50 mg kg^{-1} i.v. dose of ceftriaxone in patients with bacterial meningitis, the mean penetration of the drug into c.s.f. was 3.1%, and the elimination $t_{0.5}$ was 4 h.[446]

Ceftazidime was almost completely (> 96%) eliminated by renal excretion.[447] The mean serum $t_{0.5}$ after an i.v. or i.m. dose in healthy volunteers was 1.6 h, while total body clearance averaged 130 ml min^{-1}.

The extravascular penetration of ceftizoxime and cefotaxime was studied in a rabbit subcutaneous Visking chamber model.[448] Ceftizoxime, being only 32% bound to rabbit serum proteins, showed a penetration of 40 and 54% after single and repeated doses, respectively, much higher than the penetration of cefotaxime which is 93% protein bound. Very low serum protein binding of ceftizoxime was observed also in the rat and dog, *ca.* 32 and 17%, respectively.[449] Greater than 80% of a single parenteral dose of ceftizoxime was excreted unchanged in the urine of these species, while biliary excretion accounted for only 3.7% in the rat and 0.6% in the dog. The overall $t_{0.5}$ values in the rat and dog were 0.33 and 1.06 h, respectively.

The pharmacokinetics of ceftizoxime were dose-independent in healthy humans in the 0.5 - 4 g dosage range.[450,451] The drug was *ca.* 28% protein bound at a serum concentration of 40 µg ml^{-1}. The mean elimination $t_{0.5}$ was 1.4 - 1.7 h, and the dose was almost completely recovered in 48 h urine. Ceftizoxime was actively secreted by the renal tubules, and exhibited a prolonged $t_{0.5}$ of 2.3 h and elevated serum levels in the presence of probenecid.[452] In patients with severe renal insufficiency, ceftizoxime $t_{0.5}$ increased to *ca.* 30 h.[453] The total body clearance and 6 h urinary excretion were 6.3 ml min^{-1} and 1% of dose, respectively, compared with 179 ml min^{-1} and 76% for normal subjects. The apparent volume of ceftizoxime distribution, *ca.* 40% body weight, was not affected by renal function.

After a 2 g i.v. infusion of ceftezole in patients with normal renal function, 81% of the dose was excreted in 6 h urine and the mean ceftezole $t_{0.5}$ was 0.64 h.[454] Drug elimination was significantly impaired when kidney function was compromised, respective values being 0.6% and 10.7 h in patients with severe renal insufficiency (creatinine clearance = 0.26 ml min^{-1}).

The average $t_{0.5}$ and plasma clearance of cefonicid were 4.4 h and 0.32 ml min^{-1} kg^{-1} in healthy subjects.[455] Approximately 88% of an i.v. dose was excreted unchanged in the urine within 48 h.

The pharmacokinetics of cefotiam appear to be dose-dependent, possibly due to saturation of tubular secretion at elevated doses.[456] Increasing an i.v. dose from 0.5 g to 2.0 g resulted in reduced plasma clearance from 27 l h^{-1} to 20 l h^{-1} and prolonged $t_{0.5}$ from 0.6 h to 0.9 h. Nonetheless, urinary excretion of cefotiam was virtually complete within 4 h of all doses. The pharmacokinetics of cefmenoxime were independent of dose and dosage route following i.v. and i.m. doses of 250 mg - 2 g in 15 healthy male subjects.[457] The $t_{0.5}$ and plasma clearance averaged 0.9 h and 254 ml min^{-1}, respectively, and 68 - 75% of the cefmenoxime dose was recovered in 24 h urine.

Tetracyclines

The literature on the tetracyclines during the review period has not been as extensive as that on some other antibiotic classes. Attention is focused here on the representative compounds tetracycline, doxycycline, oxytetracycline, minocycline, and methacycline.

Tetracycline

Many studies have addressed the subject of tetracycline absorption and factors influencing its absorption efficiency.[458] One study suggested that bioavailability results obtained from single doses do not accurately predict those obtained after repeated doses.[459] Other investigators, however, have found good agreement between single-dose and multiple-dose determinations.[460]

No significant differences were observed in the urinary excretion of drug from p.o. doses of 16 tetracycline hydrochloride and tetracycline phosphate complex capsules.[461] Inadequate absorption was reported for two of nine brands of tetracycline hydrochloride tablets.[462] However, the sources of the various formulations were not identified in the latter study.

The bioavailability of p.o. tetracycline is reduced in the presence of zinc salts[463] and by solid meals,[464] but is unaffected by changes in accompanying fluid volumes. In contrast to tetracycline, the absorption of which was reduced by 50% in the presence of food, doxycycline absorption was reduced by only 20% under identical conditions. Absorption of tetracycline is also variable dependent upon whether the patient is awake or asleep after taking a p.o. dose.[465] Impaired bioavailability during sleep is possibly due to impaired dissolution of tetracycline in the relatively high gastric pH occurring at night.

Oral absorption of tetracyclines from commercial capsules decreases in the presence of bismuth subsalicylate antidiarrhoeal mixture,[466] and also may decrease with increasing doses of tetracycline.[467] Small increases observed in the bioavailability of tetracycline when this drug is administered with a small water volume, compared to water-loading conditions, are consistent with previous observations that the absorption of p.o. tetraycline and doxycycline, unlike many other compounds, is not adversely affected by reduction of fluid volume.[468]

The inhibitory effect of Fe salts on tetracycline absorption is highly dependent on the accompanying anion.[469] Tetracycline serum levels and urinary excretion were reduced 30% by ferric sodium edetate, 50% by ferrous tartrate, 70 - 80% by ferrous fumarate, ferrous succinate, and ferrous gluconate, and 80 - 90% by ferrous sulphate. The marked differences observed between the various Fe salts appeared to be related to their ability to release Fe^{2+} or Fe^{3+} ions into the upper gastrointestinal tract, and also to the absorption characteristics of the Fe compounds themselves.[470] Studies *in vitro* have demonstrated that tetracycline chelation by metallic ions is pH-dependent.[471] Tetracycline chelates with Al^{3+} and Cu^{2+}

ions as its tricarbonylmethane system becomes ionized, whereas Ca^{2+} and Mg^{2+} ions form chelates with the phenolic diketone function of tetracycline. Diffusion of tetracycline chelates across a semi-permeable membrane is depressed relative to free drug even when the chelate is water-soluble.

In a randomized crossover study using 5 normal subjects, the absorption of tetracycline from single doses of 250 mg capsules was unaffected by concomitant administration of cimetidine (300 mg) or sodium bicarbonate (2 g), but was reduced by <u>ca</u>. 90% when given with 30 ml of magnesium aluminum hydroxide gel.[472] Since all three treatments reduced gastric acidity, it was concluded that impaired absorption of tetracycline by antacids was due to chelation and not elevated pH. Conflicting results on cimetidine-tetracycline interactions have been presented by Fisher et al.[473] indicating a 30 - 40% reduction in tetracycline bioavailability by cimetidine when single doses of the two drugs were given together (Figure 3.16). However, the effect tended to diminish after chronic administration of cimetidine (Figure 3.17).

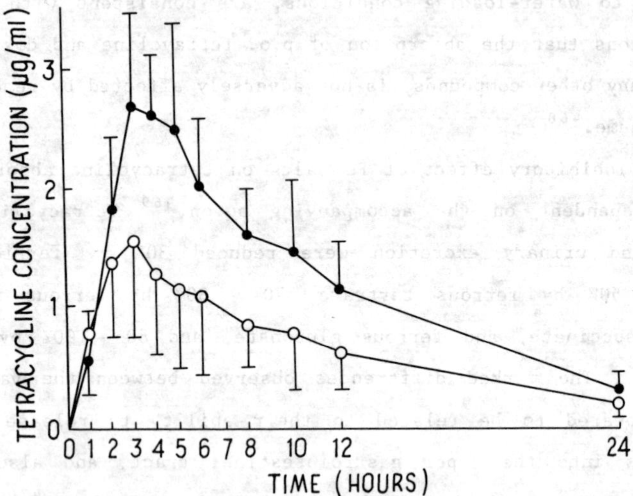

Figure 3.16   Tetracycline plasma concentrations (mean ± s.d.) for six subjects following p.o. administration of 500 mg with (o) and without (•) 400 mg cimetidine. Reproduced by permission from <u>Brit. J. Clin. Pharmacol</u>., 1980, <u>9</u>, 153.

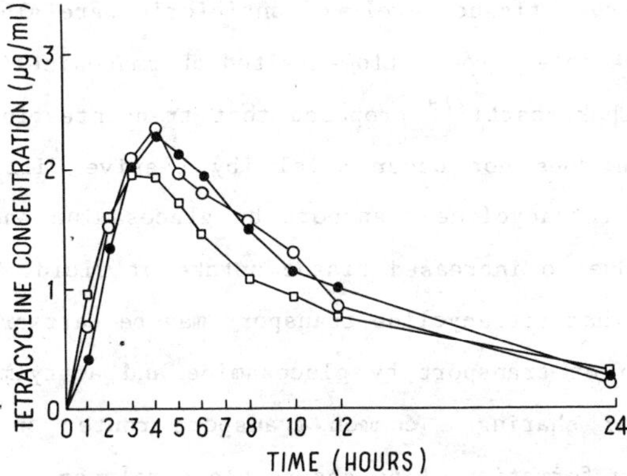

Figure 3.17   Mean tetracycline plasma concentrations
for six subjects following p.o. administration of 500
mg tetracycline (a) as tablets after cimetidine 1.6 g
daily for five days (●), (b) as suspension after cimetidine 1.6 g daily for five days (□), (c) as suspension without cimetidine pretreatment (o).   Reproduced
by permission from Brit. J. Clin. Pharmacol., 1980, 9,
153.

Serum levels of tetracycline, and also sulfamethizole and doxycycline, were considerably reduced following p.o. doses to resting subjects compared with those undergoing intensive exercise.   These results appeared to be consistent with delayed absorption during rest
and suppressed renal excretion during exercise.[474]   Absorption of
tetracycline is unaffected by the condition of achlorhydria in the
elderly[475] and Billroth gastrectomy.[476]   Contrary to previous claims,
concurrent administration of proteolytic enzymes was shown to cause no
significant increase in tetracycline absorption.[477]   Plasma levels and
urinary excretion of antibiotic were indistinguishable in healthy
volunteers who received 500 mg tetracycline in gelatin capsules or in
enteric-coated tablets which contained a proteolytic enzyme mixture.

Excellent agreement was achieved between release rates of tetracycline from implanted trilaminate 2-hydroxyethyl methacrylate-methyl
methacrylate disks in rats, and values predicted from in vitro
data.[478]   Drug release was zero-order in nature, and steady-state
tetracycline levels were achieved in plasma within 2-3 days of disk

implantation. Observed tissue levels of antibiotic were also consistent with values predicted from a flow-limited pharmacokinetic model.

Banerjee and Chakrabarti[479] proposed that transintestinal transfer of tetracycline does not occur solely by passive diffusion and
that inhibition of tetracycline transport by glucosamine and acetylmethionine is not due to increased tissue uptake of fluid. They suggest alternatively that tetracycline transport may be carrier-mediated
and that inhibition of transport by glucosamine and acetylmethionine
may be due to their sharing a common transport route, or they may
inhibit transport by formation of nonabsorbable complexes.

Transfer of tetracycline across artificial membranes, and also
across rat small intestine segments, is inhibited in the presence of a
gastric mucin dispersion, presumably due to binding of drug to the
mucin macromolecule.[480]

Although studies using _in situ_ rat intestinal preparations indicated that tetracycline absorption was unchanged in the presence and
absence of bile,[481] serum levels of p.o. dosed tetracycline were significantly reduced in the absence of bile flow in man.[482] Unlike
tetracycline, serum levels of p.o. dosed doxycycline, sulfadimidine,
and cycloserine were independent of bile flow.

Using human erythrocytes as a model system to study uptake and
release of antibiotics, Kornguth and Kunin[483] showed that tetracycline, minocycline, penicillin-G, and dicloxacillin were taken up by
cells and each drug exhibited a characteristic intracellular:extra-
cellular ratio depending on its lipid solubility. Drugs were also
distributed between cells and plasma in relation to their affinity for
plasma proteins. All four compounds were bound to human haemoglobin
and also haeme-free globin, causing a reduction in their antibacterial
activity.[484] Minocycline and tetracycline also bound to carbonic anhydrase. Interestingly, the enzymatic activity of carbonic anhydrase
was not reduced in the presence of tetracyclines. Binding of tetracyclines to human plasma at therapeutic concentrations has been exam-

ined under carefully controlled conditions.[485] Mean values for the proportion of drug bound over a concentration range of 0.1 - 10.0 µg ml^{-1} are tetracycline 35.5%, oxytetracycline 24.3%, doxycycline 60.0%, and minocycline 55.0%. Although these results agree with some previously published values, they are at variance with others, particularly in the case of doxycycline. Protein binding of minocycline is reduced at concentrations greater than 12 µg ml^{-1}, presumably due to saturation of available binding sites, but the recovery of the lipophilic minocycline molecule from serum ultrafiltrates is not effectively altered by abnormally elevated serum lipoproteins.[486] Tetracycline and minocycline effectively penetrated into sputum of patients with chronic bronchitis, achieving effective concentrations in over 60% of cases.[487] Doxycycline, on the other hand, penetrated into sputum poorly and only 20% of patients treated with this drug had satisfactory levels.

Biliary excretion of tetracycline and penicillin is increased in rats by the choleretic agents α,α-diethyl-1-naphthylacetic acid (DA 808) and α-methyl-α-(2-morpholinoethyl)-1-naphthylacetic acid (DA 1627), although the excretion of demethylchlortetracycline and rifamycin SV is unaffected.[488] DA 808 and DA 1627 appear to act as true choleretics, whereas dehydrocholic acid is a hydrocholeretic drug. Studies in lactating ewes confirm that tetracycline is actively secreted in milk.[489] However, secretion of active drug into the intestine of dogs after parenteral dosing is much less than with some other antibiotics.[490] Tetracycline administered to pregnant rats was rapidly transferred across the placenta, yielding antibiotic concentrations in foetal liver, kidney, muscle, and GI tract similar to those in the mother.[491]

Urinary excretion of both tetracycline and doxycycline is increased at high urinary pH values (Figure 3.18).[492] Alkaline treatment resulted in a 24% increase in cumulative urinary tetracycline excretion compared with acid treatment and a 54% increase for doxycy-

cline. Renal clearances of both drugs were increased during alkaline
treatment but distribution volumes were unaffected. Renal clearance
of tetracycline is unaffected by cimetidine.[473]

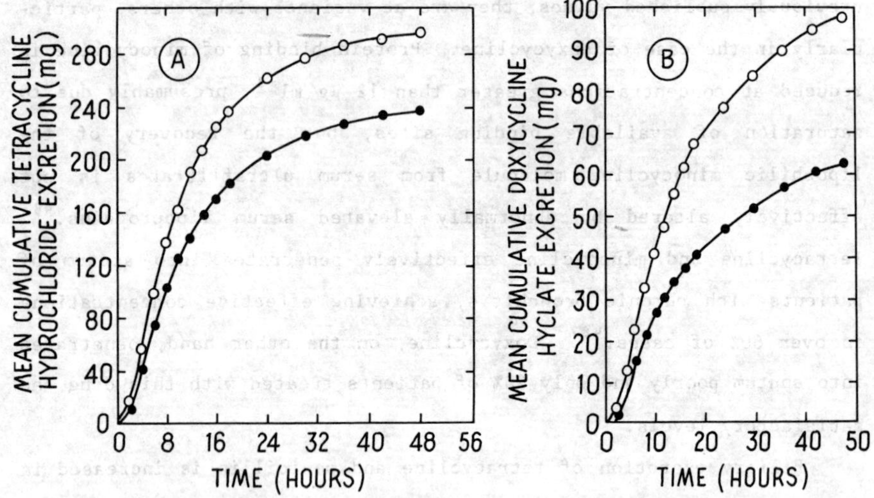

Figure 3.18   Mean cumulative amounts of tetracycline
(A, dose = 500 mg) and doxycycline (B, dose = 200 mg)
excreted in urine for eight subjects over a 48-h
period. ●, Acid treatment; o, alkaline treatment.
Reproduced by permission from *J. Pharmacokin. Biopharm.*, 1973, 1, 267.

Doxycycline

A number of studies have attested to the excellent absorption
characteristics of doxycycline. Approximately 92% of a p.o. dose of
doxycycline was absorbed in the mouse, and the absorption was unaffected by food.[493]   Doxycycline $t_{0.5}$ in this species was *ca.* 3 h
regardless of the route of administration.

The absorption efficiency of p.o. dosed doxycycline in man was
similar from solid and liquid dosage forms.[494]   However, the absorption rate of doxycyline was significantly faster from solutions and
suspensions compared with solid dosage forms. Serum antibiotic concentrations after a 200 mg p.o. dose of doxycycline hyclate were sig-

nificantly reduced when the drug was administered 2 h after ingesting 60 ml of subsalicylate bismuth.[495] Subsalicylate bismuth interference with doxycycline absorption increased when it was given concomitantly with doxycycline, and as repeated doses (q 6 h x 6 doses) prior to doxycycline administration, resulting in 37% and 51% decline, respectively, in doxycycline bioavailability. The $t_{0.5}$ of doxycycline was 17 - 22 h in all treatments.

Serum levels of doxycycline are similar whether the drug is dosed by the i.v. or p.o. route.[496] After multiple daily 200 mg i.v. doses, serum levels of antibiotic fluctuated between 5 - 6 μg ml^{-1} and 1 - 2 μg ml^{-1}, which is above the MIC for most susceptible pathogens.[497] The high lipid solubility of doxycycline results in its extensive distribution in body tissues. One hour following i.p. injection into rats, antibiotic levels in nine major organs were higher than those in serum.[498] Drug concentrations in the secretory organs, i.e. liver, renal medulla, and renal cortex, were greater than in other tissues. Doxycycline also penetrated well into lung and bronchial wall tissue[499] and into maxillary sinus mucosa and secretions.[500] However, concentrations of doxycycline, and also minocycline, in sputum of patients with chronic bronchitis were low compared to those of tetracycline.[501] Low minocycline levels were unexpected as lung tissue: serum ratios were greater than 2:1 in the dog.[502] Low doxycycline levels may have been due to poor excretion of drug by the bronchial mucosa. Poor penetration of doxycycline, minocycline, tetracycline, and oxytetracycline into saliva and tear fluids has been demonstrated after p.o. doses to man, although minocycline levels were inhibitory to meningococci in both fluids.[503] Sputum levels of doxycycline after a 200 mg dose were higher than those of tetracycline after a 500 mg dose to patients suffering from chronic bronchitis or bronchiectasis.[504] However, when the higher serum levels of doxycycline are considered, partitioning of the two drugs between plasma and sputum is almost identical. Other studies have shown that doxycycline enters thoracic duct lymph following i.v. or p.o. doses.[505] Concentrations of drug in lymph were within 30% of those in serum.

Several studies have confirmed that doxycycline is unique among the tetracyclines in that its clearance from the body is essentially unchanged, and it is free from toxic side effects at normal doses, in patients with renal failure.[506-508] Although serum levels of doxycycline are similar in normal and impaired renal function, urinary excretion of drug is considerably reduced.[509]

Unchanged blood levels of doxycycline in renal failure appear to be related to a compensatory increase in excretion of drug into the GI tract followed by chelation in the intestinal lumen.[510-513] Support for this was provided by Neuvonen and Penttila,[514] who were able to lower serum doxycycline levels by 20 - 45% and reduce elimination $t_{0.5}$ values from 17 to 11 h in man by giving p.o. doses of ferrous sulphate. Altered doxycycline kinetics were attributed to intestinal secretion of drug followed by chelation with Fe^{2+} ions, thus preventing reabsorption.

There is little evidence of significant enteral cycling of doxycycline in normal individuals.[515] Administration of either 80 mg Fe^{2+} or 4.0 g charcoal several hours after p.o. doxycycline had no effect on serum levels or urinary excretion of doxycycline following 2 x 200 mg doses, and only the Fe^{2+} treatment had any effect on doxycycline levels following 2 x 100 mg doses. The lack of interaction between charcoal and doxycycline _in vivo_ is in contrast to extensive interactions _in vitro_.

Clearance of doxycycline from serum is influenced to only a small extent by haemodialysis.[516] Urinary excretion of doxycycline is increased with increasing urinary pH.[517] However, drug $t_{0.5}$ values were increased during repeated doses under both alkaline and control conditions.

Oxytetracycline

Generic inequivalence has been demonstrated for some p.o. oxytetracycline formulations, but individual variation prevented significant differences being shown in all but the most extreme cases.[518,519] Other studies have demonstrated significant bio-availability differences between oxytetracycline dihydrate[520] and tetracycline hydrochloride[521] preparations. The serum $t_{0.5}$ of oxytetracycline in horses was reported to be 15.7 h and 10.5 h after i.v. and i.m. injections, respectively.[522] Although no explanation is offered for this difference, contributing factors may have been the influence of dose-dependent kinetics or taking an insufficient number of data points after the i.m. dose. Increased concentrations of oxytetracycline in nasal mucus due to bromhexine treatment have been attributed to evaporation of the less viscous mucus due to bromhexine treatment, rather than increased membrane permeability.[523]

Minocycline and Methacycline

Minocycline has similar pharmacokinetic properties to doxycycline in man, but is more rapidly absorbed after p.o. doses and also penetrates tissues rapidly.[524] Minocycline is partially metabolized, and renal clearance of active antibiotic is only 9 ml min^{-1}, compared with 20, 29, and 35 ml min^{-1} for doxycycline, methacycline, and demethylchlortetracycline.

A number of studies have shown that minocycline elimination from the body, like that of doxycycline, is independent of renal function.[525,526] The drug $t_{0.5}$ is only slightly elevated from a normal value of <u>ca</u>. 14 h to <u>ca</u>. 17 h in severe renal impairment.

As minocycline is eliminated from the body predominantly by metabolism its clearance might be expected to be independent of renal function. Increased incidence of toxic side-effects attributed to minocycline in renal impairment may be due to increased tissue pene-

tration of unchanged drug, or impaired renal excretion of pharmacologically active metabolites.

Serum concentrations of methacycline were similar in lung tissue
and serum after single p.o. doses in man. However, after a second
dose, lung tissue concentrations were depressed relative to those in
serum.[527]

Aminoglycosides

Introduction

The aminoglycosides constitute one of the most commonly used
classes of antibiotics. Their relatively narrow therapeutic indices
have given rise to intense interest in their activity, distribution,
and correct dosage in diseased conditions,[528,529] and in serum
level monitoring.[530,531]

Concern regarding optimal doses of gentamicin and other aminoglycosides has occasioned publications on dosage adjustment based on
individual patient parameters,[532,533] calculation of dosage regimens for multiple i.v. infusions,[534] and the risk of ototoxicity in
patients with mild-to-moderate renal impairment.[535-537]

Large interpatient variations in pharmacokinetics and drug-
related toxicity are characteristic of aminoglycoside therapy. In a
survey of 1640 patients receiving gentamicin treatment for gram-
negative infections, the daily dose necessary to obtain therapeutic
serum concentrations of antibiotic varied from 0.5 to 25.8 mg kg^{-1}
in patients with normal kidney function.[538] The use of pharmacokinetic criteria in calculating individual dose regimens resulted in a
relatively low incidence of nephrotoxicity attributable to gentamicin
and tobramycin.[539,540] It has been suggested that ideal body
weight provides the most accurate prediction of aminoglycoside serum
levels compared with methods based on actual body weight or on surface
area.[541] On the other hand, Finley et al.[542] maintained that although
pharmacokinetic dosing of aminoglycosides may provide a more reliable

means of establishing appropriate serum levels than standard recommended doses, it should not be substituted for measurement of serum levels. Schentag et al.[543] studied 201 critically ill patients and found that aminoglycoside serum concentrations in the therapeutic range were of limited value in preventing drug-induced nephrotoxicity.

Methods to detect susceptible patients and to minimize risk of nephrotoxicity have been described from both clinical[544,545] and pharmacokinetic[546] viewpoints. Clinical recommendations include continuous dosage adjustment to GFR, maintenance of an expanded extracellular fluid volume, and the use of culture results to determine how long therapy should be continued. The pharmacokinetic approach is based on the assumption of a predisposition for potentially nephrotoxic patients to accumulate aminoglycoside in tissues. This tendency is reflected in increasing 'apparent' drug biological $t_{0.5}$ values during continuous dosing, and high-risk patients can thus be identified by monitoring peak and trough aminoglycoside levels in serum during early stages of therapy.

Information regarding the relative intrarenal disposition of some aminoglycosides is conflicting. Highest levels in the cortex of healthy human kidneys are observed with netilmicin,[547] while levels of gentamicin are slightly higher than those of tobramycin.[548] In severely diseased kidneys, however, levels of tobramycin exceed those of gentamicin.[547] During repeated doses of the two aminoglycosides to patients with various infections, steady-state urinary recovery of tobramycin was essentially complete, whereas that of gentamicin was 77% of the administered dose.[549]

Gentamicin

Gentamicin is the original and most extensively used aminoglycoside, and a considerable literature has been generated on the distribution and elimination characteristics of this compound. Gentamicin is water-soluble. Like many other agents of this class it is poorly absorbed from the GI tract and must be administered parenterally.

Consistent with its high aqueous solubility, gentamicin distributes poorly into c.s.f., but c.n.s. penetration is improved in meningitis.[550] Therapeutic concentrations of gentamicin in c.s.f. were obtained in humans following combined i.m. and intrathecal doses, and the drug $t_{0.5}$ in c.s.f. was 5.5 h compared with 2 h in plasma.[551] Although this study showed that intrathecal injections yielded adequate c.s.f. gentamicin levels, the author did not prove that inadequate levels were obtained using i.m. doses alone in these subjects.[552] Gentamicin appears to enter bronchial secretions in the dog by passive diffusion across a concentration gradient after both i.v. and i.m. doses.[553] Drug concentrations in secretions were somewhat less than those in plasma, but concentrations in both fluids declined at the same rate. Artificially-induced fever caused a 25% decrease in serum gentamicin levels 30 and 60 min following i.v. injection in dogs, and a 40% decrease in levels 1, 2, and 3 h following i.m. injection to humans.[554] Decreased drug levels must be due to changes in distribution as elimination $t_{0.5}$ values were unaffected. No explanation was offered for the observed changes, but it was suggested that they may result in some febrile patients receiving inadequate doses of gentamicin.

Gentamicin has been shown to enter synovial fluid efficiently after i.m. injection.[555] Synovial fluid levels of aminoglycoside were routinely greater than 50% of those in serum and in some cases equal concentrations of drug were obtained in both fluids. Penetration of drug into interstitial fluid in rabbits was significantly improved after bolus doses compared to slow infusions, at least during a 2 h postdose period, and bolus administration may be the preferred mode of delivery for rapid extravascular penetration.[556] Uptake of gentamicin by rat-kidney cortical slices was inhibited by dinitrophenol, and also by anoxia, suggesting the requirement of aerobic phosphorylation for active transportation of gentamicin into cortical cells.[557] This type of active transport has also been shown for cephaloridine.[558] The serum extraction ratio for gentamicin from the dog renal cortex was 0.2, compared with 0.74 for p-aminohippuric acid, and the renal cortex:serum ratio for gentamicin was 12 compared with a medulla:serum ratio of 2.7.[559] Accumulation of gentamicin in the kidney appears therefore to be caused by several mechanisms including active transport, passive tubular reabsorption, and cortical cell sequestration.

The distribution of gentamicin in peritoneal fluid was studied following repeated i.v. doses in patients with cirrhotic ascites.[560] Mean diffusion into uninflammed ascites was 30 - 50%, but was 68% during episodes of bacterial peritonitis. After single 3.5 mg kg^{-1} i.v. doses, gentamicin distribution volumes averaged 0.39 1 kg^{-1} in normal infants (4 - 10 m) and 0.46 1 kg^{-1} in malnourished infants, while no significant differences were observed in the $t_{0.5}$ (1.3 - 1.4 h) and overall clearance (3.6 - 4.0 ml min^{-1} kg^{-1}) between the two groups.[561] The larger distribution space in malnourished patients was probably due to increased total body water. Gentamicin, being water soluble, distributes primarily in extracellular fluid. Lecompte et al.[562] reported a 20 - 30% decrease in distribution volume and a 40% related decrease in total body clearance of gentamicin in rats deprived of water for 4 d, compared with control animals.

The apparent volume of distribution of gentamicin tended to increase in obese patients, although with substantial interpatient variability.[563] The uptake of gentamicin in adipose tissue was 43.7% of that in the total body mass of patients with normal weight.[564] Thus the dose of gentamicin in obese patients may be calculated based on ideal body weight plus 43.7% of the fat weight. In this study, gentamicin $t_{0.5}$ was <u>ca.</u> 3 h in both normal weight and obese patients.

Inconsistencies among reports on the degree of binding by gentamicin to proteins may be related to interference by other substances. Gentamicin is normally 20% bound to serum proteins.[565] However, binding is increased in the absence of, and decreased in the presence of, excess Ca^{2+} and Mg^{2+} and is markedly increased in the presence of heparin. Binding of gentamicin to the heparin molecule appears to be the causative factor for increased apparent binding of gentamicin in plasma when heparin is used as an anticoagulant, compared with serum. Gentamicin may interfere with the binding of bilirubin to plasma albumin in infants.[566]

Unlike some other antibiotics, gentamicin and other aminoglycosides are excreted in bile to only a moderate extent.[567] Concentrations in bile are generally 30 - 80% of those in serum of individuals with normal hepatic function, but the percentage decreases in obstructive hepato-biliary disease. Comparisons of maternal and cord venous serum levels at parturition confirm that gentamicin crosses the human placenta to a limited extent.[568] Peak cord levels 60 - 120 min after dosing were 34% of maternal levels obtained 30 min after dosing.

Studies in animals indicated that the three components of gentamicin, C_1, C_{1a}, and C_2, have similar distribution characteristics in the body.[569] However studies in man have shown that component C_1 occupies a somewhat larger distribution space in the body than gentamicin.[570] The slightly lower serum levels of gentamicin C_1 compared with those of gentamicin complex, and the accumulation of both drugs during repeated doses, are indicated in Figure 3.19. In this study,

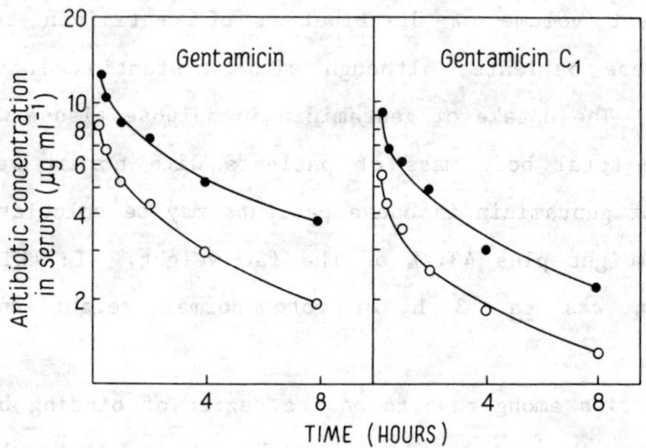

Figure 3.19 Serum levels of antibiotic after first (o —— o) and last (● —— ●) i.v. injections of gentamicin and gentamicin C_1. Reproduced by permission from <u>Antimicrob. Ag. Chemother.</u>, 1975, <u>7</u>, 328.

compounds were administered by initial i.v. injection, followed by eight-hourly i.m. injections for 7 days, and then a final i.v. injection. All doses were 1 mg kg^{-1}.

Gentamicin is generally considered to have a biological $t_{0.5}$ of 3 - 6 h in normal adults. However, development of more sophisticated analytical methods has given rise to the suggestion that gentamicin, and also tobramycin, have prolonged $t_{0.5}$ values of 110 - 120 h. Nonetheless in these studies 70 - 90% of the dose of both drugs was recovered in urine within 24 h.[571] Gentamicin $t_{0.5}$ averaged 8.2 h in 55 nonasphyxiated preterm infants and 14.6 h in 25 infants following perinatal asphyxia.[572] The respective clearance of gentamicin was 1.17 and 0.66 ml min^{-1}, while the volume of distribution was similar in the two groups. Slower elimination of gentamicin in the asphyxiated infants was apparently due to compromised renal function secondary to perinatal asphyxia.

Continuing studies on gentamicin pharmacokinetics have confirmed the persistence of this compound in the body, particularly in renal insufficiency. After repeated doses in two patients, serum and urine levels of gentamicin declined in biphasic fashion, with terminal $t_{0.5}$ values of 87 and 173 h.[573] Avid recycling of drug by the kidney caused the renal clearance to be reduced at low urinary concentrations so that clearance in urine is prolonged through 10 - 20 days. Serum levels and urinary excretion of gentamicin, together with renal clearance and output values for a patient receiving gentamicin, are shown in Figure 3.20. In 47 patients with creatinine clearances between 8 and 130 ml min^{-1}, terminal phase gentamicin $t_{0.5}$ values ranged from 27 to 693 h.[574]

Impaired elimination of gentamicin in renal insufficiency is well documented, and various dosing schedules to achieve adequate treatment without inducing toxic side-effects have been described[575-579] and reviewed.[580,581] The utility of generalized nomograms for gentamicin dose adjustment in renal failure has been questioned by Kaye et al.[582] Owing to the wide variation in pharmacokinetic parameters

among individuals, general formulae serve only as guidelines and cannot replace monitoring of individual blood levels. Most methods of

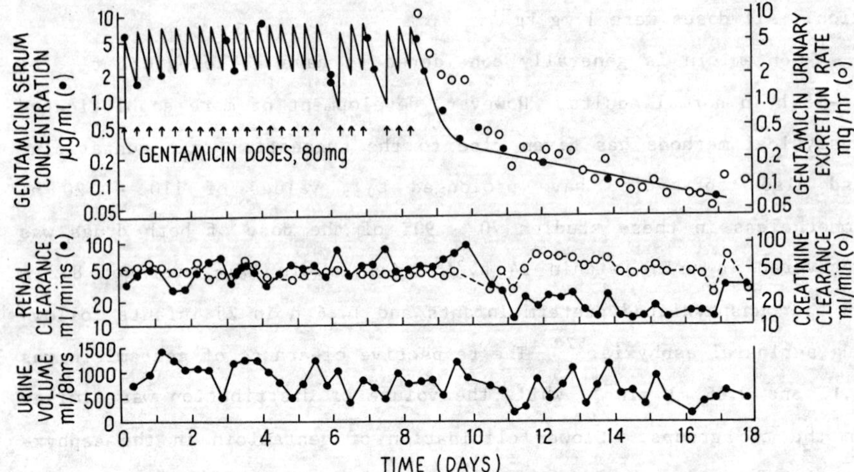

Figure 3.20   Serum concentrations and urinary excretion rates of gentamicin, clearances of creatinine and
gentamicin, and 8 h urine output of gentamicin versus
time for a patient. The solid lines in the top frame
are values simulated from two-compartment model parameters which were generated from nonlinear least-
squares regression analysis of measured serum concentrations of the washout period. Also shown in the top
frame are the times of administration of 80 mg doses.
Reproduced by permission from <u>Clin. Pharmacol. Ther.</u>,
1977, <u>22</u>, 364.

drug dose adjustment are based on mean steady-state drug levels $\overline{C}\infty$ and
use the linear relationships that exist between drug levels, the elimination rate constant k_{el}, dosing interval τ, dose size D, distribution volume V, and the $t_{0.5}$ as indicated in equation 3.5.[583] The
value of k_{el} is linearly related to creatinine clearance Cl_{CR} as

$$\overline{C}\infty = \frac{D}{Vk_{el}\tau} = \frac{1.44 \cdot t_{0.5} \cdot D}{V\tau} \qquad (3.5)$$

described in equation 3.6 where k_{nr} is the rate constant for nonrenal elimination and b is a constant. The $t_{0.5}$ for drugs cleared

$$k_{el} = k_{nr} + b \cdot Cl_{CR} \qquad (3.6)$$

predominantly via the kidneys is linearly related to serum creatinine C_{CR} as in equation 3.7,[584] where a is a constant.

$$t_{0.5} = a \cdot C_{CR} \tag{3.7}$$

Two independent studies have shown, however, that the incidence and severity of toxic side-effects due to gentamicin are highly correlated with minimum rather than mean steady-state drug levels,[585,586] thus strongly suggesting the need for reassessment of present dose-adjustment methodology for gentamicin, and perhaps other aminoglycosides. Other reports consider the accuracy of gentamicin assay procedures in biological fluids.[587,588] One of these indicates that recovery of gentamicin and tobramycin from uraemic serum may be considerably less than that from normal serum, a phenomenon not shared by streptomycin or kanamycin, and makes a case for better standardization of microbiological assay procedures.[547]

Gentamicin, tobramycin, and kanamycin were efficiently cleared from the circulation during haemodialysis, concentrations of all three drugs being reduced by approximately 50% during a 6 h dialysis period.[589-591] Clearance of tobramycin by peritoneal dialysis was more variable and also less efficient.[591,592] Christopher et al.[589] have described methods for gentamicin dose adjustment in dialysis patients.

The relative efficiency of different commercial haemodialysers has been investigated for gentamicin[593] and other agents.[594] Dialysis has been variously reported to reduce the apparent elimination $t_{0.5}$ to 10 h[593] and 5 h.[595] Dosage recommendations for gentamicin therapy were described for uraemic patients on intermittent dialysis and also in children receiving peritoneal dialysis.[596]

In patients with chronic renal failure who were on continuous ambulatory peritoneal dialysis (CAPD) administration of gentamicin in the dialysate resulted in rapid absorption of antibiotic from the peritoneal fluid into blood.[597,598] Approximately 84% of a 1 mg kg^{-1} dose was absorbed systemically during a 6 h dwell time.[598] Subsequent clearance of gentamicin from serum occurred slowly, the average $t_{0.5}$ being <u>ca</u>. 30 h. Intravenous administration of an equal dose of gentamicin in these patients resulted in little or no removal of the antibiotic by CAPD.

Conflicting data have been reported on the effect of diuretics on the renal clearance of gentamicin. In a study employing 1 mg kg^{-1} i.v. doses of gentamicin alone and simultaneously with 0.25 mg kg^{-1} furosemide or 0.1 mg kg^{-1} piretanide in healthy male volunteers, both diuretics induced a 5- to 6-fold increase in urine volume during the first 3 h postdose, and a corresponding increase in gentamicin excretion from <u>ca</u>. 20% to 50 - 60% of the dose.[599] Thus, renal clearance of gentamicin was enhanced during the period of diuresis although GFR and gentamicin $t_{0.5}$ (2 - 2.5 h) remained unaffected. On the contrary, Lawson et al.[600] reported a significant decrease in GFR caused by furosemide. Gentamicin plasma clearance averaged 69 ml min^{-1} without furosemide and 40 ml min^{-1} after furosemide.

Carbenicillin and ticarcillin chemically deactivate gentamicin and other aminoglycosides.[601,602] Studies <u>in vitro</u> have shown that gentamicin and tobramycin are inactivated to a greater extent than amikacin and netilmicin.[603] Carbenicillin has no effect on serum gentamicin $t_{0.5}$ values in subjects with normal or slightly impaired kidneys.[604] However, in severe uraemia deactivation of gentamicin by carbenicillin results in a reduced serum $t_{0.5}$ for the aminoglycoside. The mean gentamicin $t_{0.5}$ in uraemic patients was reduced from 46 h to 22 h after administration of carbenicillin, while in other patients, it was reduced from 33 h to 23 h due to ticarcillin,[605] giving rise to reduced circulating levels of aminoglycoside.[606] The gentamicin inactivation rate constants due to carbenicillin and ticarcillin are 0.016 and 0.010 h^{-1}, respectively, and these should be applied to dose calculations concerning combined therapy for uraemic individuals. Evidence that gentamicin is partially cleared from the body by metabolism is supported by observations that venous clearance of antibiotic exceeds its renal clearance in human subjects.[607]

Serum gentamicin $t_{0.5}$ values are inversely related to age in infants, decreasing from <u>ca</u>. 3.3 h in neonates to 2.5 h in infants over 20 m. In this young population, there was no relationship between serum $t_{0.5}$ and creatinine clearance values.[608] In a critical examination of gentamicin doses in children, dose adjustment based on body surface area had no advantages over dosing by body weight.[609] When two groups of children received gentamicin by i.v. injection, there were no significant differences in peak drug level variability between the two methods.

Amikacin

The absorption rate of amikacin is faster in new-born infants than in adults.[610] Amikacin penetrates into lung and cardiac tissue, and into pericardial fluid at concentrations exceeding the MIC's for most sensitive bacteria.[611] Variable levels of amikacin in bronchial secretions may reduce the effectiveness of this compound against some Gram-negative organisms, particularly <u>Psuedomonas aeruginosa</u>, at that infection site.[612] Amikacin penetrates moderately into rabbit interstitial fluid, giving rise to aminoglycoside levels after a 7.5 mg kg^{-1} dose similar to those obtained from a 1.5 mg kg^{-1} dose of gentamicin. Interstitial fluid levels obtained from both compounds were inhibitory for most susceptible organisms, and these may be relevant to the physiological situation in man. As is the case with the parent compound kanamycin, amikacin does not effectively cross the blood-brain barrier, and drug levels in human c.s.f. after i.m. injection are very low, or undetectable.[614] Other studies in rabbits suggest that amikacin penetrates some tissues less efficiently than gentamcin,[615] although the kidney is the major site for disposition of both drugs. Amikacin, tobramycin, and gentamicin accumulate to similar extents in inner ear fluids, giving rise to drug levels in these fluids many times higher than those in the brain, heart, and liver.[616]

The relatively high doses of amikacin needed to achieve and maintain therapeutic levels in children compared to adults may be due to faster clearance, altered distribution, or a combination of these. The mean serum $t_{0.5}$ in 50 patients, aged 1 - 17 yr, was 1.2 h and the total body clearance was 130 ml min^{-1} 1.73 m^{-2}.[617,618] The distribution volume in children (mean 0.26 1 kg^{-1}) is also larger than the mean value of 0.14 - 0.17 1 kg^{-1} reported in adults. The clearance of drug in the newborn was slow, however, yielding mean $t_{0.5}$ and body clearance values of 6 h and 1.4 ml min^{-1} kg^{-1}, respectively. In older children and adolescents, amikacin clearance is higher in proportion to body weight than in adults.[619] Following single 7.5 mg kg^{-1} i.v. doses of amikacin in neonates (6 - 25 d), infants (4 - 18 m), and children (3 - 11 yr), respective serum $t_{0.5}$ values averaged 2.8, 1.8, and 1.2 h, while the apparent distribution volumes were 0.43, 0.32, and 0.21 1 kg^{-1}.[620] The relatively short amikacin $t_{0.5}$ in older children compared with infants and adults was confirmed in 50 pediatric patients (age 1 - 17 yr) with malignancies and normal renal function.[621] Intravenous infusion doses of amikacin (5 mg kg^{-1} every 6 - 8 h) in children resulted in no drug accumulation after 3 to 35 days of therapy, the mean serum $t_{0.5}$ and total body clearance being 1.2 h and 131 ml min^{-1} 1.73 m^{-2}.[620]

Age-related differences in dosage requirement may be attenuated when doses are based on body surface area. Amikacin levels in fat and muscle were 13 - 16% of serum levels in children 1.5 - 3.5 h after single i.m. doses.[622] Tissue levels of drug declined at a slower rate than those in serum so that levels in fat and muscle were 71 - 77% of serum levels at 10 - 13 h. Amikacin appears to have some affinity for fat as the blood supply to fatty tissue is inferior to that to muscle.

In normal adults amikacin has similar kinetic characteristics to gentamicin. Serum levels, measured by radioenzymatic assay, declined in a biexponential manner following i.v. doses, with α and β $t_{0.5}$ values of 1 h and 2.4 h, respectively. Serum levels exceeded 10 μg ml^{-1} for 0.5 h, and 4 μg ml^{-1} for 2 h after 125 mg i.v. doses. Following a 500 mg dose, serum levels of amikacin exceeded 10 μg ml^{-1} for 3 h. Levels of antibiotic in serum were more prolonged after i.m. injection.[623] Urinary recovery (70 - 80%), and both serum and renal clearance of amikacin, are similar to those of gentamicin, but the variability in these values and also in serum levels of active drug appears to be smaller for amikacin.[624]

After parenteral administration (7.5 mg kg^{-1} i.v. or i.m) of amikacin in 17 patients with normal renal function, the average $t_{0.5}$ and serum clearance were 2.3 - 2.5 h and 73 - 74 ml min^{-1}, respectively, according to two-compartment model analysis of the 0 to 6 h blood concentration data.[625]

Prolonged elimination of amikacin was observed in a study in which the sampling period was extended to 7 d postdose.[626] These authors found no significant differences between amikacin and gentamicin kinetics and nephrotoxic potential in matched patients; the mean terminal serum $t_{0.5}$ was 7 - 8 d while the total body clearance was <u>ca.</u> 30 ml min^{-1}. It was estimated that the relatively long $t_{0.5}$ applied to approximately 10% of the total dose, a portion that distributed extensively and was not cleared completely by glomerular filtration. Approximately 69% of an i.m. dose (5.5 mg kg^{-1}) of amikacin was excreted in the 8 h urine in healthy volunteers (mean age 29 yr) compared with 44% in bedridden elderly patients (mean age 76 yr), and the respective serum $t_{0.5}$ values were 1.8 and 3.6 h.[627] Decreased renal excretion of amikacin in the elderly was probably related to impaired kidney function.

In morbidly obese patients, peak serum levels of amikacin were predictable using a volume of distribution based on ideal body weight plus a correction factor of 38% of fat weight.[628] Amikacin $t_{0.5}$ in these patients, averaging 2.1 h, was in the normal range for aminoglycosides.

Amikacin pharmacokinetics in normal and impaired renal function are similar to those for other aminoglycosides.[629-631] Linear relationships have been described between amikacin elimination and renal function,[632,633] although one study suggests the possibility of a nonlinear relationship between amikacin $t_{0.5}$ and serum creatinine.[634] The elimination $t_{0.5}$ of amikacin is related to serum creatinine concentrations in uraemic patients by the expression $t_{0.5} = -1.4 + 3.3\ C_{CR}$[631] so that the amikacin $t_{0.5}$ can be calculated approximately by multiplying the serum creatinine (mg 100 ml^{-1}) by a factor of 3. The elimination $t_{0.5}$ of amikacin may reach 60-70 h in severe renal failure.[635] Haemodialysis effectively removes amikacin from serum,[636] reducing the drug $t_{0.5}$ from 86.5 h in anephric patients, and 44.3 h in patients with minimal kidney function, to 5.6 h;[637] peritoneal dialysis resulted in a $t_{0.5}$ value of 18 h. Unlike gentamicin and tobramycin, amikacin is not appreciably inactivated by carbenicillin *in vivo*.[638] The average $t_{0.5}$ and serum clearance of i.v. amikacin in patients with severe renal failure were 65 h and 0.03 ml min kg^{-1}, respectively, when the dose was followed by infusions of carbenicillin.

Netilmicin

Netilmicin has similar pharmacokinetic characteristics to other aminoglycosides.[639,640] The pharmacokinetics of single i.m. doses of netilmicin were similar to those observed after equal doses of gentamicin.[641] Serum drug levels peaked at *ca*. 1 h (Figure 3.21) and subsequently declined with a terminal $t_{0.5}$ of 2.2 - 2.5 h. Total body clearance of netilmicin averaged 65 - 70 ml min^{-1}, and 70 - 80% of the dose was excreted in urine within 24 h, suggesting some metabolic clearance or tissue binding of drug. As previously reported for gentamicin and tobramycin,[571] a much prolonged terminal $t_{0.5}$ of 198 h was observed for netilmicin after extended blood sampling for 10 days and analysis by radioimmunoassay, and the mean total body clearance was 31 ml min^{-1}.[642] Although the long $t_{0.5}$ was associated

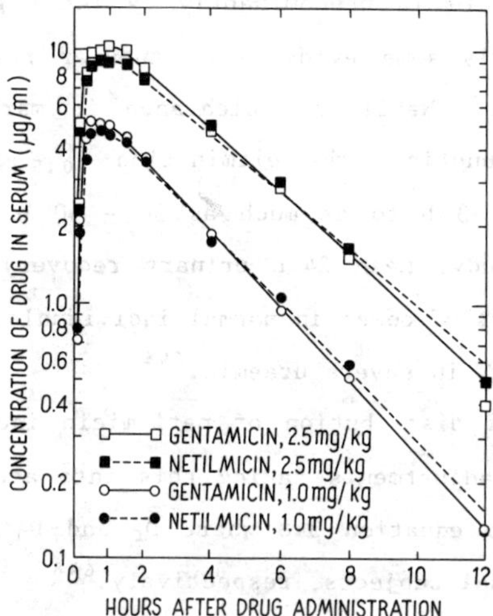

Figure 3.21   Concentrations of gentamicin and netilmicin in serum after single i.m. injections of 1.0 and
2.5 mg kg^{-1} in humans.   Reproduced by permission
from *Antimicrob. Ag. Chemother.*, 1980, *17*, 184.

with tissue accumulation of only *ca*. 5% of the netilmicin dose, it

contributed to the rising serum concentrations after multiple dosing

at 6 to 12 h intervals. Netilmicin disposition kinetics were similar

in premature and gestationally mature neonates despite considerable

interpatient variation in serum concentrations.[643]   The mean $t_{0.5}$

and total body clearance were 5.9 and 0.06 1 h^{-1} kg^{-1}, compared

with 2.5 h and 0.12 1 h^{-1} kg^{-1} in older children (3.5 m - 13 yr).

A significantly reduced $t_{0.5}$ of 1.4 h was observed in children with

cystic fibrosis, although the mean clearance remained similar to that

in control patients.[644]

In 14 patients with GI diseases who received a single 2 mg kg^{-1}

i.m. dose of netilmicin before gastric operation, maximum antibiotic

concentrations of 2.5 µg g^{-1} and 4.9 µg ml^{-1} were observed in

stomach tissue and serum, respectively, at *ca*. 1 h postdose.[645]   The

tissue:serum concentration ratio remained constant at approximately

0.5 throughout 0 - 8 h.

Elimination of netilmicin is predominantly by renal glomerular filtration, although there is some evidence of tubular reabsorption and extrarenal elimination. Netilmicin clearance is markedly reduced in impaired renal function, the elimination $t_{0.5}$ increasing from a normal value of 2 - 3 h to as much as 30 - 40 h in severe uraemia.[646-648] In one study, mean 24 h urinary recovery of antibiotic accounted for 50 - 90% of doses in normal individuals, 52 - 58% in mild uraemia, and 41 - 43% in severe uraemia.[646]

The apparent volume of distribution of netilmicin increases in severe uraemia, and dosage adjustments taking this into account have been described according to equation 3.8 where D_r and D_n are doses in renally impaired and normal subjects, respectively.[648]

$$D_r = \frac{V_d(AUC)_r \cdot \beta_r}{V_d(AUC)_n \cdot \beta_n} \cdot D_n = \frac{(serum\ clearance)_r}{(serum\ clearance)_n} \cdot D_n \qquad (3.8)$$

Tobramycin

The pharmacokinetic and antibacterial properties of tobramycin, and the influence of these on therapuetic use have been reviewed.[649] Serum levels of tobramycin are slightly lower after i.m. doses than after equivalent doses of gentamicin, although the values of most other pharmacokinetic parameters are similar for the two compounds.[650-652]

Absorption of p.o. dosed tobramycin is poor and erratic. Repeated administration of a 100 mg solution dose every 4 h resulted in variable and subtherapeutic serum antibiotic concentrations.[653] Between 0.5 and 6.7% of the tobramycin dose was recovered in urine and 35 - 79% in faeces. The pharmacokinetics of tobramycin were studied after 1 mg kg^{-1} i.v. doses in 3 healthy volunteers using a specific and sensitive HPLC assay.[654] Serum tobramycin data were characteristic of the two-compartment model, with a mean terminal $t_{0.5}$ of 68.7

h. The volume of distribution at steady state and the body clearance were 1.1 1 kg^{-1} and 91.4 ml min^{-1}, respectively, while cumulative urinary excretion over a 10 day period accounted for 91% of the dose. Tobramycin pharmacokinetics in patients with normal renal function were independent of age.[655] In this study on 77 patients (age 20 - 79 yr), serum concentrations were analyzed in terms of single-compartment kinetics, and a relatively short $t_{0.5}$ of 2.2 - 2.4 h was reported. Increased clearance of tobramycin was observed in patients with cystic fibrosis, average $t_{0.5}$ and total body clearance being 1.2 h and 181 ml min^{-1} 1.73 m^{-2}.[656]

Tobramycin penetrates into aqueous humour following single i.m. and i.v. doses, but the aqueous levels are low compared with those in serum.[657] Subconjunctival injection of tobramycin sulphate gives rise to therapeutically effective levels of drug in the aqueous humour of rabbits.[658] These levels exceed the MICs of most <u>Pseudomonas</u> species, and also other Gram-negative bacilli associated with bacterial eye infections. Studies in guinea pigs indicate that at identical dose levels tobramycin may be less ototoxic than gentamicin.[659]

Serum levels and urinary excretion of tobramycin exhibit a prolonged elimination phase similar to that of gentamicin, even in subjects with stable renal function. After repeated i.m. doses to an elderly patient, tobramycin disappearance from serum exhibited three distinct phases, with $t_{0.5}$ values of 0.3, 3.9, and 169 h, respectively.[660] Prolonged elimination of tobramycin was confirmed in 35 patients with stable renal function.[661] Serum profiles in this study were interpreted in terms of a two-compartment model and the mean β-phase $t_{0.5}$ was 146 h. Prolonged $t_{0.5}$ and also multicompartment kinetic behaviour of tobramycin predicts that drug will continue to accumulate in tissue with repeated dosing.

Two-compartment kinetics were used also to describe serum levels of tobramycin in morbidly obese patients.[662] In this study, blood samples were obtained during a 12 h postdose period. During this time the elimination $t_{0.5}$ of tobramycin was 2.1 h, which is similar to that reported for individuals with normal body weight. Tobramycin distribution is influenced by excess adipose tissue in these patients, and dosage adjustments are made to account for this.

The renal clearance of tobramycin, 92% of creatinine clearance, is unaffected by probenecid, and relationships between serum clearance of the antibiotic and serum and urinary creatinine are similar to those observed for gentamicin in renal patients[663,664] and in the newborn.[665]

The apparent elimination $t_{0.5}$ of tobramycin is increased from a normal value of 2 - 3 h to 13 - 34 h in severe uraemia.[666,667] Support for the use of nomogram-assisted dosage schedules for tobramycin in renally compromised patients is provided by Tobias et al.[668] who compared circulating levels of the drug in patients with acute leukaemia and neutropaenia receiving nomogram-assisted or standard therapy. Serum levels were higher when the nomogram was used but there was no evidence of residual drug 8 h after dosing.

Sisomicin

Sisomicin has almost identical pharmacokinetic properties to gentamicin,[669-671] and obeys two-compartment model kinetics after i.v. doses. Reported pharmacokinetic values vary somewhat, with $t_{0.5}$ values of fast and slow disposition phases in normal individuals ranging from 2 to 9 min and from 48 min to 3 h, respectively.[670,671] Intramuscular doses are efficiently and rapidly absorbed leading to equivalent, but somewhat lower, serum profiles to those after i.v. administration. Of the two aminoglycosides, sisomicin appears to have somewhat greater tissue penetration than gentamicin. Serum levels of sisomicin were somewhat lower than those from an equal dose of gentamicin after i.m. injection and i.v. infusion, although blister fluid levels of the two compounds were similar following infusion. Greater tissue sequestration and slow release of sisomicin by tissue, compared with gentamicin, is suggested also by the pattern of their urinary recovery. After i.m. injection, 24 h urinary recovery was 95% complete for gentamicin but only 76% for sisomicin. In post 24 h urine, however, an additional 21% of sisomicin was eliminated, compared with less than 1% for gentamicin.

Some accumlulation of sisomicin in serum occurred during repeated dosing at 8 h intervals, but serum levels were stable after the fourth day of dosing.[672] Steady-state levels were predictable from pharmaco-kinetic parameters calculated from the initial dose. Average serum levels from 0.5, 0.75, and 1.0 mg kg^{-1} single and multiple doses of sisomicin are given in Figure 3.22.

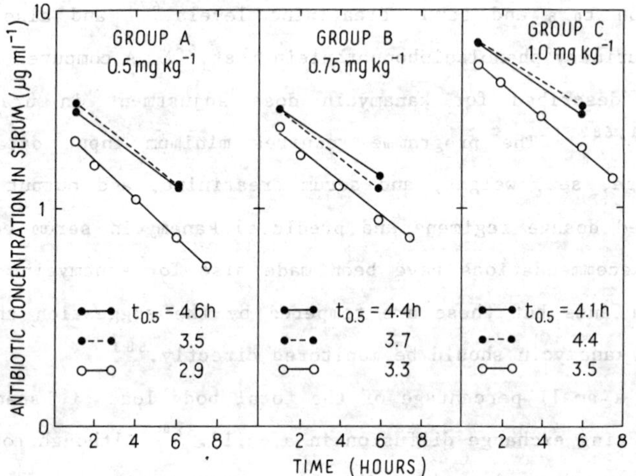

Figure 3.22   Plots of serum concentrations of siso-micin against time, after single and repeated i.m. doses: o——o = first dose, ●---● = fourth day, ●——● = seventh day of repeated dosing. Reproduced by per-mission from *J. Clin. Pharmacol.*, 1974, **14**, 567.

Sisomicin pharmacokinetics are independent of dose (25 - 100 mg) and route of administration (i.v. and i.m.).[673] Total body clearance and renal clearance of sisomicin averaged 78 and 55 ml min^{-1}, re-spectively, and 70 - 75% of a single dose was excreted in 24 h urine.

As with other aminoglycosides, sisomicin clearance is linearly related to renal function and dose adjustments are recommended based on serum creatinine levels.[674-676] Sisomicin is removed from blood by dialysis at the same rate as blood urea nitrogen and creatinine, and this relationship may be used to estimate the extent of removal of sisomicin and other aminoglycosides during dialysis.[676]

Kanamycin

Kanamycin has a renal clearance that is only <u>ca</u>. 60% of creatinine clearance in normal subjects.[677] This appears to be due to kidney tubular reabsorption, as kanamycin does not bind appreciably to plasma proteins.[678] Dose adjustments for kanamycin in patients with renal failure are proposed, based on relationship between kanamycin elimination $t_{0.5}$ and serum creatinine levels,[679] and also using a modified urinary phenolsulphonphthalein test.[680] A computer programme has been described for kanamycin dose adjustment in uraemic patients.[681,682] The programme requires minimum input data of patient's age, sex, weight, and serum creatinine, and output includes recommended dosage regimens and predicted kanamycin serum concentrations. Recommendations have been made also for kanamycin dosage in newborn infants but these are tempered by the suggestion that serum levels of kanamycin should be monitored directly.[683]

Only a small percentage of the total body load of kanamycin was removed during exchange diffusion in a child.[684] Although total blood volume was exchanged, only 3.1% of a kanamycin dose was removed by this process. A maximum removal of 10% of the dose would have occurred if the exchange had been initiated immediately after the kanamycin dose.

Neomycin and Paromomycin

The pharmacokinetics of neomycin and paromomycin were studied following single p.o. doses of the respective sulfates (16 g and 14.3 g) in healthy volunteers.[685] Serum concentrations of paramomycin reached a peak value of 3.7 μg ml^{-1} at 1.9 h and exhibited a $t_{0.5}$

of 2.6 h according to one-compartment model analysis. In contrast, neomycin data were more adequately described by the two-compartment pharmacokinetic model. Peak neomycin level in serum was 5.1 μg ml^{-1} at 2.6 h postdose, and the mean α and β phase $t_{0.5}$ values were 1.5 h and 9 h, respectively. Total recovery of paromomycin and neomycin in 0 to 32 h urine averaged 0.2 and 0.3% of the respective doses. Similar pharmacokinetic characteristics of these compounds were observed after multiple dosing in patients.

The absorption of neomycin administered by enema is similar to that after p.o. doses and absorption is not influenced by intestinal ulceration or regional enteritis.[686] Neomycin caused reduced absorption of vitamin A from the GI tract, presumably owing to disruption of the intraluminal micellar phase of fat absorption.[687]

Streptomycin

The kinetic behaviour and distribution of streptomycin are not influenced by changes in plasma albumin concentration in undernourished individuals.[688] This appears to be related to compensating increases in plasma globulin, which also binds streptomycin. However, as streptomycin is normally only 35% bound to total plasma proteins, alterations in the fraction of drug bound, however large, should not give rise to significant changes in drug disposition.[689]

Lividomycin A

Studies in animals show that the aminoglycoside lividomycin A is rapidly absorbed after i.m. injection, 70 - 90% of the dose appearing unchanged in urine.[690] Urinary recovery of p.o. doses to rabbits represented only 2% of the dose, and plasma levels of antibiotic were one-fifth of those obtained with kanamycin.

Sulfonamides

The literature on sulfonamides during the review period has been devoted primarily to the combination sulfamethoxazole-trimethroprim, and other combinations. Hence this review will focus primarily on this segment of sulfonamide kinetics, together with a brief review of the less exhaustive literature on individual sulfonamides.

The pharmacokinetics of several commonly used sulfonamides have been reviewed recently.[691] An interesting study was conducted to elucidate the relationships between molecular structure and biological disposition of the sulfonamides.[692] It appears that sulfonamides with a sulphur atom two atomic bond distances from the N_1 atom, e.g. sulfamethizole, sulfaethidole, and sulfathiazole, are excreted by active tubular secretion. When the sulfur atom is replaced by an oxygen or nitrogen atom, active secretion ceases. On the other hand, all N_4-acetylsulfonamides are excreted by active tubular secretion regardless of the substituent at the N_1 position.

Seydel and Wempe[693] studied the influence of physicochemical properties on the pharmacokinetic behaviour of a large number of sulfonamides. On the basis of observed relationships, a series of active sulfapyridines were prepared. Their kinetic behaviour was found to be in good agreement with that predicted from physicochemical properties. This paper is an excellent example of the use of physicochemical and pharmacokinetic relationships in drug design.

Sulfonamides and Benzylpyrimidones

Sulphamethoxazole (SMZ) has a smaller distribution volume in man compared to trimethoprim (TMP); hence a dose ratio consisting of 5 parts SMZ to 1 part TMP is administered to achieve the optimum SMZ: TMP concentration ratio of 20:1 in plasma. However the SMZ:TMP ratio may be considerably reduced in tissues and extravascular fluids.[694] Both drugs are efficiently absorbed from the GI tract and give peak blood levels <u>ca</u>. 2 - 4 h after dosing.[695,696]

Similar plasma levels of TMP and sulfonamide were obtained from two combination tablets containing TMP (80 mg) and SMZ (400 mg) in one and TMP (80 mg) and sulfamoxole (400 mg) in the other.[697] The pharmacokinetics of TMP/SMZ have been compared also with those of tetroxoprim/sulfadiazine after single p.o. doses in geriatric patients.[698] Both benzylpyrimidones were absorbed more rapidly than the sulfonamides, with respective half-times of 30 - 40 min and <u>ca</u>. 1 h. The elimination $t_{0.5}$ values for TMP and the sulfonamides ranged from 10 to 12 h while that for tetroxoprim was 6.7 h. Cumulative excretion in 96 h urine accounted for 61, 57, 50, and 20%, respectively, of the doses of sulfadiazine, tetroxoprim, TMP, and SMZ.

No significant differences were observed in the absorption of 250 mg TMP and 200 mg sulfametopyrazine between a combination capsule dose and separate doses of its components.[699] The plasma $t_{0.5}$ was 70 h for sulfametopyrazine and 11 h for TMP, and the plasma concentrations of sulfametopyrazine during multiple dosing were 20- to 45-fold higher than those of TMP. Approximately 20 and 60% of the sulfametopyrazine and TMP doses, respectively, were excreted intact in the urine, yielding steady-state urine concentrations of 25 - 35 $\mu g\ ml^{-1}$ sulfametopyrazine and 90 - 150 $\mu g\ ml^{-1}$ TMP.

Ten healthy subjects received orally 4 tablets containing 80 mg TMP and 400 mg SMZ or 4 tablets containing 167 mg each of sulfacarbamide, sulfadiazine, and sulfadimidine on an empty stomach.[700] Peak antibiotic concentrations were reached after 1 - 3 h in serum and 4 - 8 h in blister fluid. After repeated dosing of 2 tablets every 12 h for 4 days, blister fluid:serum peak concentration ratios were 0.89, 0.73, 0.64, 0.54, and 0.33 for TMP, sulfacarbamide, sulfadiazine, SMZ, and sulfadimidine, respectively.

Repeated doses of 800 mg SMZ and 160 mg TMP every 8 h in man resulted in plateau plasma levels of 50 - 80 $\mu g\ ml^{-1}$ total SMZ and 32 - 47 $\mu g\ ml^{-1}$ active (unchanged) SMZ after 2 - 3 d.[701] The pattern of SMZ accumulation in plasma was not influenced by the presence

of TMP. Similar accumulation patterns were observed during chronic
dosing to children aged 3 m to 10 yr.[702] Plateau serum levels of both
SMZ and TMP were obtained after 3 d. The dosing regimen used in this
study, 200 mg TMP - 1000 mg SMZ m^{-2} d^{-1} may be suboptimal for
infants as mean steady-state drug levels were below MIC values in some
cases.

Saliva:plasma concentration ratios of SMZ and TMP were 0.016 and
1.13, respectively, after p.o. doses of co-trimethoxazole to healthy
subjects,[703] and these values agree with predictions which take into
account different binding and partitioning characteristics of the two
compounds.

Studies in rats indicate that TMP crosses the placenta and equilibrates in the foetus within 30 - 60 min of an i.v. dose to the
mother.[704] Although drug was cleared faster from foetal than maternal
organs, elimination from foetal serum was delayed, owing to the slight
pH gradient between maternal and foetal blood.

Two studies have demonstrated that SMZ and TMP are excreted in
human bile at therapeutic concentrations.[705,706] The $t_{0.5}$ of
active SMZ in bile was longer than that in plasma, suggesting that
this compound may be transferred more efficiently from plasma to bile
at low plasma concentrations. In contrast, biliary $t_{0.5}$ of TMP was
shorter than that in plasma. Both SMZ and TMP penetrated the blood-
aqueous humour barrier in rabbits, achieving aqueous humour concentrations between 10 and 20% of those in serum.[707] The optimum antibacterial SMZ:TMP ratio of 20:1 was retained in aqueous humour. No
difference in the trimethoprim $t_{0.5}$ was observed in normal and
febrile rabbits, but there was greater distribution of drug to peripheral tissues in the febrile animals.[708]

A number of studies have described altered disposition of SMZ and
TMP in renal failure.[709-712] Rates of elimination and urinary concentrations of both SMZ and TMP were significantly reduced in uraemic
subjects.[713] Levels of SMZ in serum were slightly lower in uraemic

than in normal subjects. Levels of TMP in serum were similar in both
groups but tended to be higher in uraemic subjects from 5 h after dosing. Distribution of free SMZ into tissues increased during renal
insufficiency, probably due to reduced binding to serum proteins,[714]
whereas distribution of TMP into tissues showed little apparent
change. A dosage regimen involving reduced doses of both drugs, with
an interval between doses of approximately 12 h, was proposed for
patients with severe renal failure. Urine concentrations of both
drugs are markedly reduced in renal failure, as indicated in Figure
3.23.

In patients with end-stage renal disease who were on peritoneal
dialysis, simultaneous p.o. doses of 4 mg kg^{-1} TMP and 20 mg kg^{-1}

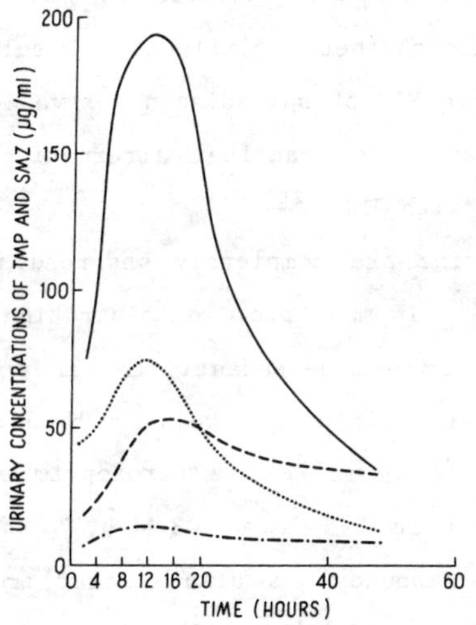

Figure 3.23   Urine concentrations of sulfamethoxazole
(SMZ) (———) and trimethoprim (TMP) (····) in normal
subjects and of SMZ (----) and TMP (-·-·) in
uraemic subjects.   Reproduced by permission from *J.
Infect. Dis.*, 1973, 128 (Suppl.), S556.

SMZ yielded peak serum concentrations of 2 and 28 µg ml^{-1}, respectively.[715]   Total plasma clearance and $t_{0.5}$ were 66.2 ml min^{-1} and
23.7 h, respectively, for TMP and 26.2 ml min^{-1} and 18.1 h, respectively, for SMZ. Peritoneal dialysis of these compounds accounted for

only 2 - 3% of the dose. Conversely, almost 90% of a TMP dose and 40% of a SMZ dose administered i.p. was absorbed, and absorption increased during peritonitis. Studies in subjects with chronic renal failure failed to provide any evidence of additional deterioration of renal function due to adjusted doses of SMZ and TMP.[716,717] These results are contrary to a previous suggestion that SMZ and TMP may be toxic to renal tissue in uraemia.[718]

Plasma levels of both SMZ and TMP were reduced to about one-half to two-thirds the normal value in subjects with varying degrees of liver damage.[719] Reduced drug levels were thought to be due to reduced drug absorption resulting from altered bile flow. The elimination $t_{0.5}$ of neither drug was affected by liver-function impairment, although prolonged excretion of TMP was observed in some cases of severe liver damage. The pharmacokinetic similarity of sulfadiazine and SMZ, and also the favourable MIC of sulfadiazine, have led to the suggestion that this agent may be a practical alternative to SMZ, either alone or in combination with TMP.[720]

Tetroxoprim and sulfadiazine are completely absorbed from p.o. doses in the rat and rabbit.[721] In man, p.o. administration of 80 mg tetroxoprim and 400 mg sulfadiazine independently and in combination resulted in virtually identical antibiotic levels in blood.[722] The mean peak concentration was 1.7 μg ml^{-1} for tetroxoprim and 16 μg ml^{-1} for sulfadiazine, reached at 2.5 h and 3.5 h, respectively. The bioavailability of these compounds was also similar from tablet and syrup dosage forms. Approximately 40 - 60% of the tetroxoprim dose and 65 - 70% of the sulfadiazine dose was excreted unchanged in the urine, yielding urinary antibiotic concentrations of 30 - 70 μg ml^{-1} and 100 - 200 μg ml^{-1}, respectively, during 0 - 4 h postdose. The plasma $t_{0.5}$ values for tetroxoprim and sulfadiazine were 5.1 and 12.6 h, respectively, and showed no changes after multiple dosing.

Tetroxoprim diffused more rapidly into prostatic tissue of patients with benign prostatic hyperplasia than sulfadiazine.[723]

Repeated administration of the two drugs for 5 days before trans-
urethral resection of the prostate resulted in an average steady-state
prostatic tissue:plasma concentration ratio of 6.9 for tetroxoprim and
0.8 for sulfadiazine.

Renal clearance of both tetroxoprim and sulfadiazine is related
to kidney function.[724] Reutter et al.[725] demonstrated a linear relationship between elimination rate constant and creatinine clearance
for both compounds. Following combined p.o. administration, $t_{0.5}$ of
tetroxoprim was 6.7 h in patients with normal renal function and 13.8
h in anuric patients, while the respective values for sulfadiazine
were 10.4 and 25.7 h. The distribution volumes of neither drug were
affected by renal impairment.

Sulfisoxazole

While no differences could be demonstrated in the systemic availability of the poorly water-soluble drug sulfisoxazole from eleven
different products in human volunteers,[726] availability of the drug
was increased in rats by polysorbate 80 and triolein.[727] Studies
with sulfisoxazole, griseofulvin, and dicoumarol, and a series of
coadministered lipids suggested that nonpolar undigestible lipids tend
to reduce the rate, but not to affect the extent, of drug absorption.
Polar, digestible lipids increase the extent of drug absorption without changing the rate. First-pass metabolism of acetylsulfisoxazole,
but not sulfisoxazole, was saturable at dose levels of 15 mg kg^{-1}
every 4 - 6 h.[728] The data suggest that acetylsulfisoxazole may be
absorbed largely intact and is presented to the site of N_4-conjugation
at a higher concentration than the more lipophilic and slowly absorbed
sulfisoxazole, giving rise to enzyme saturation. Sulfisoxazole binds
not only to albumin, but also to α-globulin and to a lesser extent to
γ-globulin and lysozyme in the rabbit eye. Such binding influences
the overall disposition of sulfisoxazole in the eye and in tear fluid,
and may change in disease states due to marked alterations in protein
fractions and binding characteristics.[729] After p.o. administration

of 75 mg kg^{-1} sulfisoxazole to well nourished adults, the drug was 88% bound to plasma proteins.[730] Binding decreased significantly to 64% in undernourished subjects, due apparently to decreased serum albumin levels in these individuals. Plasma protein binding had no effect on active tubular secretion of sulfisoxazole, as indicated by the similar overall clearance (33 - 37 ml h^{-1} kg^{-1}) and $t_{0.5}$ (6.9 - 7.7 h) values between well-nourished and undernourished subjects.

The bioavailability of sulfisoxazole from a 1 g p.o. dose was <u>ca.</u> 95%.[731] After multiple p.o. doses of 500 mg q.i.d. for 8 days, no significant change was observed in sulfisoxazole disposition despite some accumulation of the N_4-acetyl metabolite. Absorption of sulfisoxazole and other drugs into the rabbit eye is markedly influenced by the proteins present in tear fluid, cornea, and aqueous humour, and penetration of drugs into the eye after topical application might be increased by substances which inhibit drug-protein interactions.[732]

The pharmacokinetics of sulfisoxazole have been defined in man, after various routes of administration, by means of the two-compartment model.[733] After single 2 g i.m. or p.o. doses, peak plasma levels of 121 - 185 μg ml^{-1} were obtained after 2 h and the drug has a biological $t_{0.5}$ of 4.6 - 7.8 h. Plasma clearances of unbound and total drug after 1 g i.v. doses are 232 and 18.7 ml min^{-1}, respectively, and 49% of the dose is excreted in urine.[731]

Sulfamethizole

Poor correlations were obtained between dissolution and absorption rates of sulfamethizole from commercial tablets.[734] Absorption of sulfamethizole from 250 mg tablets and enteric-coated microcapsules was studied in healthy male subjects.[735] The tablet, which released sulfamethizole more rapidly <u>in vitro</u>, also resulted in faster urinary excretion of drug than the microencapsulated dosage form (Figure 3.24). Cumulative excretion of unchanged drug in 12 h urine averaged

82% of the microcapsule dose and 91% of the tablet dose. Thus, it appears that sustained absorption may be obtained from microcapsules with only a slight decrease in bioavailability.

The absorption and distribution characteristics of sulfamethizole were similar in young and old subjects, but the drug elimination $t_{0.5}$ was prolonged somewhat from 105 min in young adults to 181 min in the elderly.[736] Both the blood levels and renal clearances were correlated with creatinine clearance values. Coadministration of sulfamethizole increased elimination $t_{0.5}$ values and decreased the metabolic clearances of phenytoin, tolbutamide, and warfarin in man.[737] Reduction of warfarin metabolism in the presence of sulfamethizole may contribute to the well-known increase in warfarin anti-coagulant action in the presence of sulfonamides.

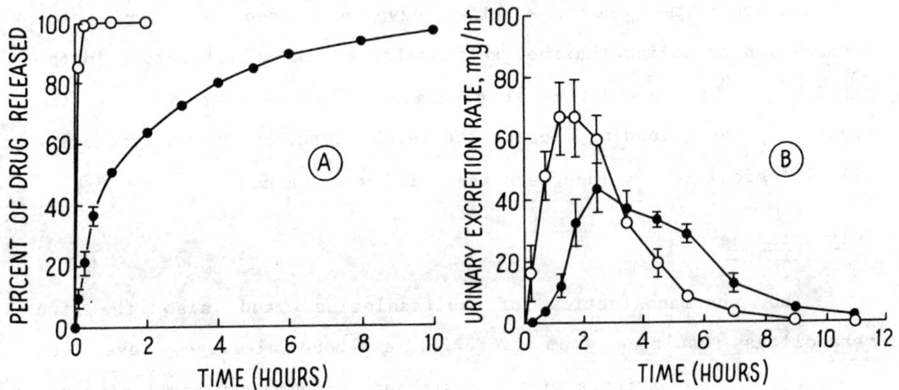

Figure 3.24 (a) Comparison between the release pattern of sulfamethizole from microcapsules (●) and the dissolution pattern of drug from tablets (o). Average of 5 experimental runs. (b) Excretion rate of sulfamethizole following administration of 250 mg of drug in tablets (●) or microcapsules (o). Average of 4 volunteers with S.E. shown by vertical bars. Reproduced by permission from Int. J. Pharmaceut., 1980, 4, 291.

Sulfamethazine

Early efforts to identify genotypes for sulfamethazine acetylation were complicated by an apparent increase in drug volume in fast acetylators, as well as low renal clearance of sulfamethazine in all subjects.[738] In a more recent study the relationship between sulfamethazine disposition and acetylator phenotype was successfully examined in 19 healthy subjects.[739] Approximately 87% of a 20 mg kg^{-1} sulfamethazine p.o. dose was bioavailable regardless of phenotype. The distribution and renal clearance of both sulfamethazine and acetylsulfamethazine did not differ significantly among phenotypes.[740] In contrast, sulfamethazine acetylation showed a well defined trimodal pattern, with metabolic clearances of 0.15, 0.75, and 1.34 ml min^{-1} kg^{-1} in slow, intermediate, and rapid acetylators, respectively.[739] The fraction of dose excreted as acetylsulfamethazine in 72 h urine averaged 0.66, 0.88, and 0.94, respectively, in slow, intermediate, and rapid acetylators.

Two-compartment model kinetics have been used to describe the disposition of sulfamethazine, sulfisomidine, and sulfathiazole in the rabbit.[741] The apparent renal clearance of these compounds was increased by water loading whereas the metabolic clearance and the overall biological $t_{0.5}$ values were essentially unchanged.

Sulfasalazine

The pharmacokinetics of sulfasalazine, and also the two metabolites resulting from bacterial azo-bond cleavage, have been reviewed.[742] In patients with and without inflammatory bowel disease, less than 12% of a 3 - 4 g p.o. dose of sulfasalazine was absorbed, and the absorbed dose was excreted in the urine and bile in an approximately 2:1 ratio.[743] A large proportion of the sulfasalazine dose was metabolized by colonic bacteria to form sulfapyridine, which in turn was almost completely absorbed and excreted in the urine. The metabolism of sulfasalazine was markedly reduced in patients after removal of the large bowel, and also in those on antibiotic therapy, resulting in decreased recovery of sulfapyridine in the urine. Sufficient absorption of unchanged sulfasalazine occurs to yield maximum serum levels at 3 - 5 h after a single p.o. dose. Steady-state serum levels vary considerably during multiple doses to human subjects, and this appears to be due to differences in absorption rates.

The rate of bacterial degradation of sulfasalazine in the human gut is slow, resulting in a 3.5 - 6 h delay between sulfasalazine dosage and appearance of sulfapyridine in plasma.[744] The disappearance $t_{0.5}$ of sulfapyridine was 6.0 - 6.3 h in two fast acetylators, and 10.6 - 16.7 h in three slow acetylators, while the apparent formation rate constants for acetylated sulfapyridine were 0.07 h^{-1} and 0.019 h^{-1} in the fast and slow acetylators, respectively. The mean saliva:plasma concentration ratio of sulfapyridine was 0.56. This value was independent of plasma drug concentration and saliva pH, and saliva levels are proposed as an alternative to plasma levels as a means of monitoring sulfapyridine intake in patients with ulcerative colitis or Crohn's disease. The clinical pharmacokinetics of sulfasalazine have been reviewed.[745]

Sulfadimidine

Polymorphic acetylation has been demonstrated for sulfadimidine in man,[746] and a method is described for the identification of fast and slow acetylator genotypes for sulfadimidine in normal and uraemic individuals.[747] Contrary to earlier findings, renal excretion of sulfadimidine has been shown to be reduced in uraemic subjects.[748-750] Two studies demonstrated reduced plasma protein binding of sulfadimidine in uraemia,[748,750] and this may be due to displacement by an endogenous substance rather than drug metabolite(s).[751]

Sulfacetamide

The distribution kinetics of sulfacetamide were changed in rats bearing a Walker carcinosarcoma compared with control animals, but changes were dependent on the route of administration.[752] In tumour-bearing animals, the fraction of circulating drug bound to plasma

proteins decreased, although this was partly due to an overall decrease in plasma proteins. Different temporal relationships were
observed between various tissue and plasma levels of drug in tumour-
bearing and control animals. Plasma drug levels were reduced in
tumour-bearing rats compared with controls after p.o. doses, but the
reverse was the case after i.v. doses. These results reflect both
impaired drug absorption and elimination in tumour-bearing animals.
Renal excretion of sulfacetamide by the rat kidney is reduced by pretreatment with SKF-525A.[753] This appears to be the first reported
case of SKF-525A directly altering drug distribution or renal excretion.

Sulfametrole

Sulfametrole is metabolized primarily to N_4-acetylsulfametrole,
and the acetylation occurs in a unimodal way indicating no acetylator
phenotype in man.[754] Renal clearance of sulfametrole is dependent on
urine flow and pH, and ranged from 0.13 to 1.23 ml min^{-1} at pH 5.0 -
5.5 and from 4.59 to 11.9 ml min^{-1} at pH 7.0 - 8.0. The respective
$t_{0.5}$ values were 10 h and 7.5 h indicating decreased reabsorption
from alkaline urine. Active tubular secretion was not involved in
sulfametrole excretion but was the primary excretory route for the
N_4-acetyl metabolite. Coadministration of probenecid reduced tubular
secretion of N_4-acetylsulfametrole, yielding $t_{0.5}$ and renal clearance values of 44 h and 12.9 ml min^{-1}, respectively, compared with
3.2 h and 31.7 ml min^{-1} under control conditions.

Sulfaclomide

The mean elimination $t_{0.5}$ of the long-acting sulfonamide sulfa-
clomide was increased from 84 h to 120 h in patients with impaired
renal function, while sulfamerazine $t_{0.5}$ was unchanged at 20 - 24
h.[755] After repeated doses for 11 days, $t_{0.5}$ values of both drugs
were prolonged by about one-fifth the single dose value in uraemic
patients, but were unchanged in normal individuals. Although no

explanation was offered for this, it is reasonable to suspect inhibition of metabolism on repeated doses, due to accumulation of metabolites in uraemic patients but not in individuals with normal renal function.

Sulfametopyrazine

The pharmacokinetics of the long-acting sulfonamide sulfametopyrazine and its N_1- and N_4-conjugates were studied after single p.o. doses to man.[756] Absorption, distribution, elimination, and excretion coefficients were calculated, as well as concentrations in plasma water and interstitial fluid. Good agreement was obtained between drug concentrations in urine and those calculated from excretion coefficients. Concentrations of active drug in all body compartments exceeded therapeutic levels 7 days after dosing.

Sulfameter

Of the two crystal forms of sulfameter, the more energetic crystal form II is absorbed at a faster rate and is <u>ca</u>. 1.4 times more bioavailable than the water-stable form III.[757,758] These observations support previous dissolution studies and it is proposed that, provided the metastable form II is stabilized, then this would be a better choice for p.o. dosage preparations than form III which is currently used. Further studies showed that measurement of urinary excretion is a useful alternative to blood level measurements when comparing rate and extent of sulfameter absorption.[759] Seventy-two-hour urinary excretion data confirmed that crystal form II is absorbed at a faster rate than crystal form III in man, but there was no significant difference in the overall absorption efficiency of the two forms. Drug absorption kinetics were generally first-order, but in some cases, zero-order kinetics were obtained, indicating rate-limiting drug dissolution.

Other Sulfonamides and Combinations

Bioavailability studies on different brands of the triple-sulfonamide combination sulfadiazine, sulfamethazine, and sulfamerazine in man have shown that, although *in vitro* T_{50} dissolution times varied from 4 to 253 min, there were no significant differences in physiological availability between brands.[760] In all cases, however, total sulfonamide was more slowly absorbed than from a control solution and in most cases no detectable blood levels occurred until 2 h after dosing.

The bioavailability of sulfamethoxydiazine was increased by concomitant administration of food, the effect being greater after a high-lipid meal than after a high-protein or high-carbohydrate meal.[761] Concomitant intake of food had no effect on the bioavailability of the short-acting sulfonamide sulfaisodimidine in human volunteers.[762] Absorption of sulfaethidole was reduced following reduction of mesenteric blood flow to the intestine in dogs.[763] However, the reduction in absorption rate was not linear, and the rate was still 27% of normal at zero blood flow. It is suggested that residual absorption may be due to drainage by the lymphatic system. Sulfafurazole absorption was retarded in patients with small-intestinal villous damage, although absorption of isoniazid, chloramphenicol, salicylate, and cycloserine in the same patients appeared to be unaffected.[764] Studies in children indicate that sulfaguanol is poorly absorbed after p.o. doses.[765]

The elimination $t_{0.5}$ of sulfadiazine after i.v. injection increased from 10 h in normal renal function to 22 h in renal failure.[766] The overall distribution volume was about 0.36 l kg^{-1} in all subjects. This value is considerably smaller than those reported previously and it is suggested that earlier values, obtained following p.o. doses, were overestimates due to incomplete drug absorption. Simultaneous administration of sulfadiazine and nitrofurantoin had little effect on the pharmacokinetics of either compound in experimental animals and man.[767]

Erythromycin, Its Salts, and Esters

Much of the literature on erythromycin has centered on claims regarding the relative bioavailability of various formulations of erythromycin base, its salts, and esters.[768-772] A bioavailability monograph has been presented for erythromycin[773] and its clinical pharmacology has been reviewed.[774]

Absorption of erythromycin from an encapsulated enteric-coated dosage form of erythromycin base was superior to that of encapsulated erythromycin stearate following p.o. doses to volunteers.[775] Serum concentrations of antibiotic were significantly higher from the base than from the stearate at most sampling times, and mean areas under plasma level curves were almost threefold higher from the base than the stearate. Unprotected and film-coated erythromycin base tablets were reported to be absorbed more rapidly than enteric-coated tablets in fasting conditions.[776] However, enteral absorption of erythromycin from nonenteric-coated erythromycin preparations can be reduced due to gastric acid.[777] The extent of this sensitivity is indicated by 70 - 90% destruction of erythromycin in nonenteric-coated products within 30 min. Erythromycin absorption characteristics may also be complicated by secretion of drug from the circulation into the intestinal lumen.[778] This is an active process in rabbits and occurs against a concentration gradient. Absorption of p.o. erythromycin base or erythromycin estolate was erratic in pregnant women, and peak serum levels of antibiotic varied from 0.3 to 7.2 μg ml^{-1} following a single 500 mg dose.[779] Colburn et al.[780] used a computer program to fit multiple-dose erythromycin data, and concluded that the pharmacokinetics of erythromycin are adequately described by a simple one-compartment model incorporating a lag time. Superior fits of the data by the model were obtained also by incorporating zero-order rather

than first-order absorption kinetics. This is demonstrated in Figure
3.25, in which solid lines represent lines of best fit to mean data
points during repeated doses of erythromycin to 22 healthy male
volunteers.

Mather et al.[781] also found a single first-order rate constant
inadequate to describe erythromycin absorption and suggested as
alternatives a zero-order process, a sequence of first-order processes, or a combination of zero-order and first-order processes.

Food retards stomach emptying and increases the gastric inactivation of unprotected and film-coated erythromycin while having little
effect on the enteric-coated form.[776] Thus, under postprandial condi-

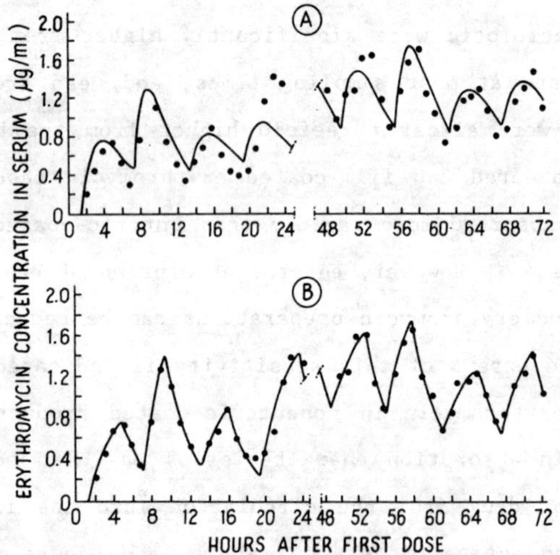

Figure 3.25   Curve fits to mean serum erythromycin
concentrations during repeated p.o. doses of 250 mg
enteric-coated erythromycin tablets every 6 hours to
22 healthy male volunteers. A: variable first-order
absorption is assumed, and B: variable zero-order
absorption is assumed. Reproduced by permission from
J. Clin. Pharmacol., 1977, 17, 592.

tions during multiple dosing, the absorption of film-coated erythromycin base and stearate formulations was 40 - 60% less than that of
enteric-coated base tablets. However, a great deal of conflicting
data exist, and the confused situation regarding the effects of food

on the bioavailability of oral erythromycin has been discussed in a recent review.[782]

Following single 500 mg p.o. doses of erythromycin base to normal subjects and to patients with alcoholic liver disease and ascites, serum drug levels were characterized by a two-compartment open model with zero-order absorption.[783] Mean serum concentrations were higher in the patients than in the healthy subjects; C_{max} values in the respective groups averaged 2.0 and 1.5 µg ml^{-1} and were reached at 4 - 6 h postdose.

The bioavailability of erythromycin stearate has been shown to differ between commercial tablets. A twofold variation was reported between peak plasma levels and also between AUC values from single p.o. doses of similar dosage forms of erythromycin stearate from five different commercial sources.[784] Previous claims of enhanced GI absorption of erythromycin-2'-propionate ester relative to erythromycin were examined in terms of serum-protein binding and, although serum levels of antibiotic are greater from the propionate ester, the difference could be accounted for by greater binding of the ester to serum proteins and its reduced distribution space in the body.[785]

Other studies, based on both serum levels and urinary excretion of antibiotic, show that erythromycin estolate is considerably more bioavailable than erythromycin stearate in nonfasting subjects.[786] Orally dosed erythromycin estolate gives rise to higher levels of erythromycin activity in aqueous humour than equivalent p.o. doses of erythromycin base after repeated doses.[787]

Increased circulating levels of unchanged erythromycin estolate in the presence of food following single and repeated doses to 10 healthy male volunteers are shown in Figures 3.26 and 3.27.[772] These figures show also circulating levels of erythromycin base that are obtained from _in vivo_ hydrolysis of the ester. Circulating levels of free base comprise _ca_. 20% of circulating levels of total antibiotic in both the single and repeated dose situations. After repeated

doses, free base levels are relatively insensitive to the absence or
presence of food. In this study, partial support was provided for the
contention that the absorption of erythromycin may be zero-order in
nature.[780] After single doses of the estolate and stearate forms of
erythromycin, plasma levels were best described using a zero-order
absorption model. Following repeated doses, the first-order absorption model appeared more appropriate.[768]

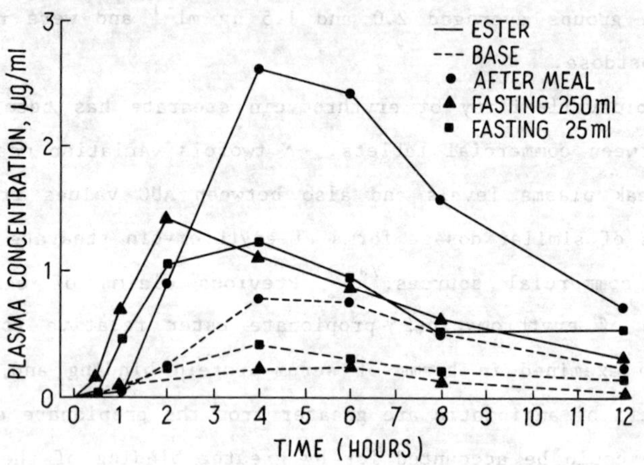

Figure 3.26   Plasma levels of erythromycin 2'-propan-
oate and erythromycin base following single doses of
erythromycin estolate capsules. Reproduced by permission from J. Pharm. Sci., 1979, 68, 150.

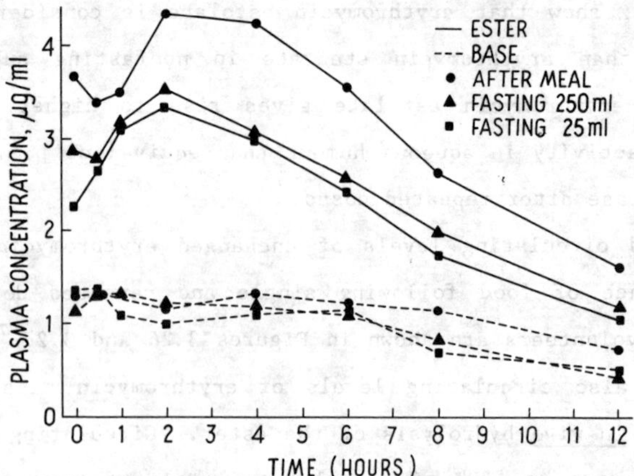

Figure 3.27   Plasma levels of erythromycin 2'-propan-
oate and erythromycin base following repeated doses of
erythromycin estolate capsules. Reproduced by permission from J. Pharm. Sci., 1979, 68, 150.

DiSanto et al.[788] reported similar circulating levels of bioactive erythromycin base during multiple dosing, 250 mg every 6 h, of erythromycin enteric-coated tablets and erythromycin estolate capsules, although total erythromycin (base plus propionate) plasma levels from the estolate were <u>ca</u>. 3 times higher than those of the base. Similarly, the serum AUC of total erythromycin (base plus propionate) obtained from an erythromycin estolate suspension was 3 times greater than that obtained from an equal dose of erythromycin ethylsuccinate.[789] Another study, however, showed the absorption from erythromycin estolate and stearate to be only 36% and 55%, respectively, of that from enteric-coated erythromycin base.[790] The difference between formulations became insignificant after repeated administration.

Serum antibiotic levels in 6 - 65 month old children from p.o. erythromycin ethylsuccinate were increased when taken after food.[791] The ethylsuccinate ester also yielded higher serum levels when taken with milk.[792] Under these conditions the absorption of erythromycin estolate and ampicillin was unchanged, while serum levels of cephalexin, penicillin V, and penicillin G were reduced.[792] Circulating levels of total erythromycin, which comprised both the original ester and hydrolysed base, were between 3- and 10-fold higher from the estolate than from the ethylsuccinate. However, dosed ethylsuccinate is rapidly hydrolysed <u>in vivo</u>, and circulates predominantly as the free base. Erythromycin ethylsuccinate was absorbed more rapidly than the stearate, although the overall bioavailability was not significantly different from equivalent doses of the two esters.[793]

The stability and bioavailability in man of erythromycin lactobionate have been studied from formulations with and without lipid coatings.[794] The absorption of p.o. dosed erythromycin lactobionate protected with cholesteryl acetate was greater than from the unprotected material, and from film-coated erythromycin stearate.

Erythromycin is extensively bound to α_1-acid glycoprotein in serum.[795] The binding is concentration-dependent, varying (at 38°C) from 74% at 1 µg ml^{-1} to 46% at 24 µg ml^{-1}, and appears to decrease with decreasing temperature.[796] Erythromycin concentrations in various tissues were higher than corresponding serum levels. After p.o. dosing as the propionate or stearate to rats, similar levels of erythromycin were observed in the brain and plasma, whereas concentrations in the lung, liver, kidney, and ileum were considerably higher.[797] Erythromycin diffuses readily into the lungs in humans. Data obtained from patients who had undergone surgery for bronchopulmonary cancer showed tissue:serum concentration ratios of _ca_. 5:1 in healthy lung tissues and 3:1 in tumoral lung tissues.[798]

Penetration of erythromycin into human skin blister fluid occurred slowly, reaching a peak concentration of _ca_. 0.3 µg ml^{-1} at 5 h after a 500 mg p.o. dose of microencapsulated erythromycin base.[799] Antibiotic levels in blister fluid were sustained for more than 12 h, and the fluid:serum AUC ratio was 0.1 - 0.2. Erythromycin also penetrates slowly into peritoneal fluid.[800] The fluid:serum AUC ratio in a group of female patients with pelvic inflammatory disease averaged 0.33 and 0.65 from p.o. erythromycin doses given as the stearate and enteric-coated base granules, respectively. In peripheral lymph, peak erythromycin concentration was _ca_. 24% of the corresponding serum level.[801]

After repeated doses of erythromycin ethylsuccinate (30 - 60 mg kg^{-1} d^{-1}) in patients with secretory otitis media, erythromycin concentrations in middle ear effusions slowly increased to a plateau of 1.1 - 1.2 µg ml^{-1} at 26 h, which was similar to the concomitant plasma level and exceeded MIC's of most susceptible pathogens.[802] Therapeutic erythromycin concentrations similar to plasma levels also were achieved in adenoid and tonsil tissues,[803] and in sinus membranes.[804]

Erythromycin is eliminated primarily by hepatic metabolism. After single i.v. administration of 250 mg base equivalents of erythromycin lactobionate to healthy subjects, erythromycin pharmaco-kinetics obeyed classical two-compartment model kinetics with little intersubject variability.[805,806] The terminal $t_{0.5}$ and serum clearance were 1.5 - 2 h and 0.42 1 h^{-1} kg^{-1}, respectively, and only 12% of the dose was excreted unchanged in urine. Increasing the dose from 125 or 250 mg to 900 mg prolonged the $t_{0.5}$ to 2 - 3 h but had little effect on serum clearance, probably due to concentration-dependent binding of erythromycin to serum proteins. In a study using enteric-coated erythromycin base in the dose range of 250 - 1000 mg, Josefsson et al.[807] reported a similar increase in $t_{0.5}$ with in-creasing dose. However, these investigators also observed a dose-related increase in the urinary recovery of erythromycin, which would suggest capacity-limited saturation of metabolic enzymes at elevated doses. Multiple dosing of erythromycin (1 g d^{-1}) at 6 to 12 h in-tervals for 7 d resulted in similarly prolonged $t_{0.5}$ values compared to single dose data.[808] Erythromycin metabolism in the rat was stimu-lated by pretreatment with phenobarbital, resulting in significantly reduced serum and tissue levels of parent drug.[809] Phenobarbital also increased biliary excretion of unchanged erythromycin, although the mechanism by which this occurred is unclear.

The disposition of erythromycin is influenced to only a minor degree by renal impairment,[810] the terminal elimination $t_{0.5}$ in-creasing from a normal value of 2 h to 4 - 7 h in patients with severe renal impairment.[805] The overall distribution volume of erythromycin, V_{dss}, increases from 57% to 109% of body weight with declining renal function. However, this value was calculated from serum levels of total drug. In view of the extensive binding of erythromycin to plas-ma proteins, the true distribution volume is probably far greater than these calculated values. Erythromycin is actively secreted in bile following parenteral doses, and antibiotic levels in bile fluid are approximately 8-times higher than levels in serum obtained at the same time.[811]

Other Antimicrobial Agents

This section is devoted to some antimicrobial agents that do not fit into the previously described categories.

Clindamycin

The bioavailability and pharmacokinetics of clindamycin have been reported in some detail. After p.o. doses of the hydrochloride salt the antibiotic is rapidly absorbed, yielding peak serum levels within 45 min, and is cleared from serum with a $t_{0.5}$ of <u>ca</u>. 2.5 h in human adults.[812] In another study, clindamycin was rapidly absorbed following single 300 mg p.o. doses in healthy volunteers.[813] Blood antibiotic levels reached a peak of 1.9 µg ml^{-1} at <u>ca</u>. 0.5 h, and rapidly declined to below 1.0 µg ml^{-1} within 2 h of dosing. The rate of p.o. clindamycin absorption is reduced 20-fold by the presence of kaolin-pectin suspension, but the extent of absorption is unaffected.[814] This type of interaction is similar to that involving ampicillin and warfarin, but not with that of lincomycin, tetracycline, and digoxin, the bioavailability of which was significantly reduced by kaolin-pectin interactions.

The palmitate ester of clindamycin is absorbed as efficiently as, and yields similar kinetic constants to, the hydrochloride salt but the 2-hexadecylcarbonate is poorly absorbed and yields much lower antibiotic levels in serum.[815] Enteral absorption of clindamycin palmitate, like the hydrochloride, is not reduced by the presence of food,[816] but may be delayed if dosed shortly after a meal. This is in direct contrast to lincomycin, where food caused a marked reduction in serum levels of antibiotic.[817] Peak serum levels of clindamycin after i.m. injection of clindamycin phosphate are slightly higher than those obtained from oral preparations, but the time of peak height is delayed to <u>ca</u>. 3 h after dosing. This is due, apparently, to delayed hydrolysis of the ester to free clindamycin after the i.m. dose.[818,819] Serum levels of clindamycin increased linearly with increasing doses of all dosage forms, but areas under serum-level curves were not dose-proportional. Studies in animals have indicated that slower absorption, and also prolonged plasma levels, of clidamycin hydrochloride after i.m. compared to p.o. doses may be due to precipitation and slow redissolution of antibiotic at the injection site.[820]

Steady-state serum levels of clindamycin are attained after 4 or 5 doses given every 6 h, and there is no evidence of enzyme induction. Although the disposition of clindamycin in the body can be described by a one-compartment model, therapeutic antibiotic levels are obtained in most tissues including lung, bone, and synovial fluid.[821] Following single 300 mg p.o. doses, clindamycin concentration in gingival crevicular fluid was highest (2.0 μg ml^{-1}) at <u>ca</u>. 1.5 h, and remained above 1.0 μg ml^{-1} for <u>ca</u>. 6 h.[813] After repeated i.m. doses to rabbits, the penetration of clindamycin into capsules implanted in the peritoneal cavity was <u>ca</u>. 30%.[822] Infection of the capsules with <u>Bacteroides fragilis</u> did not affect clindamycin penetration, although more than half of the antibiotic in infected capsules was found to be inactive, possibly due to bacterial or leukocyte enzyme degradation. Both clindamycin and lincomycin are actively secreted into the milk of lactating ewes; milk levels exceed serum levels within 30 min and continue until at least 11 h after a single i.m. dose.[823] Clindamycin is transferred into human breast milk.[824] However, large interindividual variations were found in milk concentrations, which ranged from one-tenth to several times the corresponding clindamycin level in plasma. Clindamycin is rapidly excreted in bile and appears in therapeutic concentrations in bile of patients with radiologically nonfunctioning gallbladders.[825] Clindamycin has been shown also to cross the placental barrier in pregnant women and to concentrate in the foetal liver.[826] Clindamycin penetrates human bone tissue after repeated i.m. doses, with bone:serum concentration ratios averaging 0.4.[827]

Clindamycin has an elimination $t_{0.5}$ of <u>ca</u>. 2 h in normal adults, elimination is somewhat faster in children but the $t_{0.5}$ varies considerably among individuals.[828] The literature on the relative pharmacokinetics of clindamycin in normal and impaired renal function is conflicting. The drug is cleared predominantly by hepatic metabolism so that impaired renal function might be expected to have little influence on its elimination kinetics. This was confirmed by Eastwood and Gower,[829] who obtained serum drug $t_{0.5}$ values of 2.2 h and 1.6 h in normal and severely impaired renal function, respectively. Other reports, however, have shown that clindamycin $t_{0.5}$ may be prolonged to 6 - 8 h in impaired renal function,[830,831] i.e., three times normal values, although data from uraemic subjects are often erratic.[832] Slower elimination of clindamycin in renal failure may be due to metabolite product inhibition but more studies are obviously needed on this drug. Clindamycin $t_{0.5}$ in uraemic subjects is not changed by haemodialysis.

In 15 patients with liver disease without ascites or biliary obstruction, the $t_{0.5}$ of clindamycin after i.v. doses ranged from 0.63 to 4.7 h.[833] A correlation was found between clindamycin $t_{0.5}$ and indirect bilirubin levels in the 0.2 - 1.55 mg dl^{-1} range, as shown in equation 3.9.

$$t_{0.5} \text{ (h)} = 3.2 \times \text{(indirect bilirubin)} + 0.48 \qquad (3.9)$$

However in another study clindamycin elimination was largely unaffected by hepatitis or cirrhosis and it is suggested that dose adjustment may be unnecessary in some types of liver disease provided drug levels are monitored.[834]

Vancomycin

Because of interindividual variations in vancomycin disposition kinetics, serum concentration monitoring and dose adjustments are essential to optimize vancomycin therapy.[835] Blouin et al.[836] compared serum vancomycin profiles in normal (66 - 89 kg) and morbidly obese (111 - 226 kg) subjects after 1 g i.v. infusions. Despite a shorter $t_{0.5}$ of 3.2 h in the obese subjects compared with 4.8 h in normal weight subjects, the two groups had virtually identical total body clearances of 1.1 ml min^{-1} kg^{-1} and also similar absolute volumes of the central compartment (6.4 - 7.7 1). Thus, total body weight should be used to calculate vancomycin dose for morbidly obese patients, although the relatively large total dose in these patients may be divided into more frequent doses than in normal weight subjects in order to avoid excessive transient concentrations in serum.

After single 500 to 1000 mg i.v. infusions of vancomycin over 30 min, serum drug levels declined triexponentially, with a terminal $t_{0.5}$ of 4.7 - 11.2 h.[837] Total clearance was consistent among subjects and ranged from 1.09 to 1.37 ml min^{-1} kg^{-1}. Vancomycin was 55% bound to proteins at serum concentrations of 10 - 100 µg ml^{-1}, and the drug appeared to be excreted primarily by passive glomerular filtration. Vancomycin was shown to penetrate into the c.s.f. of rabbits; the c.s.f.:serum concentration ratio was 0.02 in normal rabbits but increased to _ca_. 0.04 in rabbits with experimental pneumococcal meningitis.[838]

Elimination of vancomycin was significantly impaired in rats with renal damage induced by uranyl nitrate; mean vancomycin clearance and $t_{0.5}$ were 0.2 ml min^{-1} and 23 h, respectively, compared with 3.2 ml min^{-1} and 1.4 h in control animals.[839] Total 72 h urinary excretion of vancomycin decreased from 50.5% of dose in control animals to 35.6% in rats with kidney failure. In man 90% of vancomycin is cleared through the kidneys and elimination is markedly reduced in renal impairment.[840] Vancomycin clearance is linearly related to creatinine clearance and methods for dose adjustment have been presented based on this relationship. In anuric patients adequate serum levels are maintained by _ca_. 7% of the normal dose. In 4 patients with renal failure who were on chronic intermittent peritoneal dialysis the mean $t_{0.5}$ of vancomycin was 30 h during dialysis.[841] Penetration of the antibiotic from serum into peritoneal fluid was erratic, yielding peritoneal concentrations ranging from 0 to 96% of the simultaneous serum level. Intraperitoneal administration of vancomycin thus appears to be necessary for treating peritonitis in these patients.

Lincomycin

In a 3-way crossover study, 15 normal adults received single i.m. doses of 600, 1000, and 1500 mg lincomycin at weekly intervals.[842] The drug was rapidly absorbed from the injection site, reaching peak concentrations in serum at 1 - 1.5 h and in saliva at ca. 4 h. While the lincomycin $t_{0.5}$, approximately 5 h, was independent of dose size, total clearance of lincomycin increased with increasing dose, possibly due to saturable serum protein binding. Novak et al.[843] infused i.v. doses of lincomycin ranging from 4800 - 8400 mg d^{-1} for 7 d into human volunteers. Drug was administered on a q.i.d. basis. Despite the dose size, no accumulation in serum levels was observed after the 5th infusion, and equilibrium serum levels averaged 24 - 37 $\mu g \, ml^{-1}$ (peak) and 10 - 12 $\mu g \, ml^{-1}$ (nadir) for the low- and high-dose groups, respectively. Very low levels of lincomycin in spinal fluid in one subject indicated that lincomycin does not cross the blood-brain barrier to any extent.

Coumermycin A₁

After p.o. and i.v. doses to man, plasma levels of coumermycin A_1 were interpreted in terms of a two-compartment model with the central compartment having a volume equivalent to plasma water.[844] Although only four subjects were used in this study, dose-dependent kinetics appeared to be operative, as indicated by decreased elimination rates with increasing doses. Improved absorption efficiency of coumermycin A_1 has been obtained by administering a 1:4 ratio of the monosodium salt of coumermycin A_1 together with N-methylglucamine in dogs and humans.[845,846] Absorption efficiencies of 20 - 25% were obtained, which were 5 - 15 times greater than from the antibiotic alone.

Virginiamycin

Virginiamycin is rapidly, but only partially, absorbed from p.o. doses in man[847] and experimental animals.[848] After a rapid distribution phase, circulating levels of antibiotic decline exponentially with a $t_{0.5}$ of 20 h in man and 5 h in rats.

Chloramphenicol

Absorption of p.o. chloramphenicol was similar in both fasted and nonfasted dogs.[849] However, the absorption rate was increased in the presence of food, resulting in earlier, but not significantly higher peak chloramphenicol levels. The absorption $t_{0.5}$ of chloramphenicol was 1 h from capsules and 20 min from a powder after p.o. doses to man.[850] Differences in absorption rates are attributed to storage conditions, chloramphenicol particle size, and the presence of adjuvants in the capsule formulations. In this study, reasonable correlations were obtained between *in vitro* disintegration and dissolution data, and *in vivo* absorption rates.

In 18 children aged between 2 m and 14 yr, the bioavailability of i.v. dosed chloramphenicol succinate was 70% relative to that of p.o. administered chloramphenicol palmitate.[851] Incomplete bioavailability of the i.v. dose was due to incomplete hydrolysis of the succinate to chloramphenicol. Large interindividual variability was observed in the hydrolysis of chloramphenicol succinate as well as in chloramphenicol clearance, resulting in poor correlation between serum concentration and chloramphenicol dose.[851,852]

Chloramphenicol was absorbed faster via the rat lung than doxycycline, erythromycin, tetracycline, or benzylpenicillin.[853] This is demonstrated in Figure 3.28 which shows that chloramphenicol absorption was virtually complete at about 6 min, at which time benzylpenicillin, the most slowly absorbed drug, was about 10% absorbed. Comparison of molecular weights and chloroform-water partition coefficients suggest that lipid solubility was the main determinant of absorption rates.

The binding of chloramphenicol to plasma proteins is reduced from a mean value of 53% to 42% in cirrhosis patients, and to 32% in premature neonates.[854] Although the reduction observed in cirrhosis is of little clinical significance, reduced binding in premature infants implies the need for reduced chloramphenicol doses in this population.

After i.v. infusion of 25 mg kg^{-1} chloramphenicol succinate into 12 young patients (2.5 m - 20 yr), the mean $t_{0.5}$ of chloramphenicol succinate was 2.7 h while that of chloramphenicol was 4.0 h.[852] The total clearance and renal clearance of chloramphenicol were 6.81 - 98.2 and 2.54 - 26.9 ml min^{-1} m^{-2}, respectively.   In 3 - 24 m

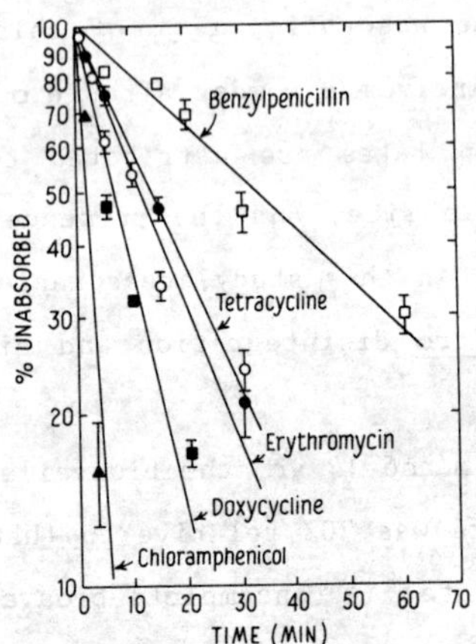

Figure 3.28 Absorption rates of antibiotics from the rat lung. Krebs-Ringer phosphate solution (0.1 ml) containing a compound was administered intrathecally to rats. Initial concentrations were ^{14}C-chloramphenicol 1 mmol l^{-1}, ^{3}H-doxycycline 0.06 mmol l^{-1}, ^{14}C-erythromycin 1 mmol l^{-1}, ^{3}H-tetracycline 1 mmol l^{-1}, and ^{14}C-benzylpenicillin 1 mmol l^{-1}. Each point is a mean from 3 to 16 animals. Vertical bars indicate S.E. Reproduced by permission from *Proc. Soc. Exp. Biol. Med.*, 1974, <u>145</u>, 752.

infants who received the same succinate dose, chloramphenicol clearance ranged from 0.058 to 0.236 l h^{-1} kg^{-1}.[855] Since chloramphenicol is extensively metabolized prior to excretion, its clearance is impaired in patients with liver disease.[856,857] In patients with chronic pyelonephritis, glomerular nephritis, and polycystic kidneys, decrease in renal clearance of chloramphenicol is related to inulin clearance.[858] However the decrease in chloramphenicol clearance is smaller than that of inulin, indicating increased excretion of chloramphenicol by residual nephrons. Increased excretion by residual nephrons has been demonstrated also for the arylamino and nitro metabolites of chloramphenicol.[859] Plasma $t_{0.5}$ values of chloramphenicol in domestic animals vary from 0.9 h in ponies to 5.1 h in cats, and there is an inverse relationship between $t_{0.5}$ and distribution volumes in the different species.[860]

Thiamphenicol

Results of numerous studies have shown that the serum $t_{0.5}$ of thiamphenicol is prolonged in renal insufficiency and also in impaired liver function.[861-863] Typical serum drug $t_{0.5}$ values are 80 min in normal renal function and 320 min in severe renal failure. Haemodialysis reduced the drug $t_{0.5}$ in severe uraemia to about 180 min. A more palatable synthetic ester for paediatric use, thiamphenicol palmitate, was completely hydrolysed _in vitro_ by pancreatic lipase and this process was markedly accelerated in the presence of the surfactant Tween 80.[864] Serum thiamphenicol levels in rats peaked later after dosing the ester, and concentrations obtained from this dosage form were more prolonged than those obtained after dosing nonesterified thiamphenicol.

Nitrofurantoin

Nitrofurantoin is reported to be well absorbed from p.o. doses and absorption is improved further when it is administered after food.[865-867] Increased absorption of drug in the presence of food may have been due to the increased time that the drug was in the stomach, permitting greater dissolution prior to passage into the duodenum. This hypothesis is supported by the observation that coadministration of propantheline, which reduces gastric motility and hence the gastric emptying rate, caused a marked increase in nitrofurantoin bioavailability in man.[868]

Despite its apparently acceptable absorption profile, considerable differences have been observed in the relative bioavailability of nitrofurantoin from a number of commercial preparations.[869-871] Many of these preparations conformed to standard uniformity and *in vitro* dissolution and disintegration requirements. Typical variations observed between formulations are: absorption rate, 0.56 - 0.97 h^{-1}; 14 h urinary excretion, 22.3 - 34.6 mg and peak plasma levels, 0.7 - 1.5 $\mu g \ ml^{-1}$. Comparison of *in vitro* and *in vivo* data indicated that neither the USP combined disintegration-dissolution test nor other dissolution tests accurately predicted drug absorption characteristics.[872]

Two nitrofurantoin products containing macrocrystalline drug were less bioavailable after p.o. doses to man than some other nitrofurantoin products although, again, all formulations conformed to official specifications.[873] Nitrofurantoin is inefficiently absorbed rectally, yielding lower drug concentrations in urine than equivalent p.o. doses.[874] Nitrofurantoin absorption is significantly increased in man from a drug-deoxycholic acid coprecipitate compared with a physical mixture, and faster absorption of drug from the coprecipitate is associated with a faster *in vitro* dissolution rate.[875]

Nitrofurantoin is excreted in the bile of dogs and about one-third of the amount excreted is reabsorbed from the intestine within 3 h.[876] Nitrofurantoin has a hydrocholeretic effect, <u>ca</u>. 10 times greater than an equimolar dose of dehydrocholic acid. Nitrofurantoin was 62.7% and 60.3% bound to plasma proteins at plasma concentrations of 100 and 500 ng ml^{-1}, respectively. After i.v. infusion, 47% of the dose was excreted in the urine intact and 1.4% as the metabolite aminofurantoin. The terminal plasma $t_{0.5}$ of nitrofurantoin was _ca._ 1 h. Maier-Lenz et al.[877] reported a nitrofurantoin elimination $t_{0.5}$ of 0.7 h after p.o. dosing with both conventional tablets and sustained-release dosage forms.

Concentrations of nitrofurantoin, sulfamethizole, and cephalexin were compared in urine obtained from diseased and relatively normal kidneys in humans and primates with unequally functioning pyelonephretic kidneys.[878] While sulfamethizole and cephalexin reached adequate peak urine concentrations in the poorly functioning kidneys, nitrofurantoin concentrations were generally below antibacterial values. With all three agents, drug excretion through the impaired kidney was greater than that predicted from renal blood flow or creatinine clearance values.

Rifampin

The p.o. absorption of rifampin has been examined under a variety of conditions.[879] Serum levels of rifampin in man were similar from p.o. gelatin capsules and tablet dosage forms.[880] Peak drug levels of 8 - 9 µg ml^{-1} were obtained 2 h after a single 450 mg dose. In subjects who had previously received repeated rifampin doses, however, peak drug levels were reduced to 6 µg ml^{-1}, presumably due to enzyme induction. Absorption of rifampin from oral syrup preparations was double that from equivalent encapsulated doses, while absorption from different tablet formulations was erratic, with 24 h urinary excretion accounting for between 7.4 and 21.0% of dose.[881] It is proposed that equiactive doses of rifampin in syrups should be 25 - 50% lower than capsules and tablets.

Rifampin absorption from p.o. doses was considerably reduced by the presence of food, resulting in both lower and later peak drug levels in serum.[882] Absorption of rifampin was also inhibited in man at high p.o. doses, presumably owing to saturation of some absorption mechanism, while drug metabolism in the liver was also saturated at high doses, resulting in nonexponential decay of unchanged drug in serum.[883] Administration of 10 mg kg^{-1} rifampin as a suspension, a suspension-apple sauce mixture, and a powder-apple sauce mixture in 38 infants and children yielded peak serum concentrations of 9 - 11.5 µg ml^{-1} at 1 h, regardless of the formulation.[884] Concomitantly administered preoperative opiates and anticholinergics significantly reduced rifampin absorption by delaying gastric emptying and decreasing bowel motility.[885] However, this drug interaction diminished when rifampin was given 2 h before the preoperative medication.

Both rifampin and rifamycin SV obeyed two-compartment model kinetics following i.v. doses to lactating ewes.[886] Disposition of drugs between compartments and appearance in milk were functions of their relative oil-water partition coefficients and pKa values. Rifamycin SV is a strong acid and is almost completely ionized at physiological pH whereas rifampin (pKa 7.9) is about 70% unionized. Thus the less ionized and more lipid soluble rifampin has a greater overall distribution volume in the body than rifamycin SV and is also secreted into milk to a greater extent.

Rifampin levels in human pleural fluid were generally lower than those in plasma up to about 12 h postdose.[887] After this time, however, pleural fluid drug levels tended to exceed those in plasma. Although prolonged drug levels in pleural fluid were attributed to a complex distribution mechanism, they can also be rationalized if one considers pleural fluid to be associated with the tissue compartment of a two-compartment model system,[886] with slow diffusion of drug back from the tissue compartment to the central compartment during postabsorption and postdistribution phases. Rifampin penetrates readily into tears and saliva of children,[887] and also into cardiac valve tissue of patients undergoing cardiac surgery for valve replacement. Circulating levels of rifampin were reported to be significantly increased by probenecid.[888] However, a later study showed that increased levels were too inconsistent and occurred too infrequently to be of therapeutic value.[889] The metabolism and pharmacokinetics of rifampin have been reviewed.[890,891]

The elimination kinetics of rifampin in man are dose-dependent and also change with repeated dosing. The serum $t_{0.5}$ remains constant at <u>ca</u>. 2.5 h at doses up to 12 mg kg^{-1} but increases to 6.5 h at a dose of 16 mg kg^{-1}.[892,893] After repeated doses, the serum drug $t_{0.5}$ is reduced, and the extent of reduction is proportional to dose size.[894-896] Decreased elimination rates after large single doses appear to be due to saturation of hepatic enzymes which facilitate transfer of drug from blood to bile, whereas increased elimination rates after multiple doses may be due to induction of these enzymes.[897] Serum levels of rifampin and isoniazid were higher in patients with impaired renal function,[898] but neither drug influenced the serum levels, $t_{0.5}$, or urinary excretion of the other. Whereas serum levels of rifampin decreased in patients with normal liver function during multiple dosing, they tended to increase in patients with chronic liver disease.[899] The mean $t_{0.5}$ of rifampin was 3.8 h, and 34% of the dose was excreted in the urine of patients with pulmonary tuberculosis.[900]

Conflicting reports have appeared on the effect of repeated dosing on the elimination kinetics of rifampin and trimethoprim when administered in combination. In one study,[901] the elimination $t_{0.5}$ of rifampin was reduced from 2.7 to 1.5 h during repeated doses, while the trimethoprim elimination rate was unchanged. In another study,[902] the serum $t_{0.5}$ of both compounds was reduced by approximately 50% after repeated dosing. In both reports, reduced serum $t_{0.5}$ values are attributed to enzyme induction by rifampin. Disproportionate increases in rifampin plasma AUC values, and also the percentage of drug recovered in urine, from increasing p.o. rifampin doses are attributed to saturation of first-pass metabolism at high dose levels.[903] Combined use of fluorimetric and microbiological assays has shown that dogs excrete rifampin less efficiently than humans, and a biological $t_{0.5}$ of *ca.* 8 h is obtained after a 10 mg kg^{-1} dose.[904]

Cinoxacin

Cinoxacin is well absorbed from p.o. doses[905] but its pharmacokinetics and elimination are influenced by urinary pH, kidney function, and also by the inhibitory effects of probenecid. The serum $t_{0.5}$ of cinoxacin, which is cleared 60 - 70% as unchanged drug in urine, increases from a normal value of 1.5 - 2.0 h to 8 - 10 h in severe renal insufficiency.[906-908] However, when dosed at 12-hourly intervals, no undue accumulation of drug occurs in normal or impaired renal function, and the pharmacokinetic characteristics of cinoxacin are also unchanged with repeated doses.[908] The elimination $t_{0.5}$ of cinoxacin is increased almost 3-fold, but the distribution volume is not significantly altered, by probenecid.[909,910] While inhibition of cinoxacin renal excretion by probenecid suggests that cinoxacin is actively secreted into the kidney tubules, the mean ratio of cinoxacin renal clearance to creatinine clearance in normal individuals is only 1.3:1, indicating tubular reabsorption subsequent to secretion. Evidence of extensive renal tubular absorption is provided by a study in dogs, in which the cinoxacin elimination $t_{0.5}$ was increased from a normal value of 3.8 h to 15.8 h when urine was acidified by ingestion of ammonium chloride, and was reduced to 0.9 h when urine was made alkaline by ingestion of sodium bicarbonate.[911] These observations are consistent with renal tubular reabsorption of the weakly acidic cinoxacin molecule from acidic urine, but not from alkaline urine where it would exist predominantly in the ionized form. Acidification also reduces the concentration of cinoxacin in dog urine, and lowers the mean 24 h urinary recovery to less than 10% of a 10 mg kg^{-1} i.v. dose.

The pH dependency of cinoxacin pharmacokinetics has been demonstrated also in man. Acidification and alkalinization of urine by ammonium chloride and sodium bicarbonate, respectively, had no effect on cinoxacin absorption or distribution but significantly altered its elimination (Figure 3.29).[905] Mean plasma $t_{0.5}$ values of cinoxacin were 1.1, 2.0, and 0.6 h in controls and in acidification and alkalinization treated subjects, respectively. Renal clearance of cinoxacin was highly correlated with urine pH and averaged 76, 118, and 278 ml min^{-1} under acidic, control, and alkaline urine conditions.

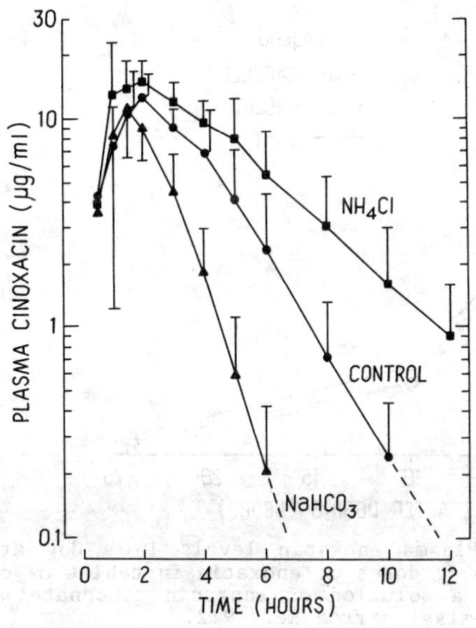

Figure 3.29 Mean concentrations of cinoxacin in plasma after control (●), ammonium chloride (■), and sodium bicarbonate (▲) treatments. Error bars indicate one standard deviation (n = 9). Reproduced by permission from <u>Antimicrob. Ag. Chemother.</u>, 1982, <u>21</u>, 472.

Enoxacin

The pharmacokinetics of the new quinolone antibacterial agent enoxacin have been studied extensively in experimental animals. Enoxacin is well absorbed from p.o. doses as the free base or the gluconate salt in dogs, with systemic bioavailability varying between 67 and 100%.[912] In dogs enoxacin has a distribution volume of 1.7 –

2.2 l kg^{-1}, is eliminated from plasma with a $t_{0.5}$ of 4 - 5 h, and has a total body clearance of 4.5 - 6.2 ml min^{-1} kg^{-1}. The bio-availability of i.m. dosed enoxacin, 10 mg kg^{-1}, was 100% relative to an i.v. dose in beagle dogs.[913] The formulation in which enoxacin is administered appears not to influence its absorption as virtually identical plasma profiles were obtained following single 200 mg p.o. doses of enoxacin free base in capsules, tablets, or as a solution of the gluconate salt.[914] Typical plasma enoxacin profiles obtained in a dog that received all three dosages are shown in Figure 3.30.

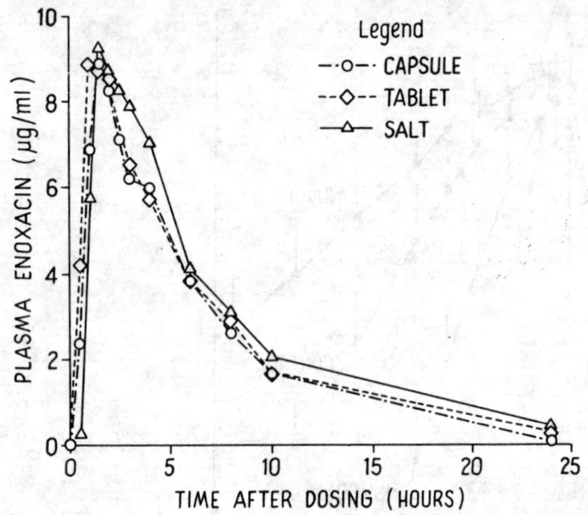

Figure 3.30   Plasma enoxacin levels in a dog after single 200 mg p.o. doses of enoxacin in tablet or capsule form, and a solution of enoxacin gluconate. Reproduced by permission from Ref. 912.

Following multiple twice-daily doses of 50 mg kg^{-1}, mean plasma levels of enoxacin in dogs 4 h postdose were 20 µg ml^{-1}. Tissue levels in heart, lung, liver, kidney, spleen, and muscle exceeded the levels in plasma, indicating excellent tissue distribution of anti-bacterial activity.[914] Following 10 mg kg^{-1} and 20 mg kg^{-1} i.v. doses to monkeys, plasma enoxacin levels declined in biexponential fashion with mean distribution and elimination $t_{0.5}$ values of 6 min and 3 - 5 h, respectively. Areas under plasma curves were dose-proportional.[915]

Rosoxacin

Following single 300 mg p.o. doses of rosoxacin in healthy males, a mean peak plasma level of 4.7 µg ml^{-1} was attained at 2.6 h.[916] The decline in rosoxacin concentration was monoexponential with a mean $t_{0.5}$ of 3.4 h.

Nalidixic and Oxolinic Acids

Peak serum levels of total (free and conjugated) nalidixic acid were 34 µg ml^{-1} following a single 1 g dose to healthy women.[917] Levels were almost double this initial value following repeated q.i.d. doses. At steady-state 24 h urinary recovery accounted for <u>ca</u>. 80% of the daily dose. Oxolinic acid accumulated to a greater extent than nalidixic acid, serum levels increasing 4- to 5-fold after repeated twice-daily doses.

The average $t_{0.5}$ of nalidixic acid after a 1 g p.o. dose was 2.7 h in young adults (21 - 36 yr) but increased to 11.5 h in elderly subjects (64 - 89 yr), probably due to declining renal function in the latter.[918] Consequently, plasma levels of both nalidixic acid and the active metabolite 7-hydroxynalidixic acid were higher in the older group.

Methenamine

The absorption of methenamine from a 1 g methenamine hippurate tablet was rapid and extensive; mean peak serum concentration in 10 healthy subjects was 30 µg ml^{-1} at <u>ca</u>. 1 h.[919] Approximately 82% of a single dose was excreted in 24 h urine, and the overall $t_{0.5}$ was <u>ca</u>. 4 h. Repeated dosing of 1 g methenamine hippurate, twice daily for 7 days, resulted in no drug accumulation or altered pharmaco-kinetic parameters. Antibiotic concentrations greater than 150 µg ml^{-1} were constantly maintained in the urine during this regimen.

Isoniazid

The bioavailability of isoniazid (INH) was virtually identical from three commercial formulations in fasted subjects,[920] but absorption is markedly reduced in the presence of food.[921,922] In one study, all test meals significantly impaired INH absorption in both slow and rapid acetylators, although the effect was greatest after carbohydrate meals, possibly due to the formation of nonabsorbable condensation products between INH and various sugars.[922] There was no significant food effect on INH elimination $t_{0.5}$, which averaged 3 - 4 h in slow acetylators and 1 - 2 h in rapid acetylators. Serum concentrations of the metabolite acetyl-INH in rapid acetylators were 2-fold higher compared to those in slow acetylators, regardless of treatment. Studies in rats have indicated that aspirin and ethanol delay INH absorption from the GI tract, although the extent of absorption is unaffected.[923]

The pharmacokinetics of INH metabolism have been described in two independent studies.[924,925] Both studies are complex and differ in their assumption of one-compartment[924] and two-compartment[925] disposition kinetics of INH and its metabolites. Both models are also acknowledged to be insufficient in assuming first-order kinetics throughout when saturable kinetics are implied by the data. Despite the different approaches, however, the overall parameter values common to both studies are in good agreement. The disposition of INH was unaltered in patients with idiopathic systemic lupus erythematosus.[926] Isoniazid crosses the placenta into the foetus.[927] After repeated administration to the mother during late pregnancy, similar concentrations of the antibiotic were found in maternal and newborn serum.

A number of methods have been proposed to screen INH acetylator phenotypes. In one study five such methods were examined. All gave similar discrimination, but with different levels of efficiency.[928] Greatest discrimination efficiency was obtained with the SpM urine test, based on spectrophotometric determination of INH and acetyl-INH, while poorest discrimination was obtained with a CD procedure which is similar to the SpM test but omits a sample acidification step. Other tests gave intermediate results. Application of the urine test to populations of eskimos and caucasians showed that the majority of the former group were fast acetylators whereas the majority of the latter group were slow acetylators.[929] Frequency patterns in both populations indicated a trimodal distribution of fast, medium, and slow INH acetylators. One method of rapid phenotype identification is based on relative quantities of acetyl-INH and INH excreted in urine in the 6 to 8 h time interval following a single dose of INH.[930] The proportion of acetylated metabolite and unchanged INH excreted in this period is directly related to the plasma $t_{0.5}$ of INH.

A number of methods have been proposed for dosing INH to fast and slow acetylator phenotypes. One method involves the use of p.o. matrix formulations.[931] One 30 mg dose of INH in the slow-release matrix is reported to give similar blood levels of INH in fast acetylators to those in slow acetylators receiving 10 mg of INH in a conventional dosage form. An alternative suggestion is that of once-weekly therapy for fast acetylators of 15 mg kg^{-1} INH in conventional dosage form together with 15 mg kg^{-1} of an enteric-coated preparation, while slow acetylators receive only the 15 mg kg^{-1} conventional dose of INH. Sustained-release preparations seem to be appropriate for INH as the drug is absorbed from the entire intestine and probably also from the colon and rectum.[932]

Slow-release formulations for maintenance of fast acetylators have been evaluated by Eidus et al.[933,934] Although similar blood levels of INH could be obtained in fast and slow acetylators by using conventional and slow-release dosage forms in some cases, considerable variations between individuals and also the need for immediate fast drug input in the fast-acetylator population indicate the need for further study of this intriguing problem. Increased susceptibility of fast INH inactivators to hepatitis has been rationalized in terms of the faster rate of metabolism of INH to isonicotinic acid.[935] The free hydrazine moiety liberated in this metabolic step may be converted into a potent acetylating agent, which may cause liver injury in man.

Ethambutol

Plasma levels of ethambutol peaked at 2 - 4 h after p.o. doses to volunteers and subsequently declined during the 12 h postdose period with a $t_{0.5}$ of 4 - 5 h.[936] However, inclusion of 24 h plasma levels, and 72 h urine data, indicated that the true terminal ethambutol $t_{0.5}$ is <u>ca</u>. 10 h. The fractional increase in ethambutol accumulation during repeated dosing due to prolonged $t_{0.5}$ is <u>ca</u>. 10% in patients with normal renal function, which is probably not clinically significant.

Successful treatment of tuberculosis meningitis with ethambutol requires an adequate concentration of drug in the c.s.f., and inconsistent results previously reported in this respect may have been due to inadequate assay procedures.[937] Studies using a chemical assay have shown that a daily dose of 20 - 30 mg kg^{-1} to human patients will yield c.s.f. levels > 1.0 $\mu g\ ml^{-1}$, and serum and c.s.f. levels of ethambutol are linearly related when serum levels reach this value.[938]

p-Aminosalicylic Acid

The bioavailability of p-aminosalicylic acid (PAS) and its salts from various formulations has been studied in man.[939-942] Absorption of PAS and its Na^+, K^+, and Ca^{2+} salts from aqueous suspensions or solutions was essentially complete. Absorption rates were faster from the PAS salts, and areas under plasma level curves were greater than from PAS, possibly due to saturation of first-pass metabolism of PAS from the more rapidly absorbed forms. A higher proportion of circulating unmetabolized PAS following a large p.o. dose, compared with

a somewhat smaller dose (4 g versus 2.9 g as the free acid), was similarly attributed to saturation of metabolizing enzymes during absorption of the larger dose.[942]

Two studies have challenged the validity of USP disintegration
tests for uncoated and enteric-coated tablets containing PAS.
Schirmer et al.[943] showed that the tests would pass uncoated tablets,
which were 30.4% available, and enteric-coated tablets, which were
0.0 - 35.5% available. Wagner et al.[944] demonstrated that an enteric-
coated PAS formulation, although passing the USP test, was voided
intact in faeces after p.o. dosing, still containing 98% of the
labelled dose. These studies suggest that the time allowed for disintegration or the intensity of agitation in the USP tests should be reduced in order to give better prediction of _in vivo_ bioavailability.
Further evidence was presented that PAS, like neomycin sulphate and
colchicine, inhibits intestinal mucosal transport processes and can
cause weight loss and malabsorption symptoms in patients regularly
receiving this drug.[945]

Pyrizinamide

The antituberculosis drug pyrizinamide is extensively metabolized
in the dog and man, and renal clearance of both unchanged drug and
metabolites involves both filtration and active or passive reabsorption.[946] The experimental evidence strongly suggests that marked
urate retention, associated with pyrizinamide, is due mainly to the
action of pyrizinoate.

References

1. L.W. Dittert, W.O. Griffin, Jr., J.C. La Piana, F.J. Shainfield, and J.T. Doluisio, 'Antimicrobial Agents and Chemotherapy - 1969,' ed. G. L. Hobby, American Society for Microbiology, Bethesda, 1970, p. 42.

2. J.W. Poole, J. Pharm. Sci., 1970, 59, 1255.

3. J.W. Poole, Rev. Canad. Biol., 1973, 32, Suppl., 43.

4. C.F. Speirs, D. Stenhouse, K.W. Stephen, and E.T. Wallace, Brit. J. Pharmacol., 1971, 43, 242.

5. W.G. Crouthamel, J. Amer. Pharm. Assoc., 1977, NS17, 243.

6. M. Barza and L. Weinstein, Clin. Pharmacokin., 1976, 1, 297.

7. A. Hedges, C.M. Kaye, W.P. Maclay, and P. Turner, J. Clin. Pharmacol., 1974, 14, 363.

8. H. Rollag, Jr., T. Midtvedt, and S. Wetterhus, Acta Paediatr. Scand., 1975, 64, 421.

9. Th. Dimmling, H.G. Bredehorst, and E. Vander Elst, Eur. J. Clin. Pharmacol., 1976, 10, 55.

10. P. Bolme and M. Erikkson, Acta Paediatr. Scand., 1976, 65, 253.

11. T. Bergan, B.P. Berdal, and V. Holm, Acta Pharmacol. Toxicol., 1976, 38, 308.

12. Y. Finkel, P. Bolme, and M. Eriksson, Acta Pharmacol. Toxicol., 1981, 49, 301.

13. S.I. Terry, J.C. Gould, J.P.A. McManus, and L.F. Prescott, Eur. J. Clin. Pharmacol., 1982, 23, 245.

14. J.S. Tan, J.C. Holmes, N.O. Fowler, G.T. Manitsas, and J.P. Phair, J. Clin. Invest., 1974, 53, 7.

15. M. Barza, J. Brusch, M.G. Bergeron, O. Kemmotsu, and L. Weinstein, J. Infect. Dis., 1975, 131, S86.

16. R.G. Dacey and M.A. Sande, Antimicrob. Ag. Chemother., 1974, 6, 437.

17. S.E. Holm and C. Ekedahl, J. Antimicrob. Chemother., 1982, 10, 121.

18. J. Hulbert, J. Clin. Pathol., 1972, 25, 73.

19. L.D. Rollins, R.H. Teske, R.J. Condon, and G.G. Carter, J. Amer. Vet. Med. Assoc., 1972, 161, 490.

20. F.C. Wilson, J.N. Worcester, P.D. Coleman, and W.E. Byrd, J. Bone Joint Surgery, 1971, 53-A, 1622.

21. J.O. Klein, M.J. Schaberg, M. Buntin, and H.M. Gezon, J. Pediat., 1973, 82, 1065.

22. R.E. Kauffman, B.M. Boulos, and D.L. Azarnoff, Amer. J. Obstet. Gynecol., 1973, 117, 64.

23. P.L. Whyatt, G.W.A. Slywka, A.P. Melikian, and M.C. Meyer, <u>J. Pharm. Sci.</u>, 1976, <u>65</u>, 652.

24. C. MacLeod, H. Rabin, J. Ruedy, M. Caron, D. Zarowny, and R.O. Davies, <u>Canad. Med. Assoc. J.</u>, 1972, <u>107</u>, 203.

25. E.J. Triggs, J.M. Johnson, and B. Learoyd, <u>Eur. J. Clin. Pharmacol.</u>, 1980, <u>18</u>, 195.

26. H.M. Ali and A.M. Farouk, <u>Int. J. Pharmaceut.</u>, 1980, <u>6</u>, 301.

27. P.G. Welling, H. Huang, P.A. Koch, W.A. Craig, and P.O. Madsen, <u>J. Pharm. Sci.</u>, 1977, <u>66</u>, 549.

28. J. Silverio and J. W. Poole, <u>Pediatrics</u>, 1973, <u>51</u>, 578.

29. J.W. Poole, G. Owen, J. Silverio, J.N. Freyhof, and S.B. Rosenman, <u>Curr. Ther. Res.</u>, 1968, <u>10</u>, 292.

30. S.A. Hill, K.H. Jones, H. Seager, and C.B. Taskis, <u>J. Pharm. Pharmacol.</u>, 1975, <u>27</u>, 594.

31. R. Dugal, J. Brodeur, and G. Caille, <u>J. Clin. Pharmacol.</u>, 1974, <u>14</u>, 513.

32. A. Sahra, F. Metrau, N. Feitosa, J.M. Santi, and L.R. Trabulsi, <u>Curr. Ther. Res.</u>, 1973, <u>15</u>, 866.

33. J.D. Nelson, S. Shelton, H.T. Kusmiesz, and K.C. Haltalin, <u>Clin. Pharmacol. Ther.</u>, 1972, <u>13</u>, 879.

34. J.T. Doluisio, J.C. La Piana, and L.W. Dittert, <u>J. Pharm. Sci.</u>, 1971, <u>60</u>, 715.

35. C. Henning and O. Cars, <u>Chemotherapy</u>, 1982, <u>28</u>, 185.

36. R.M. Brown, R. Wise, J.M. Andrews, and J. Hancox, <u>Antimicrob. Ag. Chemother.</u>, 1982, <u>21</u>, 565.

37. J. Sjövall, <u>J. Antimicrob. Chemother.</u>, 1981, <u>8</u>, 41.

38. E. Rubinstein, J. Haspel, E. Klein, G. Ben-Ari, R. Schwarzkopf, and A. Tadmor, <u>Antimicrob. Ag. Chemother.</u>, 1980, <u>17</u>, 905.

39. P.L. Parsons, J.P. Beavis, M. Laurence, J.A. David, G.M. Paddock, and J.R. Trounce, <u>Brit. J. Clin. Pharmacol.</u>, 1978, <u>6</u>, 135.

40. O.M.J. Driessen, N. Sorgedrager, M.F. Michel, K.F. Kerrebijn, and J. Hermans, <u>Eur. J. Clin. Pharmacol.</u>, 1978, <u>13</u>, 449.

41. J. Fabre, P. Blanchard, and M. Rudhardt, <u>Chemotherapy</u>, 1977, <u>23</u>, 129.

42. A. Philipson, <u>J. Infect. Dis.</u>, 1977, <u>136</u>, 370.

43. R.N. Brogden, T.M. Speight, and G.S. Avery, <u>Drugs</u>, 1975, <u>9</u>, 88.

44. W.W. Karney, M. Turck, and K.K. Holmes, <u>Antimicrob. Ag. Chemother.</u>, 1974, <u>5</u>, 114.

45. W.J. Jusko, G.P. Lewis, and G.W. Schmitt, <u>Clin. Pharmacol. Ther.</u>, 1973, <u>14</u>, 90.

46. Å. Ryrfeldt, N.O. Bodin, and E. Hansson, <u>Acta Pharmacol. Toxicol.</u>, 1973, 33, 219.

47. J.M. Brogard, M. Pinget, C. Meyer, M. Dorner, and J. Lavillaureix, Chemotherapy, 1977, 23, 213.

48. J. Kampmann, F. Lindahl, J.M. Hansen, and K. Siersbaek-Nielsen, Brit. J. Pharmacol., 1973, 47, 782.

49. P. Naumann, H. Lode, and E. Reintjens, Arzneim.-Forsch., 1973, 23, 218.

50. M. Rozencweig, M. Staguet, and J. Klastersky, Clin. Pharmacol. Ther., 1976, 19, 592.

51. T.B. Kjaer, P.G. Welling, and P.O. Madsen, J. Pharm. Sci., 1977, 66, 345.

52. T. Bergan, Antimicrob. Ag. Chemother., 1978, 13, 971.

53. J. Sjövall, L. Magni, and T. Bergan, Antimicrob. Ag. Chemother., 1978, 13, 90.

54. P.T. Männistö, U. Repo and M. Malkki, J. Antimicrob. Chemother., 1979, 5, 236.

55. T. Bergan, A. Engeset, W. Olszewski, and R. Solberg, Lymphology, 1979, 12, 85.

56. T. Bergan, D. Bratlid, and A. Brøndbo, J. Antimicrob. Chemother., 1978, 4, 79.

57. T. Bergan, Antibiot. Chemother., 1978, 25, 1.

58. J.B. Wilcox, R.N. Brogden, and G.S. Avery, Drugs, 1973, 6, 94.

59. F. Jeppesen and P. Illum, Antibiotics (Japan), 1972, 73, 428.

60. J.C.K. Loo, E.L. Foltz, H. Wallick, and K.C. Kwan, Clin. Pharmacol. Ther., 1974, 16, 35.

61. W.M.M. Kirby, R.C. Gordon, and C. Regamey, J. Infect. Dis., 1974, 129, S154.

62. G. Gothoni, P. Pentikäinen, H.I. Vapaatalo, R. Hackman, and K. af Björksten, Ann. Clin. Res., 1972, 4, 228.

63. L. Pedersen-Bjergaard and K.E. Petersen, Clin. Pharmacokin., 1977, 2, 451.

64. A. Fedorcak, H. Mielenz, and G. Bozler, Arzneim.-Forsch., 1977, 27, 659.

65. A. Swahn, Eur. J. Clin. Pharmacol., 1976, 9, 299.

66. B. Lund, J.P. Kampmann, F. Lindahl, and J.M. Hansen, Clin. Pharmacol. Ther., 1976, 19, 587.

67. A. Philipson, Amer. J. Obstet. Gynecol., 1978, 130, 674.

68. M.W. Kunst and H. Mattie, Antimicrob. Ag. Chemother., 1975, 8, 11.

69. R. Sutherland, S. Elson, and E.A.P. Croydon, Chemotherapy, 1972, 17, 145.

70. A. Philipson, L.D. Sabath, and B. Rosnar, Antimicrob. Ag. Chemother., 1975, 8, 311.

71. G. Kienel, <u>Arzneim.-Forsch.</u>, 1976, <u>26</u>, 781.

72. R. Kahrimanis and P. Pierpaoli, <u>New Engl. J. Med.</u>, 1971, <u>285</u>, 236.

73. F. Modr and F. Dvoracek, <u>Rev. Czech. Med.</u>, 1970, <u>16</u>, 84.

74. W.J. Jusko and G.P. Lewis, <u>Lancet</u>, 1972, <u>i</u>, 690.

75. W.J. Jusko and G.P. Lewis, <u>J. Pharm. Sci.</u>, 1973, <u>62</u>, 69.

76. A. Arancibia, J. Guttmann, G. González, and C. González, <u>Antimicrob. Ag. Chemother.</u>, 1980, <u>17</u>, 199.

77. A. Dalhoff, P. Koeppe, and D. von Kobyletzki, <u>Arzneim.-Forsch.</u>, 1981, <u>31</u>, 1148.

78. L. Okolicsanyi, M. Venuti, R. Orlando, G. Benoni, M.T. Dorigo, T. Berti, M. Serembe, A. Porro, and G. Vettori, <u>Drugs Exptl. Clin. Res.</u>, 1981, <u>7</u>, 725.

79. I.D. Farrell, A.P. Ball, G. Brookes, P.G. Davey, T.J. Muscroft, and I. Gonda, <u>J. Antimicrob. Chemother.</u>, 1981, <u>7</u>, 110.

80. F.N. Eshelman and D.A. Spyker, <u>Antimicrob. Ag. Chemother.</u>, 1978, <u>14</u>, 539.

81. P.G. Welling, H. Huang, P.A. Koch, W.A. Craig, and P.O. Madsen, <u>J. Pharm. Sci.</u>, 1977, <u>66</u>, 549.

82. C.M. Ginsburg, G.H. McCracken, M.L. Thomas, and J. Clahsen, <u>Pediatrics</u>, 1979, <u>64</u>, 627.

83. R.N. Brogden, A. Carmine, R.C. Heel, P.A. Morley, T.M. Speight, and G.S. Avery, <u>Drugs</u>, 1981, <u>22</u>, 337.

84. J. Haginaka, T. Nakagawa, T. Hoshino, K. Yamaoka, and T. Uno, <u>Chem. Pharm. Bull.</u>, 1981, <u>29</u>, 3342.

85. J.D. Nelson, H. Kusmiesz, and S. Shelton, <u>Antimicrob. Ag. Chemother.</u>, 1982, <u>21</u>, 681.

86. D.H. Staniforth, R.J. Lillystone, and D. Jackson, <u>J. Antimicrob. Chemother.</u>, 1982, <u>10</u>, 131.

87. D. Zarowny, R. Ogilvie, D. Tamblyn, C. MacLeod, and J. Ruedy, <u>Clin. Pharmacol. Ther.</u>, 1974, <u>16</u>, 1045.

88. J. Hermans, O. Driessen, N. Sorgedrager, and M. Spoor, <u>Arzneim.-Forsch.</u>, 1975, <u>25</u>, 947.

89. R.C. Rudoy, N. Goto, D. Pettit, and H. Uemura, <u>Antimicrob. Ag. Chemother.</u>, 1979, <u>15</u>, 628.

90. I.J. Kiss, E. Faragó, J. Schnitzler, and I. Varhélyi, <u>Int. J. Clin. Pharmacol. Ther. Toxicol.</u>, 1981, <u>19</u>, 69.

91. L. Weingärtner, U. Sitka, R. Patsch, H.-H. Thiemann, W. Brömme, and I. Richter, <u>Int. J. Clin. Pharmacol. Ther. Toxicol.</u>, 1980, <u>18</u>, 185.

92. N. Clumeck, J.P. Thys, R. Vanhoof, M.P. Vanderlinden, J.P. Butzler, and E. Yourassowsky, <u>Antimicrob. Ag. Chemother.</u>, 1978, <u>14</u>, 531.

93. R. Münch, R. Lüthy, J. Blaser, and W. Siegenthaler, J. Antimicrob. Chemother., 1981, 8, 29.

94. L. Mizen, K. Bhandari, J. Sayer, and E. Catherall, Drugs Exptl. Clin. Res., 1981, 7, 263.

95. G. Humbert, D.A. Spyker, J.P. Fillastre, and A. Leroy, Antimicrob. Ag. Chemother., 1979, 15, 28.

96. E.L. Francke, G.B. Appel, and H.C. Neu, Clin. Pharmacol. Ther., 1979, 26, 31.

97. P. Chelvan, J.M.T. Hamilton-Miller, and W. Brumfitt, J. Antimicrob. Chemother., 1979, 5, 232.

98. C. Watanakunakorn, Antimicrob. Ag. Chemother., 1977, 11, 1007.

99. R. Yogev, W.E. Schultz, and S.B. Rosenman, Antimicrob. Ag. Chemother., 1981, 19, 545.

100. W. Banner, Jr., W.M. Gooch, III, G. Burckart, and S.B. Korones, Antimicrob. Ag. Chemother., 1980, 17, 691.

101. E.S. Waller, M.A. Sharanevych, and G.J. Yakatan, J. Clin. Pharmacol., 1982, 22, 482.

102. M. Rudnick, G. Morrison, B. Walker, and I. Singer, Clin. Pharmacol. Ther., 1976, 20, 413.

103. C.R. Diaz, J.G. Kane, R.H. Parker, and F.R. Pelsor, Antimicrob. Ag. Chemother., 1977, 12, 98.

104. M.A.L. Evans, P. Wilson, T. Leung, and J.D. Williams, J. Antimicrob. Chemother., 1978, 4, 255.

105. T.B. Tjandramaga, A. Mullie, R. Verbesselt, P.J. de Schepper, and L. Verbist, Antimicrob. Ag. Chemother., 1978, 14, 829.

106. V.K. Batra, J.A. Morrison, K.C. Lasseter, and V.A. Joy, Clin. Pharmacol. Ther., 1979, 26, 41.

107. J. Russo, Jr., M.I.B. Thompson, M.E. Russo, B.A. Saxon, J.M. Matsen, F.G. Moody, and L.F. Rikkers, Antimicrob. Ag. Chemother., 1982, 22, 488.

108. G.M. Dickinson, D.G. Droller, R.L. Greenman, and T.A. Hoffman, Antimicrob. Ag. Chemother., 1981, 20, 481.

109. B.R. Meyers, S.Z. Hirschman, L. Strougo, and E. Srulevitch, Antimicrob. Ag. Chemother., 1980, 17, 608.

110. C.B. Wilson, J.R. Koup, K.E. Opheim, L.A. Adelman, J. Levy, T.L. Stull, C. Clausen, and A.L. Smith, Antimicrob. Ag. Chemother., 1982, 22, 442.

111. J.A. Giron, B.R. Meyers, and S.Z. Hirschman, Antimicrob. Ag. Chemother., 1981, 19, 309.

112. J.A. Giron, B.R. Meyers, S.Z. Hirschman, and E. Srulevitch, Antimicrob. Ag. Chemother., 1981, 19, 279.

113. M.I.B. Thompson, M.E. Russo, J.M. Matsen, and E. Atkin-Thor, Antimicrob. Ag. Chemother., 1981, 19, 450.

114. J.A. Morrison, A.C. Dornbush, S.S. Sathe, and P.G. Gooding, Drugs Exptl. Clin. Res., 1981, 7, 415.

115. E.L. Francke, G.B. Appel, and H.C. Neu, <u>Antimicrob. Ag. Chemother.</u>, 1979, 16, 788.

116. L.D. Sarff, G.H. McCracken, Jr., M.L. Thomas, L.J. Horton, and N. Threlkeld, <u>J. Pediatr.</u>, 1977, 90, 1005.

117. L.J. Strausbaugh, T.W. Murray, and M.A. Sande, <u>J. Antimicrob. Chemother.</u>, 1980, 6, 363.

118. F.M. Gengo and J.J. Schentag, <u>Antimicrob. Ag. Chemother.</u>, 1981, 19, 836.

119. B. Gradnik and L. Fleischmann, <u>Farmaco Ed. Pr.</u>, 1971, 26, 116.

120. C.M. Ginsburg, G.H. McCracken, Jr., T.C. Zweighaft, and J.C. Clahsen, <u>Antimicrob. Ag. Chemother.</u>, 1981, 19, 1086.

121. A. Tsuji, E. Nakashima, I. Kagami, and T. Yamana, <u>J. Pharm. Sci.</u>, 1981, 70, 772.

122. C. Simon, V. Malerczyk, U. Müller, and G. Müller, <u>Deut. Med. Woch.</u>, 1972, 97, 1999.

123. A.K. Knirsch, D.C. Hobbs, and J.J. Korst, <u>J. Infect. Dis.</u>, 1973, 127, Suppl., S105.

124. K. Butler, A.R. English, B. Briggs, E. Gralla, R.B. Stebbins, and D.C. Hobbs, <u>J. Infect. Dis.</u>, 1973, 127, Suppl., S97.

125. A. Whelton, G.G. Carter, H.H. Bryant, L.A. Porteous, and W.G. Walker, <u>Ann. Intern. Med.</u>, 1973, 78, 659.

126. M. Hatala, J. Morávek, and O. Schuck, <u>Int. J. Clin. Pharmacol. Ther. Toxicol.</u>, 1974, 10, 179.

127. L. Madacsy, M. Bokor, and G. Kozocsa, <u>Int. J. Clin. Pharmacol.</u>, 1976, 14, 155.

128. L. Madacsy, L. Matusovits, and M. Bokor, <u>Acta Paediat. Acad. Sci. Hung.</u>, 1973, 14, 43.

129. Z. Modr, K. Dvordcek, I. Janku, and V. Krebs, <u>Int. J. Clin. Pharmacol.</u>, 1977, 15, 81.

130. C.D. Morehead, S. Shelton, H. Kusmiesz, and J.D. Nelson, <u>Antimicrob. Ag. Chemother.</u>, 1972, 2, 267.

131. R.R. Bailey, J.B. Eastwood, and R.B. Vaughan, <u>Postgrad. Med. J.</u>, 1972, 48, 422.

132. J.D. Nelson and E.W. Reimold, <u>Lancet</u>, 1973, i, 486.

133. T.A. Hoffman, R. Cesteso, and W.E. Bullock, <u>Ann. Intern. Med.</u>, 1970, 73, 173.

134. R.D. Libke, J.T. Clarke, E.D. Ralph, R.P. Luthy, and W.M.M. Kirby, <u>Clin. Pharmacol. Ther.</u>, 1975, 17, 441.

135. F.D. Daschner, G. Thoma, H. Langmaack, and A. Dalhoff, <u>Antimicrob. Ag. Chemother.</u>, 1980, 17, 738.

136. A. Gouyette, M.D. Kitzis, J. Guibert, and J.F. Acar, <u>J. Antimicrob. Chemother.</u>, 1982, 10, 419.

137. B.E. Davies, M.J. Humphrey, P.F. Langley, L. Lees, B. Legg, and G.A. Wadds, <u>Eur. J. Clin. Pharmacol.</u>, 1982, 23, 167.

138. M. Higi, L. Essers, G. Linzenmeier, and S. Seeber, Int. J. Clin. Pharmacol. Ther. Toxicol., 1982, 20, 514.

139. D. Höffler, A. Dalhoff, and P. Koeppe, Deut. Med. Woch., 1978, 103, 931.

140. M.F. Parry and H.C. Neu, J. Infect. Dis., 1976, 133, 46.

141. R. Wise, D.S. Reeves, and A.S. Parker, Antimicrob. Ag. Chemother., 1974, 5, 119.

142. M. Davies, J.R. Morgan, and C. Anand, Chemotherapy, 1974, 20, 339.

143. Y. Murai, T. Nakagawa, K. Yamaoka, and T. Uno, Chem. Pharm. Bull., 1981, 29, 3290.

144. D.N. Gerding, L.R. Peterson, J.K. Salomonson, W.H. Hall, and E.A. Schierl, J. Infect. Dis., 1978, 138, 166.

145. R.H. Fitzgerald, P.J. Kelly, R.J. Snyder, and J.A. Washington, Antimicrob. Ag. Chemother., 1978, 14, 723.

146. L.R. Peterson, D.N. Gerding, D. McLinn, and W.H. Hall, J. Antimicrob. Chemother., 1979, 5, 219.

147. G.J. Burckart, W.E. Evans, and G.L. Whitington, Amer. J. Hosp. Pharm., 1978, 35, 1380.

148. E.H. Nauta and H. Mattie, Clin. Pharmacol. Ther., 1976, 20, 98.

149. M.M. Uwaydah, B.M. Faris, I.N. Samara, H.F. Shammas, and K.F. To'Mey, Amer. J. Ophthalmol., 1976, 82, 114.

150. G.J. Schwartz, T. Hegyi, and A. Spitzer, J. Pediatr., 1976, 89, 310.

151. G. Ziv and F.G. Sulman, Arch. Int. Pharmacodyn. Ther., 1974, 207, 373.

152. E.H. Nauta, H. Mattie, and W.R.O. Goslings, Antimicrob. Ag. Chemother., 1974, 6, 300.

153. R.D. Lee, J.L. Brusch, M.J. Barza, and L. Weinstein, Antimicrob. Ag. Chemother., 1975, 8, 105.

154. O. Cars, S. Ögren, and H. Erlendsdóttir, J. Antimicrob. Chemother., 1982, 9, 201.

155. K.A. DeSante, L.W. Dittert, S. Stavchansky, and J.T. Doluisio, J. Clin. Pharmacol., 1980, 20, 534.

156. R. Sutherland, E.A.P. Croydon, and G.N. Rolinson, Brit. Med. J., 1970, iv, 455.

157. L. Herngren, M. Ehrnebo, and L.O. Boréus, Eur. J. Clin. Pharmacol., 1982, 22, 351.

158. I.J. Kiss, E. Faragó, A. Gömöry, and J. Szamaránszky, Int. J. Clin. Pharmacol. Ther. Toxicol., 1980, 18, 405.

159. H.H.W. Thijssen Dand J. Wolters, Eur. J. Clin. Pharmacol., 1982, 22, 429.

160. P.L. Oe, S. Simonian, and J. Verhoef, Chemotherapy, 1973, 19, 279.

161. D.H. Lawson, A.K. Henderson, and R.R. McGeachy, Postgrad. Med. J., 1974, 50, 500.

162. J. Verhoef, P.L. Oe, and S. Simonian, Chemotherapy, 1973, 19, 272.

163. E.H. Nauta and H. Mattie, Brit. J. Clin. Pharmacol., 1975, 2, 111.

164. M.F. Michel, J.P. van Waardhuizen, and K.F. Kerrebijn, Chemotherapy, 1973, 18, 77.

165. C.-H. Ramsay, N.-O. Bodin, and E. Hansson, Arzneim.-Forsch., 1972, 22, 1962.

166. G.R. Hodges and S.E. Worley, Antimicrob. Ag. Chemother., 1982, 22, 909.

167. J. Modai, J. Pierre, E. Bergogne-Berezin, and M.F. Avril, Arzneim.-Forsch., 1979, 29, 1967.

168. D.H. Wittmann, H.-H. Schassan, and H. Seidel, Arzneim.-Forsch., 1981, 31, 1157.

169. D. Adam, K. Wilhelm, and V. Chyský, Arzneim.-Forsch., 1981, 31, 1972.

170. J. Welter, D.-H. Wittmann, and H.-H. Schassan, Int. J. Clin. Pharm. Res., 1982, 2, 265.

171. A. Georgopoulos and E. Schütze, Antimicrob. Ag. Chemother., 1980, 17, 779.

172. L. Verbist, T.B. Tjandramaga, R. Verbesselt, and P.J. De Schepper, Arzneim.-Forsch., 1979, 29, 1962.

173. U. Gundert-Remy, D. Föster, P. Schacht, and E. Weber, J. Antimicrob. Chemother., 1982, 9, 65.

174. U. Gundert-Remy and E. Weber, Eur. J. Clin. Pharmacol., 1982, 22, 435.

175. J.M. Brogard, J. Kopferschmitt, J.P. Arnaud, M. Dorner, and J. la Villaureix, Antimicrob. Ag. Chemother., 1980, 18, 69.

176. L. Weingärtner, U. Sitka, R. Patsch, I. Richter, and H.H. Thiemann, Arzneim.-Forsch., 1979, 29, 1952.

177. G. Heimann, B. von Heereman, and E. Gladtke, Arzneim.-Forsch., 1979, 29, 1949.

178. G. Heimann and D. Föster, Drugs Exptl. Clin. Res., 1981, 7, 287.

179. T. Rubio, F. Wirth, and E. Karotkin, J. Antimicrob. Chemother., 1982, 9, 241.

180. T. Bergan and H. Michalsen, Arzneim.-Forsch., 1979, 29, 1955.

181. T. Bergan, S.B. Thorsteinsson, and O. Steingrimsson, Chemotherapy, 1982, 28, 160.

182. A. Leroy, G. Humbert, M. Godin, and J.P. Fillastre, Antimicrob. Ag. Chemother., 1980, 17, 344.

183. R. Schurig, D. Kampf, H. Becker, and D. Föster, Arzneim.-Forsch., 1979, 29, 1944.

184. J.M. Aletta, E.F. Francke, and H.C. Neu, Clin. Pharmacol. Ther.,
      1980, 27, 563.

185. A. Mangione, F.D. Boudinot, R.M. Schultz, and W.J. Jusko,
      Antimicrob. Ag. Chemother., 1982, 21, 428.

186. G.R. Aronoff, R.S. Sloan, R.A. Stanish, and N.S. Fineberg, Eur.
      J. Clin. Pharmacol., 1982, 21, 505.

187. S.J. Pancoast and H.C. Neu, Clin. Pharmacol. Ther., 1978, 24,
      108.

188. G.R. Aronoff, R.S. Sloan, F.C. Luft, R.L. Nelson, D.R. Maxwell,
      and S.A. Kleit, Clin. Pharmacol. Ther., 1980, 28, 523.

189. N. Frimodt-Möller, S. Maigaard, R.D. Toothaker, R.W. Bundtzen,
      M.V. Brodey, W.A. Craig, P.G. Welling, and P.O. Madsen,
      Antimicrob. Ag. Chemother., 1980, 17, 599.

190. T. Bergan, E.K. Brodwall and E. Wiik-Larsen, Antimicrob. Ag.
      Chemother., 1979, 16, 651.

191. T. Bergan, Antimicrob. Ag. Chemother., 1978, 14, 801.

192. D. Kampf, R. Schurig, K. Weihermüller, and D. Föster,
      Antimicrob. Ag. Chemother., 1980, 18, 81.

193. G.R. Aronoff, J. Antimicrob. Chemother., 1982, 9, 77.

194. D.M. Janicke, A. Mangione, R.W. Schultz, and W.J. Jusko,
      Antimicrob. Ag. Chemother., 1981, 20, 590.

195. J. Kosmidis, P. Doundoulaki, Ch. Stathakis, N. Zerefos, A.
      Bounia, and G.K. Daikos, Arzneim.-Forsch., 1979, 29, 1960.

196. S. Hartley and R. Wise, J. Antimicrob. Chemother., 1982, 10, 49.

197. A. Montanari, L. Borghi, M. Canali, P. Coruzzi, A. Novarini, and
      A. Borghetti, Int. J. Clin. Pharmacol. Ther. Toxicol., 1980, 18,
      225.

198. R.M. Brown, R. Wise, and J.M. Andrews, J. Antimicrob.
      Chemother., 1982, 10, 295.

199. M. Mitchard, J. Andrews, M.J. Kendall, and R. Wise, J.
      Antimicrob. Chemother., 1977, 3, (Suppl. B), 83.

200. K. Josefsson, T. Bergan, L. Magni, B.G. Pring, and D.
      Westerlund, Eur. J. Clin. Pharmacol., 1982, 23, 249.

201. K. Roholt, J. Antimicrob. Chemother., 1977, 3, (Suppl. B), 71.

202. J.G. Gambertoglio, S.L. Barriere, E.T. Lin, and J.E. Conte, Jr.,
      Antimicrob. Ag. Chemother., 1980, 18, 952.

203. M.M. Hares, A. Hegarty, J. Tomkyns, D.W. Burdon, and M.R.B.
      Keighley, J. Antimicrob. Chemother., 1982, 9, 217.

204. J. Andrews, M.J. Kendall, and M. Mitchard, Brit. J. Clin.
      Pharmacol., 1976, 3, 627.

205. G. Levy, J. Pharm. Sci., 1967, 56, 928.

206. A.P. Ball, A.K. Viswan, M. Mitchard, and R. Wise, J.
      Antimicrob. Chemother., 1978, 4, 241.

207.   R. Wise, A. Dyas, A. Hegarty, and J.M. Andrews, Antimicrob. Ag. Chemother., 1982, 22, 969.

208.   P. Patamasucon and G.H. McCracken, Jr., Antimicrob. Ag. Chemother., 1982, 21, 390.

209.   G.J. Miraglia, K.J. Renz, and H.H. Gadebusch, Antimicrob. Ag. Chemother., 1973, 3, 270.

210.   J.P. Phair, J. Carleton, and J.S. Tan, Antimicrob. Ag. Chemother., 1972, 2, 329.

211.   W.M.M. Kirby and C. Regamey, J. Infect. Dis., 1973, 128, Suppl., S341.

212.   T.M. Speight, R.N. Brogden, and G.S. Avery, Drugs, 1973, 3, 9.

213.   C.H. Nightingale, D.S. Greene, and R. Quintiliani, J. Pharm. Sci., 1975, 64, 1899.

214.   J.L. DeYoung, H.G.H. Tan, H.E. Huber, and M.A. Zoglio, J. Pharm. Sci., 1978, 67, 320.

215.   A. Tsuji, E. Nakashima, T. Asano, R. Nakashima, and T. Yamana, J. Pharm. Pharmacol., 1979, 31, 718.

216.   E.R. Finkelstein, R. Quintiliani, and C.H. Nightingale, J. Pediatr., 1978, 92, 902.

217.   M. Chow, R. Quintiliani, B.A. Cuncha, M. Thompson, E. Finkelstein, and C.H. Nightingale, J. Clin. Pharmacol., 1979, 19, 85.

218.   E. Finkelstein, R. Quintiliani, R. Lee, A. Bracci, and C.H. Nightingale, J. Pharm. Sci., 1978, 67, 1447.

219.   T.R. Tetzlaff, G.H. McCracken, and M.L. Thomas, J. Pediatr., 1978, 92, 292.

220.   S. Dean, L.K. Harding, R. Wise, and N. Wright, Eur. J. Clin. Pharmacol., 1976, 16, 73.

221.   C. Harvengt, P. DeSchepper, F. Lamy, and J. Hansen, J. Clin. Pharmacol., 1973, 13, 36.

222.   P.E. Gower, C.H. Dash, and C.H. O'Callaghan, J. Pharm. Pharmacol., 1973, 25, 376.

223.   P. Nicholas, B.R. Meyers, and S.Z. Hirschman, J. Clin. Pharmacol., 1973, 13, 463.

224.   R. Boothman, M.M. Kerr, M.J. Marshall, and W.L. Burland, Arch. Dis. Childhood, 1973, 48, 147.

225.   T.W. Mischler, A.A. Sugerman, D.A. Willard, L.J. Brannick, and E.S. Neiss, J. Clin. Pharmacol., 1974, 14, 604.

226.   S. Barrios, J.H. Sorensen, and R.G.W. Spickett, J. Pharm. Pharmacol., 1975, 27, 711.

227.   A. Kohonen, M. Paavolainen, and C.-V. Renkonen, Ann. Clin. Res., 1975, 7, 50.

228.   J.M. Symes, J.D. Jarvis, and G.C. Tresidder, Chemotherapy, 1974, 20, 257.

229. G.M. Halprin, and S.M. McMahon, Antimicrob. Ag. Chemother.,
      1973, 3, 703.

230. J. Duval, M. Mora, M. Chartier, and N. Mansour, La Nouvelle
      Presse Medicale, 1972, 1, 1419.

231. D.O. Kanyuck, J.S. Welles, J.L. Emmerson, and R.C. Anderson,
      Proc. Soc. Exp. Biol. Med., 1971, 136, 997.

232. D.S. Greene, D.R. Flanagan, R. Quintiliani, and C.H.
      Nightingale, J. Clin. Pharmacol., 1976, 16, 257.

233. J.G. Wagner, J. Pharmacokin. Biopharm., 1974, 2, 469.

234. C.H. O'Callaghan, J.P.R. Tootill, and W.D. Robinson, J. Pharm.
      Pharmacol., 1971, 23, 50.

235. J.A. Davies and J.M. Holt, J. Clin. Pathol., 1972, 25, 518.

236. J.E.L. Sales, M. Sutcliffe, and F. O'Grady, Brit. Med. J.,
      1972, iii, 441.

237. J.-M. Brogard, F. Kuntzmann, M. Dorner, P.L. Haegele, and J.
      Lavillaureix, Pathologie Biologie, 1971, 19, 1121.

238. B.R. Meyers, S.Z. Hirschmann, G. Wormser, G. Gartenberg, and E.
      Srulevitch, J. Clin. Pharmacol., 1978, 18, 174.

239. P.G. Welling, S. Dean, A. Selen, M.J. Kendall, and R. Wise,
      Int. J. Clin. Pharmacol. Biopharm., 1979, 17, 397.

240. G.H. McCracken, C.M. Ginsberg, J.C. Clahsen, and M.L. Thomas,
      J. Antimicrob. Chemother., 1978, 4, 515.

241. I. Weliky, H.H. Gadebusch, K. Kripalani, P. Arnow, and E.C.
      Schreiber, Antimicrob. Ag. Chemother., 1974, 5, 49.

242. T.W. Mischler, A.A. Sugerman, D.A. Willard, L.J. Brannick, and
      E.S. Neiss, J. Clin. Pharmacol., 1974, 14, 604.

243. E.S. Rattie, P.D. Bernardo, and L.J. Ravin, Antimicrob. Ag.
      Chemother., 1976, 10, 283.

244. R.A. Vukovich, L.J. Brannick, A.A. Sugerman, and E.S. Neiss,
      Clin. Pharmacol. Ther., 1975, 18, 215.

245. S.A. Sahn, J.T. Good, Jr., and L.B. Reller, J. Antimicrob.
      Chemother., 1981, 8, 345.

246. D.A. Taryle, J.T. Good, Jr., L.B. Reller, and S.A. Sahn,
      Antimicrob. Ag. Chemother., 1980, 6, 143.

247. B. Hoffstedt and M. Walder, Antimicrob. Ag. Chemother., 1981,
      20, 783.

248. M.W. Kunst and H. Mattie, J. Infect. Dis., 1978, 137, 830.

249. D.H. Roberts, M.J. Kendall, D.B. Jack, and P.G. Welling, Brit.
      J. Clin. Pharmacol., 1981, 11, 561.

250. F.L. Minn, A.A. Sugerman, and G.E. Bernfeld, J. Clin.
      Pharmacol., 1976, 16, 171.

251. A.E. Solomon, J.D. Briggs, R. McGeachy, and J.D. Sleigh, Brit.
      J. Clin. Pharmacol., 1975, 2, 443.

252. J.C. Rotschafer, K.B. Crossley, T.S. Lesar, D. Zaske, and K. Miller, Antimicrob. Ag. Chemother., 1982, 21, 170.

253. H. Lode, R. Stahlman, G. Dzwillo, and P. Koeppe, Arzneim.-Forsch., 1980, 30, 505.

254. J.P. Fillastre, A. Leroy, G. Humbert, and M. Godin, J. Antimicrob. Chemother., 1980, 6, 155.

255. P.G. Welling, S. Dean, A. Selen, M.J. Kendall, and R. Wise, Brit. J. Clin. Pharmacol., 1979, 8, 491.

256. G. Gartenberg, B.R. Meyers, S.Z. Hirschmann, and E. Srulevitch, J. Antimicrob. Chemother., 1977, 12, 730.

257. R. Bloch, J.J. Szwed, R.S. Sloan, and F.C. Luft, Antimicrob. Ag. Chemother., 1977, 12, 730.

258. J.-M. Brogard, M. Pinget, F. Comte, M. Adloff, and J. Lavillaureix, Chemotherapy, 1982, 28, 189.

259. E.L. Mariño, A. Dominguez-Gil, and C. Muriel, Int. J. Clin. Pharmacol. Ther. Toxicol., 1982, 20, 73.

260. E.L. Mariño and A. Dominguez-Gil, Eur. J. Clin. Pharmacol., 1980, 18, 505.

261. M. Prenna and S. Ripa, Chemotherapy, 1980, 26, 98.

262. E.L. Mariño and A. Dominguez-Gil, Int. J. Clin. Pharmacol. Ther. Toxicol., 1981, 19, 506.

263. C.M. Ginsburg, J. Antimicrob. Chemother., 1982, 10, 27.

264. A. Windorfer and P. Bauer, J. Antimicrob. Chemother., 1982, 10, 85.

265. B. Hampel, H. Lode, J. Wagner, and P. Koeppe, Antimicrob. Ag. Chemother., 1982, 22, 1061.

266. C. Simon, Arzneim.-Forsch., 1980, 30, 502.

267. A.M. Brisson and J.B. Fourtillan, J. Antimicrob. Chemother., 1982, 10, 11.

268. A. Leroy, G. Humbert, M. Godin, and J.P. Fillastre, J. Antimicrob. Chemother., 1982, 10, 39.

269. G. Humbert, A. Leroy, J.P. Fillastre, and M. Godin, Chemotherapy, 1979, 25, 189.

270. R.E. Cutler, A.D. Blair, and M.R. Kelly, Clin. Pharmacol. Ther., 1979, 25, 514.

271. T. Bergan, Chemotherapy, 1980, 26, 225.

272. A. Gerardin, J.B. Lecaillon, J.P. Schoeller, G. Humbert, and J. Guibert, J. Pharmacokin. Biopharm., 1982, 10, 15.

273. P. Actor, D.H. Pitkin, G. Lucyszyn, J.A. Weisbach, and J.L. Bran, Antimicrob. Ag. Chemother., 1976, 9, 800.

274. T. Bergan, Chemotherapy, 1977, 23, 389.

275. C. Harvengt, H. Meunier, and F. Lamy, J. Clin. Pharmacol., 1977, 17, 128.

276. M. Barza, S. Melethil, S. Berger, and E.C. Ernst, *Antimicrob. Ag. Chemother.*, 1976, 10, 421.

277. C. Regamey, R.C. Gordon, and W.M.M. Kirby, *Arch. Int. Med.*, 1974, 133, 407.

278. G.R. Hodges and S. Saslaw, *Amer. J. Med. Sci.*, 1973, 265, 23.

279. P. Nicholas, B.R. Meyers, and S.Z. Hirschman, *J. Clin. Pharmacol.*, 1973, 13, 325.

280. P. DeSchepper, C. Harvengt, C. Vranckx, B. Boon, and F. Lamy, *J. Clin. Pharmacol.*, 1973, 13, 83.

281. J.M. Brogard, M. Dorner, M. Pinget, M. Adloff, and J. Lavillaureix, *J. Infect. Dis.*, 1975, 131, 625.

282. M. Nishida, T. Murakawa, T. Matsubara, Y. Kohno, Y. Yolota, T. Yasutomi, and M. Okamoto, *Chemotherapy*, 1976, 22, 30.

283. K.R. Ratzan, C. Ruiz, and G.L. Irvin, *Antimicrob. Ag. Chemother.*, 1974, 6, 426.

284. M.D. Ram and S. Watanatittan, *Arch. Surgery*, 1974, 108, 187.

285. I. Polacek and H. Mühlbauer, *Biopharm. Drug Dispos.*, 1980, 1, 127.

286. R.C. Daly, R.H. Fitzgerald, Jr., and J.A. Washington, II, *Antimicrob. Ag. Chemother.*, 1982, 22, 461.

287. R.E. Polk, B.J. Kline, and S.M. Markowitz, *Antimicrob. Ag. Chemother.*, 1981, 20, 576.

288. N.G. Watermann, M.J. Raff, L. Scharfenberger, and P.A. Barnwell, *J. Infect. Dis.*, 1976, 113, 642.

289. C. Carbon, A. Contrepois, N. Brion, and S. Lamotte-Barrillon, *Antimicrob. Ag. Chemother.*, 1977, 11, 594.

290. H.P. Bassaris, R. Quintiliani, E.G. Maderazo, R.C. Tilton, and C.H. Nightingale, *Curr. Ther. Res.*, 1976, 19, 110.

291. L.B. Reller, W.W. Karney, H.N. Beaty, K.K. Holmes, and M. Turck, *Antimicrob. Ag. Chemother.*, 1973, 3, 488.

292. G. Wewalka and M. Endler, *Arzneim.-Forsch.*, 1978, 28, 72.

293. H. Yoshioka, K. Cho, M. Takimoto, S. Maruyama, and T. Shimizu, *J. Pediatr.*, 1979, 94, 151.

294. B. Bernard, L. Barton, M. Abate, and C.A. Ballard, *J. Infect. Dis.*, 1977, 136, 377.

295. J. Kozatoni, M. Okui, K. Noda, T. Ogino, and H. Noguchi, *Chem. Pharm. Bull. (Japan)*, 1972, 6, 135.

296. A.J. Khan, *Curr. Ther. Res.*, 1973, 15, 727.

297. K. Seiga, K. Yamaji, K. Miyoshi, and M. Minagawa, *Int. J. Clin. Pharmacol.*, 1972, 6, 135.

298. M.F. Rein, F.B. Westervelt, and M.A. Sande, *Antimicrob. Ag. Chemother.*, 1973, 4, 366.

299. M.E. Levison, S.P. Levison, K. Ries, and D. Kaye, J. Infect. Dis., 1973, 128, Suppl., S354.

300. A. Leroy, M.-A. Canonne, J.-P. Fillastre, and G. Humbert, Cur. Ther. Res., 1974, 16, 878.

301. T. Madhavan, K. Yaremchuk, N. Levin, E. Fisher, F. Cox, K. Burch, E. Haas, D. Pohland, and E.L. Quinn, Antimicrob. Ag. Chemother., 1975, 8, 63.

302. A.W. Czerwinski, J.A. Pederson, and J.P. Barry, J. Clin. Pharmacol., 1974, 14, 560.

303. W.A. Craig, P.G. Welling, T.C. Jackson, and C.M. Kunin, J. Infect. Dis., 1973, 128, (Suppl.), S347.

304. R.V. McCloskey, M.F. Forland, M.J. Sweeney, and D.N. Lawrence, J. Infect. Dis.,]973, 128, (Suppl.), S358.

305. C.P. Craig and S.I. Rifkin, Clin. Pharmacol. Ther., 1976, 19, 825.

306. T. Bergan, A. Digranes, and A. Schreiner, Chemotherapy, 1978, 24, 277.

307. H. Otaya and Y. Hayashi, Int. J. Clin. Pharmacol., 1974, 10, 117.

308. C.W. Norden and E. Kennedy, J. Infect. Dis., 1971, 124, 565.

309. G.L. Boyle, R. Abel, G.W. Lazachek, and I.H. Leopold, Amer. J. Ophthalmol., 1972, 74, 868.

310. D. Höffler, P. Koeppe, E. Fuchs, and P. Fiegel, Int. J. Clin. Pharmacol., 1972, 5, 450.

311. K.W. Miller, K.K.H. Chan, H.G. McCoy, R.P. Fischer, W.G. Lindsay, and D.E. Zaske, Clin. Pharmacol. Ther., 1979, 26, 54.

312. T.F. Rolewicz, B.L. Mirkin, M.J. Cooper, and M.W. Anders, Clin. Pharmacol. Ther., 1977, 22, 928.

313. M.J. Cooper, M.W. Anders, and B.L. Mirkin, Drug Metab. Dispos., 1973, 1, 659.

314. R.M. Kluge, F.M. Calia, J.S. McLaughlin, and R.B. Hornick, Antimicrob. Ag. Chemother., 1973, 4, 270.

315. J.B. Hook and H.E. Williamson, J. Pharmacol. Exp. Ther., 1965, 149, 404.

316. J.M. Leheri and L.G. Wesson, Amer. J. Physiol., 1964, 206, 1379.

317. A.D. Tice, M. Barza, M.G. Bergeron, J.L. Brusch, and L. Weinstein, Antimicrob. Ag. Chemother., 1975, 7, 168.

318. L.D. Bechtol, Curr. Ther. Res., 1972, 14, 790.

319. H.P. Erhlich, V. Licko, and T.K. Hunt, Amer. J. Med. Sci., 1973, 265, 33.

320. B.E. Cabana, D.R. Van Harken, and G.H. Hottendorf, Antimicrob. Ag. Chemother., 1976, 10, 307.

321. J. Axelrod, B.R. Meyers, and S.Z. Hirschman, J. Clin. Pharmacol., 1972, 12, 84.

322. A. Arvidsson, O. Borgå, and G. Alván, <u>Clin. Pharmacol. Ther.</u>, 1979, <u>25</u>, 870.

323. T. Bergan, O. Ørjavik, and E.K. Brodwall, <u>Arzneim.-Forsch.</u>, 1981, <u>31</u>, 1773.

324. J.J. Schrogie, R.O. Davies, K.C. Yeh, D. Rogers, G.I. Holmes, H. Skeggs, and C.M. Martin, <u>J. Antimicrob. Chemother.</u>, 1978, <u>4</u> (Suppl. B), 69.

325. J.J. Schrogie, J.D. Rogers, K.C. Yeh, R.O. Davies, G.I. Holmes, H. Skeggs, and C.M. Martin, <u>Rev. Infect. Dis.</u>, 1979, <u>1</u>, 90.

326. P.F. Sonneville, K.S. Albert, H. Skeggs, H. Gentner, K.C. Kwan, and C.W. Martin, <u>Eur. J. Clin. Pharmacol.</u>, 1977, <u>12</u>, 273.

327. A.K. Miller, E. Celozzi, Y. Kong, B.A. Pelak, D. Hendlin, and E.O. Stapley, <u>Antimicrob. Ag. Chemother.</u>, 1974, <u>5</u>, 33.

328. A.P. Gillet and R. Wise, <u>Lancet</u>, 1978, <u>i</u>, 962.

329. Z. Landau, E. Rubinstein, and H. Halkin, <u>J. Antimicrob. Chemother.</u>, 1980, <u>6</u>, 657.

330. V. Herlitz, H. Langmaack, M. Metzger, and F.D. Daschner, <u>J. Antimicrob. Chemother.</u>, 1980, <u>6</u>, 717.

331. R. Wise, I.A. Donovan, N.S. Ambrose, and J.E. Allcock, <u>J. Antimicrob. Chemother.</u>, 1981, <u>8</u>, 453.

332. M.J. Garcia, A. Dominguez-Gil, F.D. Perez, F.P. Rodriguez, and F.D. Moronta, <u>Eur. J. Clin. Pharmacol.</u>, 1981, <u>20</u>, 371.

333. C.H. Nightingale, N. Olson, and R. Quintiliani, <u>Curr. Ther. Res.</u>, 1981, <u>29</u>, 444.

334. R. Massip, M.D. Kitzis, V.T. Tran, M.J. Armengaud, and M. Armengaud, <u>Rev. Infect. Dis.</u>, 1979, <u>1</u>, 132.

335. S. Ramachandran Nair, C.E. Cherubin, and M. Weinstein, <u>Rev. Infect. Dis.</u>, 1979, <u>1</u>, 134.

336. P.A.A. Galvao, A.V. Lomar, W. Francisco, C.V.F. deGodoy, and R. Norrby, <u>Antimicrob. Ag. Chemother.</u>, 1980, <u>17</u>, 526.

337. W.E. Feldman, S. Moffitt, and N.S. Manning, <u>Antimicrob. Ag. Chemother.</u>, 1982, <u>21</u>, 468.

338. G. Humbert, A. Leroy, J.-P. Rogez, and C. Cherubin, <u>Antimicrob. Ag. Chemother.</u>, 1980, <u>17</u>, 675.

339. D.L. Hemsell, I. Birkett, L. Reveley, and J.A. Bland, <u>Obstet. Gynecol.</u>, 1982, <u>59</u>, 149.

340. J.F. Hansbrough and J.E. Clark, <u>Antimicrob. Ag. Chemother.</u>, 1982, <u>22</u>, 709.

341. M. Dubois, D. Delapierre, L. Chanteux, J. Demonty, R. Lambotte, R. Kramp, and A. Dresse, <u>J. Clin. Pharmacol.</u>, 1981, <u>21</u>, 477.

342. W. Brumfitt, J. Kosmidis, J.M.T. Hamilton-Miller, and J.N.G. Gilchrist, <u>Antimicrob. Ag. Chemother.</u>, 1974, <u>6</u>, 290.

343. P.F. Sonneville, R.R. Kartodirdjo, H. Skeggs, A.E. Till, and C.M. Martin, <u>Eur. J. Clin. Pharmacol.</u>, 1976, <u>9</u>, 397.

344. D.P. Thornhill and D.S. Reeves, J. Antimicrob. Chemother., 1981, 8, 421.

345. P.H. Vlasses, A.M. Holbrook, J.J. Schrogie, J.D. Rogers, R.K. Ferguson, and W.B. Abrams, Antimicrob. Ag. Chemother., 1980, 17, 847.

346. W.E. Feldman, S. Moffitt, and N. Sprow, Antimicrob. Ag. Chemother., 1980, 17, 669.

347. M.J. Garcia, A. Garcia, M.J. Nieto, A. Dominguez-Gil, G. Alonso, and L. Mellado, Int. J. Clin. Pharmacol. Ther. Toxicol., 1980, 18, 503.

348. W.L. Greaves, J.H. Kreeft, R.L. Ogilvie, and G.K. Richards, Antimicrob. Ag. Chemother., 1981, 19, 253.

349. D. Kampf, R. Schurig, I. Korsukewitz, and O. Bruckner, Antimicrob. Ag. Chemother., 1981, 20, 741.

350. J.P. Fillastre, A. Leroy, M. Godin, G. Oksenhendler, and G. Humbert, J. Antimicrob. Chemother., 1978, 4 (Suppl. B), 79.

351. M.J. Garcia, A. Dominguez-Gil, J.M. Tabernero, and J.A. Sanchez Tomero, Eur. J. Clin. Pharmacol., 1979, 16, 119.

352. G. Humbert, J.P. Fillastre, A. Leroy, M. Godin, and C. Van Winzum, Rev. Infect. Dis., 1979, 1, 118.

353. M.J. Garcia, A.A. Dominguez-Gil, M. Cepeda, and A. Dominguez-Gil, Biopharm. Drug Dispos., 1981, 2, 205.

354. H.C. Neu, J. Infect. Dis., 1978, 137, S80.

355. N.S. Aziz, J.G. Gambertoglio, E.T. Lin, H. Grausz, and L.Z. Benet, J. Pharmacokin. Biopharm., 1978, 6, 153.

356. H.N. Beaty and E. Walters, Antimicrob. Ag. Chemother., 1979, 16, 584.

357. F. Daschner, E. Blume, H. Langmaack, and W. Wolfart, J. Antimicrob. Chemother., 1979, 5, 474.

358. J.G.N. Studley, J.J. Schentag, and W.G. Schenk, Jr., Antimicrob. Ag. Chemother., 1982, 22, 262.

359. B.R. Meyers and S.Z. Hirschman, Antimicrob. Ag. Chemother., 1977, 11, 248.

360. J.M. Brogard, J. Koferschmitt, M.L. Spach, O. Grudet, and J. Lavillaureix, J. Clin. Pharmacol., 1979, 19, 366.

361. J.G. Gambertoglio, N.S. Aziz, E.T. Lin, H. Grausz, J.L. Naughton, and L.Z. Benet, Clin. Pharmacol. Ther., 1979, 26, 592.

362. G.B. Appel, H.C. Neu, M.F. Parry, M.J. Goldberger, and G.B. Jacob, Antimicrob. Ag. Chemother., 1976, 10, 623.

363. J.A. Campillo, J.M. Lanao, A. Dominguez-Gil, J.M. Tabernero, and F. Rubio, Int. J. Clin. Pharmacol. Biopharm., 1979, 17, 416.

364. G. LaGreca, S. Biasioli, S. Chiaramonte, A. Fabris, M. Feriani, E. Pisani, C. Ronco, and L. Xerri, Int. J. Clin. Pharmacol. Ther. Toxicol., 1982, 20, 92.

365. A. Lechi, E. Arosio, L. Xerri, C. Mengoli, G. Montesi, and O. Ghidini, Int. J. Clin. Pharmacol. Ther. Toxicol., 1982, 20, 493.

366. B. Hoffstedt, B. Ode, M. Walder, A. Hanson, P. Christensson, and S. Cronberg, J. Antimicrob. Chemother., 1980, 6, 153.

367. D.A. Leigh, J. Marriner, D. Nisbet, H.D.W. Powell, J.C.T. Church, and K. Wise, J. Antimicrob. Chemother., 1982, 9, 303.

368. H. Friedrich, G. Haensel-Friedrich, H. Langmaak, and F.-D. Daschner, Chemotherapy, 1980, 26, 91.

369. M. de los A. del Rio, D.F. Chrane, S. Shelton, G.H. McCracken, Jr., and J.D. Nelson, Antimicrob. Ag. Chemother., 1982, 22, 990.

370. S.M. Harding, L.A. Eilin, and A.M. Harris, J. Antimicrob. Chemother., 1979, 5, 87.

371. C.W.H. Havard, A. Fernando, B. Bannister, W. Brumfitt, and J.M. T. Hamilton-Miller, J. Antimicrob. Chemother., 1981, 8, 401.

372. J. Broekhuysen, F. Deger, J. Douchamps, E. Freschi, N. Mal, P. Neve, R. Parfait, G. Siska, and M. Winand, Brit. J. Clin. Pharmacol., 1981, 12, 801.

373. J.G. Douglas, R.P. Bax, and J.F. Munro, J. Antimicrob. Chemother., 1980, 6, 543.

374. R.D. Foord, Antimicrob. Ag. Chemother., 1976, 9, 741.

375. R. Norrby, R.D. Foord, and P. Hedlund, J. Antimicrob. Chemother., 1977, 3, 355.

376. P.E. Gower and C.H. Dash, Eur. J. Clin. Pharmacol., 1977, 12, 221.

377. R.W. Bundtzen, R.D. Toothaker, O.S. Nielson, P.O. Madsen, P.G. Welling, and W.A. Craig, Antimicrob. Ag. Chemother., 1981, 19, 443.

378. K.P. Fu, P. Aswapokee, I. Ho, C. Matthijssen, and H.C. Neu, Antimicrob. Ag. Chemother., 1979, 16, 592.

379. R.F. Frongillo, L. Galuppo, and A. Moretti, Antimicrob. Ag. Chemother., 1981, 19, 22.

380. A. Karimi, K. Seeger, D. Stolke, and H. Knothe, J. Antimicrob. Chemother., 1980, 6, 119.

381. D.A. Kafetzis, C.V. Lazarides, C.A. Siafas, P.A. Georgakopoulos, and C.J. Papadatos, J. Antimicrob. Chemother., 1980, 6, 135.

382. M. Grabe, K.-E. Andersson, A. Forsgren, and S. Hellsten, Infection, 1981, 9, 154.

383. F. Esmieu, J. Guibert, H.C. Rosenkilde, I. Ho, and A. LeGo, J. Antimicrob. Chemother., 1980, 6, 83.

384. R. Wise, S. Baker, and R. Livingston, Antimicrob. Ag. Chemother., 1980, 18, 369.

385. H.C. Neu, P. Aswapokee, K.P. Fu, I. Ho, C. Matthijssen, Clin. Pharmacol. Ther., 1980, 27, 677.

386. R. Luthy, J. Blaser, A. Bonetti, H. Simmen, R. Wise, and W. Siegenthaler, Antimicrob. Ag. Chemother., 1981, 20, 567.

387. H.M. von Hattingberg, W. Marget, B.H. Belohradsky, and R. Roos, J. Antimicrob. Chemother., 1980, 6, 113.

388. G.H. McCracken, Jr., N.E. Threlkeld, and M.L. Thomas, Antimicrob. Ag. Chemother., 1982, 21, 683.

389. D.A. Kafetzis, D.C. Brater, J. Kanarios, C.A. Sinaniotis, and C.J. Papadatos, Antimicrob. Ag. Chemother., 1981, 20, 487.

390. Y. Usuda, O. Sekine, N. Aoki, T. Shimizu, Y. Hirasawa, T. Aoki, and K. Fujimoto, Drugs Exptl. Clin. Res., 1981, 7, 249.

391. T. Bergan, E.W. Larsen, and E.K. Brodwall, Chemotherapy, 1982, 28, 35.

392. R. Wise, N. Wright, and P.J. Wills, Antimicrob. Ag. Chemother., 1981, 19, 526.

393. J.P. Fillastre, A. Leroy, G. Humbert, and M. Godin, J. Antimicrob. Chemother., 1980, 6, 103.

394. K. Dvořáček, Z. Modr, O. Schmidt, and A. Nécásková, Arzneim.-Forsch., 1974, 24, 1468.

395. Y. Nakai, Y. Kanai, T. Fugono, and S. Tanayama, J. Antibiotics, 1976, 29, 81.

396. K.G. Naber and P.O. Madsen, Antimicrob. Ag. Chemother., 1973, 3, 81.

397. A.R. Nissenson, N.W. Levin, and R.H. Parker, Clin. Pharmacol. Ther., 1972, 13, 887.

398. F. Reutter and N.P. Maurice, Arzneim.-Forsch., 1974, 24, 1466.

399. A. Dominguez-Gil, M.C. Castineiras, J.M. Tabernero, J.L. Rodriguez Commes, and D. deCastro, Eur. J. Clin. Pharmacol., 1978, 13, 445.

400. A. Dominguez-Gil, J.M. Lanoa, J.M. Tabernero, J.L. Rodriguez Commes, and S. deCastro, Eur. J. Clin. Pharmacol., 1979, 16, 49.

401. V.T. Androile, J. Infect. Dis., 1978, 137, S88.

402. J.M. Brogard, M. Dorner, C. Brandt, and J. Lavillaureix, Int. J. Clin. Pharmacol., 1976, 13, 168.

403. J.-M. Brogard, H. Ruscher, J. Frankhauser, F. Kuntzmann, and J. Lavillaureix, Pathologie Biologie, 1973, 21, 671.

404. J.M. Brogard, P. Haegele, M. Dorner, and J. Lavillaureix, Antimicrob. Ag. Chemother., 1973, 3, 19.

405. M. Pfeffer, R.C. Gaver, and D.R. Van Harken, J. Pharm. Sci., 1980, 69, 398.

406. E.H. Estey, S.S. Weaver, B.M. LeBlanc, N. Brown, D.H. Ho, and G.P. Bodey, Clin. Pharmacol. Ther., 1981, 30, 398.

407. J.F. Jovanovich, L.D. Saravolatz, K. Burch, and D.J. Pohlod, Antimicrob. Ag. Chemother., 1981, 20, 530.

408. S.S. Hawkins, R.H. Alford, W.J. Stone, R.D. Smyth, and M. Pfeffer, Clin. Pharmacol. Ther., 1981, 30, 468.

409. F.H. Lee, R.D. Smyth, and D.R. van Harken, <u>Antimicrob. Ag.</u> <u>Chemother.</u>, 1981, <u>19</u>, 625.

410. F.H. Lee, M. Pfeffer, D.R. van Harken, R.D. Smyth, and G.H. Hottendorf, <u>Antimicrob. Ag. Chemother.</u>, 1980, <u>17</u>, 188.

411. Y. Harada, S. Matsubara, M. Kakimoto, T. Noto, T. Tehashi, N. Kimura, S. Suzuki, H. Ogawa, and K. Koyama, <u>J. Antibiotics</u>, 1976, <u>29</u>, 1071.

412. K.S. Israel, H.R. Black, G.L. Brier, J.D. Wolny, and K.A. DeSante, <u>Antimicrob. Ag. Chemother.</u>, 1982, <u>22</u>, 94.

413. R. Latif, M.C. Thirumoorthi, J.A. Buckley, D.M. Kobos, M.K. Aravind, R.E. Kauffman, and A.S. Dajani, <u>Dev. Pharmacol. Ther.</u>, 1981, <u>3</u>, 222.

414. K.A. DeSante, K.S. Israel, G.L. Brier, J.D. Wolny, and B.L. Hatcher, <u>Antimicrob. Ag. Chemother.</u>, 1982, <u>21</u>, 58.

415. S. Srinivasan, K.P. Fu, and H.C. Neu, <u>Antimicrob. Ag.</u> <u>Chemother.</u>, 1981, <u>19</u>, 302.

416. W.M. Scheld, D.A. Spyker, G.R. Donowitz, W.K. Bolton, and M.A. Sande, <u>Antimicrob. Ag. Chemother.</u>, 1981, <u>19</u>, 613.

417. O.V. Matinez, J.U. Levi, A. Livingstone, T.I. Malinin, R. Zeppa, D. Hutson, and N. Einhorn, <u>Antimicrob. Ag. Chemother.</u>, 1981, <u>20</u>, 231.

418. M.F. Romagnoli, K. Flynn, G.R. Siber, and D.A. Goldmann, <u>Antimicrob. Ag. Chemother.</u>, 1982, <u>22</u>, 47.

419. R.E. Polk, J.E. Smith, K. Ducey, and R.R. Lower, <u>Antimicrob.</u> <u>Ag. Chemother.</u>, 1982, <u>22</u>, 201.

420. U.B. Schaad, G.H. McCracken, Jr., C.A. Loock, and M.L. Thomas, <u>J. Infect. Dis.</u>, 1981, <u>143</u>, 156.

421. J. Modai, M. Wolff, J. Lebas, A. Meulemans, and C. Manuel, <u>Antimicrob. Ag. Chemother.</u>, 1982, <u>21</u>, 551.

422. W.K. Bolton, W.M. Scheld, D.A. Spyker, T.L. Overby, and M.A. Sande, <u>Antimicrob. Ag. Chemother.</u>, 1980, <u>18</u>, 933.

423. P. Garzone, J. Lyon, V.L. Yu, J. Zuravleff, W. Diven, and W. Pasculle, <u>Clin. Pharmacol. Ther.</u>, 1981, <u>30</u>, 86.

424. A. Leroy, G. Humbert, and J.P. Fillastre, <u>Antimicrob. Ag.</u> <u>Chemother.</u>, 1981, <u>19</u>, 965.

425. G.R. Aronoff, R.S. Sloan, and F.C. Luft, <u>J. Infect. Dis.</u>, 1982, <u>145</u>, 365.

426. G.R. Aronoff, R.S. Sloan, S.A. Mong, F.C. Luft, and S.A. Kleit, <u>Antimicrob. Ag. Chemother.</u>, 1981, <u>19</u>, 575.

427. E.J. Jacobson, J.J. Zahrowski, and A.R. Nissenson, <u>Clin.</u> <u>Pharmacol. Ther.</u>, 1981, <u>30</u>, 487.

428. M. Lam, C.V. Manion, and A.W. Czerwinski, <u>Antimicrob. Ag.</u> <u>Chemother.</u>, 1981, <u>19</u>, 461.

429. N. Wright, P.J. Wills, and R. Wise, <u>J. Antimicrob. Chemother.</u>, 1981, <u>8</u>, 395.

430. M. Ohkawa, M. Orito, T. Sugata, M. Shimamura, M. Sawaki, E. Nakashita, K. Kuroda, and K. Sasahara, Antimicrob. Ag. Chemother., 1980, 18, 386.

431. J.R. Perfect and D.T. Durack, J. Antimicrob. Chemother., 1981, 8, 49.

432. S. Srinivasan, E.L. Francke, and H.C. Neu, Antimicrob. Ag. Chemother., 1981, 19, 298.

433. W.K. Bolton, W.M. Scheld, D.A. Spyker, and M.A. Sande, Antimicrob. Ag. Chemother., 1981, 19, 821.

434. O. Sekine, Y. Usuda, T. Shimizu, N. Aoki, Y. Hirasawa, and T. Aoki, Drugs Exptl. Clin. Res., 1981, 7, 209.

435. T. Nakamura, I. Hashimoto, Y. Sawada, J. Mikami, E. Bekki, S. Hirasawa, H. Abe, and Y. Watanabe, Antimicrob. Ag. Chemother., 1980, 18, 980.

436. A.W. Maksymiuk, B.M. LeBlanc, N.S. Brown, D.-H. Ho, and G.P. Bodey, Antimicrob. Ag. Chemother., 1981, 19, 1037.

437. D. Adam, R.R. Wittke, and F. Eisenberger, Drugs Exptl. Clin. Res., 1981, 7, 227.

438. H. Giamarellou, A. Koumaditis, K. Dispiraki, H. Xefteri, and G.K. Daikos, Drugs Exptl. Clin. Res., 1981, 7, 219.

439. P. Federspil, E. Tiesler, and N. Weides, Int. J. Clin. Pharm. Res., 1982, 2, 247.

440. T.P. Gibson, G.R. Granneman, J.E. Kallal, and L.T. Sennello, Clin. Pharmacol. Ther., 1982, 31, 602.

441. H. Giamarellou, A. Koumaditis, and G.K. Daikos, Drugs Exptl. Clin. Res., 1981, 7, 425.

442. P.J. McNamara, K. Stoeckel, and W.H. Ziegler, Eur. J. Clin. Pharmacol., 1982, 22, 71.

443. K. Stoeckel, P.J. McNamara, R. Brandt, H. Plozza-Nottebrock, and W.H. Ziegler, Clin. Pharmacol. Ther., 1981, 29, 650.

444. I.H. Patel, S. Chen, M. Parsonnet, M.R. Hackman, M.A. Brooks, J. Konikoff, and S.A. Kaplan, Antimicrob. Ag. Chemother., 1981, 20, 634.

445. A.A. Pollock, P.E. Tee, I.H. Patel, J. Spicehandler, M.S. Simberkoff, and J.J. Rahal, Jr., Antimicrob. Ag. Chemother., 1982, 22, 816.

446. M. Del Rio, G.H. McCracken, Jr., J.D. Nelson, D. Chrane, and S. Shelton, Antimicrob. Ag. Chemother., 1982, 22, 622.

447. T.B. Tjandramaga, A. Van Hecken, A. Mullie, R. Verbesselt, P.J. De Schepper, and L. Verbist, Antimicrob. Ag. Chemother., 1982, 22, 237.

448. D.N. Gerding, L.L. Van Etta, and L.R. Peterson, Antimicrob. Ag. Chemother., 1982, 22, 844.

449. T. Murakawa, H. Sakamoto, S. Fukada, S. Nakamoto, T. Hirose, N. Itoh, and M. Nishida, Antimicrob. Ag. Chemother., 1980, 17, 157.

450. N. Nakashima, K. Suzuki, H. Hashimoto, and K. Nishijima, J. Clin. Pharmacol., 1981, 21, 388.

451. L.R. Peterson, D.N. Gerding, L.L. Van Etta, J.H. Eckfeldt, and T.A. Larson, Antimicrob. Ag. Chemother., 1982, 22, 878.

452. J. Dubb, P. Actor, D. Pitkin, F. Alexander, R. Familiar, S. Ehrlich, and R. Stote, Clin. Pharmacol. Ther., 1982, 31, 516.

453. M. Ohkawa, A. Okasho, T. Sugata, and K. Kuroda, Antimicrob. Ag. Chemother., 1982, 22, 308.

454. M. Ohkawa and K. Kuroda, Chemotherapy, 1980, 26, 242.

455. S.L. Barriere, G.J. Hatheway, J.G. Gambertoglio, E.T. Lin, and J.E. Conte, Jr., Antimicrob. Ag. Chemother., 1982, 21, 935.

456. F.D. Daschner, K.A. Hemmer, P. Offermann, and J. Slanicka, Antimicrob. Ag. Chemother., 1982, 22, 958.

457. G.R. Granneman, L.T. Sennello, F.J. Steinberg, and R.C. Sonders, Antimicrob. Ag. Chemother., 1982, 21, 141.

458. M. Garty and A. Hurwitz, Clin. Pharmacol. Ther., 1980, 28, 203.

459. C.M. Davis, J.V. Candersarl, and E.W. Kraus, Amer. J. Med. Sci., 1973, 265, 69.

460. W.H. Barr, L.M. Gerbracht, K. Letcher, M. Plaut, and N. Strahl, Clin. Pharmacol. Ther., 1972, 13, 97.

461. M.C. Meyer, R.E. Dann, P.L. Whyatt, and G.W.A. Slywka, J. Pharmacokin. Biopharm., 1974, 2, 287.

462. A. Hart, H.E. Barber, and T.N. Calvey, Brit. J. Clin. Pharmacol., 1975, 2, 277.

463. K.-E. Andersson, L. Bratt, H. Dencker, C. Kamme, and E. Lanner, Eur. J. Clin. Pharmacol., 1976, 10, 59.

464. P.G. Welling, P.A. Koch, C.C. Lau, and W.A. Craig, Antimicrob. Ag. Chemother., 1977, 11, 462.

465. J. Adir and W.H. Barr, J. Pharm. Sci., 1977, 66, 1000.

466. K.S. Albert, R.D. Welch, K.A. DeSante, and A.R. DiSanto, J. Pharm. Sci., 1979, 68, 586.

467. J. Adir and W.H. Barr, J. Pharmacokin. Biopharm., 1978, 6, 99.

468. P.G. Welling, J. Pharmacokin. Biopharm., 1977, 5, 291.

469. P.J. Neuvonen and H. Turakka, Eur. J. Clin. Pharmacol., 1974, 7, 357.

470. H. Brise and L. Halberg, Acta Med. Scand., 1962, 171, 23.

471. T.-F. Chin and J.L. Lach, Amer. J. Hosp. Pharm., 1975, 32, 625.

472. M. Garty and A. Hurwitz, Clin. Pharmacol. Ther., 1980, 28, 203.

473. P. Fisher, F. House, P. Inns, P.J. Morrison, H.J. Rogers, and I.D. Bradbrook, Brit. J. Clin. Pharmacol., 1980, 9, 153.

474. P. Ylitalo, H. Hinkka, and P.J. Neuvonen, Eur. J. Clin. Pharmacol., 1977, 12, 367.

475. P.A. Kramer, D.J. Chapron, J. Benson, and S.A. Mercik, <u>Clin. Pharmacol. Ther.</u>, 1978, <u>23</u>, 467.

476. H.R. Ochs, D.J. Greenblatt, and H.J. Dengler, <u>J. Pharmacokin. Biopharm.</u>, 1978, <u>6</u>, 295.

477. I.D. Bradbrook, P.J. Morrison, and H.J. Rogers, <u>Brit. J. Clin. Pharmacol.</u>, 1978, <u>6</u>, 552.

478. L. Olanoff and J.M. Anderson, <u>J. Pharm. Sci.</u>, 1979, <u>68</u>, 1151.

479. S. Banerjee and K. Chakrabarti, <u>J. Pharm. Pharmacol.</u>, 1976, <u>28</u>, 133.

480. M.P. Braybooks, B.W. Barry, and E.T. Abbs, <u>J. Pharm. Pharmacol.</u>, 1975, <u>27</u>, 508.

481. J. Adir, <u>J. Pharm. Sci.</u>, 1975, <u>64</u>, 1847.

482. S. Aukee, V.M.K. Venho, J. Jussila, and P. Karjalainen, <u>Ann. Clin. Res.</u>, 1975, <u>7</u>, 42.

483. M.L. Kornguth and C.M. Kunin, <u>J. Infect. Dis.</u>, 1976, <u>133</u>, 175.

484. M.L. Kornguth and C.M. Kunin, <u>J. Infect. Dis.</u>, 1976, <u>133</u>, 185.

485. R.G. Greene, J.R. Brown, R.T. Calvert, <u>J. Pharm. Pharmacol.</u>, 1976, <u>28</u>, 514.

486. M.J. Raff, J.T. Summersgill, F.J. Fontana, P.A. Barnwell, N.G. Waterman, and L. Scharjenberger, <u>J. Antibiotics</u>, 1977, <u>30</u>, 593.

487. R.W. Ruhen and M.K. Tandon, <u>Med. J. Austral.</u>, 1976, <u>1</u>, 151.

488. G. Coppi, L. Monti, and R. Genova, <u>Chemotherapy</u>, 1971, <u>16</u>, 345.

489. G. Ziv, E. Bogin, J. Shani, and F.G. Sulman, <u>Antimicrob. Ag. Chemother.</u>, 1973, <u>3</u>, 607.

490. K. Fukaya, <u>Jap. J. Exp. Med.</u>, 1972, <u>42</u>, 435.

491. L.S. Olanoff and J.M. Anderson, <u>J. Pharmacokin. Biopharm.</u>, 1980, <u>8</u>, 599.

492. J.M. Jaffe, J.L. Colaizzi, R.I. Poust, and R.H. McDonald, <u>J. Pharmacokin. Biopharm.</u>, 1973, <u>1</u>, 267.

493. R. Böcker, and C.-J. Estler, <u>Arzneim.-Forsch.</u>, 1981, <u>31</u>, 2116.

494. E.J. Antal, J.M. Jaffe, R.I. Poust, and J.L. Colaizzi, <u>J. Pharm. Sci.</u>, 1975, <u>64</u>, 2015.

495. C.D. Ericsson, S. Feldman, L.K. Pickering, and T.G. Cleary, <u>J. Amer. Med. Assoc.</u>, 1982, <u>247</u>, 2266.

496. B.J. Leibowitz, J.L. Hakes, M.M. Cahn, and E.J. Levy, <u>Curr. Ther. Res.</u>, 1972, <u>14</u>, 820.

497. J. Klastersky, R. Cappel, B. Rens, and D. Daneau, <u>Curr. Ther. Res.</u>, 1972, <u>14</u>, 49.

498. P. Blanchard, M. Rudhardt, and J. Fabre, <u>Chemotherapy</u>, 1975, <u>21</u>, 8.

499. J. Gartmann, <u>Chemotherapy</u>, 1975, <u>21</u>, 19.

500. C.M. Eneroth, C. Lundberg, and B. Wretlind, Chemotherapy, 1975, 21, 1.

501. R.W. Ruhen and M.K. Landon, Pathology, 1975, 7, 193.

502. R.G. Kelly and L.A. Kanegis, Toxicol. Appl. Pharmacol., 1967, 11, 1971.

503. P.D. Hoeprich and D.M. Warshauer, Antimicrob. Ag. Chemother., 1974, 5, 330.

504. C.G.C. MacArthur, A.J. Johnson, M.V. Chadwick, and H.J. Wingfield, J. Antimicrob. Chemother., 1978, 4, 509.

505. K.-E. Andersson, H. Dencker, P.-A. Mardh, and M. Akerlund, Chemotherapy, 1976, 22, 277.

506. P. Lee, E.R. Crutch, and R.B.I. Morrison, NZ Med. J., 1972, 75, 355.

507. A. Whelton, M. Schach von Wittenau, T.M. Twomey, W. Walker, and J.R. Bianchine, Kidney Internat., 1974, 5, 365.

508. N.K. Ao, O.P. Taneja, V.N. Bhatia, and D.S. Aggarwal, Chemotherapy, 1974, 20, 129.

509. A. Kasanen, T. Raines, H. Sundqvist, and R. Tikkanen, Curr. Ther. Res., 1974, 16, 243.

510. M. Schach von Wittenau and T.M. Twomey, Chemotherapy, 1971, 16, 217.

511. A. Welton, M. Schach von Wittenau, T.M. Twomey, W.G. Walker, and J.R. Bianchine, 'Doxycycline, A Compendium of Clinical Evaluations', Pfizer, New York, 1973, pp 53-60.

512. W.A. Mahon, G.E. Johnson, M.F. Kelly, and S.S.A. Fenton, Rev. Canad. Biol., 1973, 32, Suppl., 107.

513. M. Schach von Wittenau, T.M. Twomey, and A. Swindell, Chemotherapy, 1972, 17, 26.

514. P.J. Neuvonen and O. Penttila, Eur. J. Clin. Pharmacol., 1974, 17, 361.

515. W.M.K. Venho, R.O. Salonen, and M.J. Matilla, Eur. J. Clin. Pharmacol., 1978, 14, 277.

516. J.F. Mahoney and D. Lloyd-Jones, Med. J. Austral., 1975, 2, 673.

517. J.M. Jaffe, R.I. Poust, S.L. Feld, and J.L. Colaizzi, J. Pharm. Sci., 1974, 63, 1256.

518. T. Bergan, B. Øydvin, and L. Lunde, Acta Pharmacol. Toxicol., 1973, 33, 138.

519. E.G. Lovering, I.J. McGilveray, I. McMillan, W. Tostowaryk, T. Matula, and G. Marier, Canad. J. Pharm. Sci., 1975, 10, 36.

520. H.E. Barber, T.N. Calvey, K. Muir, and A. Hart, Brit. J. Clin. Pharmacol., 1974, 1, 405.

521. K. Butler, Rev. Canad. Biol., 1973, 32, Suppl., 53.

522. R.H. Teske, L.D. Rollins, R.J. Condon, and G.G. Carter, J. Amer. Vet. Med. Assoc., 1973, 162, 119.

523. J. Offermeier, R. Miller, and H.D. Brandt, <u>S. African Med. J.</u>, 1972, <u>46</u>, 1509.

524. H. MacDonald, R.G. Kelly, E.S. Allen, J.F. Noble, and L.A. Kanegis, <u>Clin. Pharmacol. Ther.</u>, 1973, <u>14</u>, 852.

525. P.G. Welling, W.R. Shaw, S.J. Uman, F.L.S. Tse, and W.A. Craig, <u>Antimicrob. Ag. Chemother.</u>, 1975, <u>8</u>, 532.

526. D. Heaney and G. Eknoyan, <u>Clin. Pharmacol. Ther.</u>, 1978, <u>24</u>, 233.

527. J.J. Timmes, N.J. Demos, and S.I. Chong, <u>Clin. Pharmacol. Ther.</u>, 1971, <u>12</u>, 920.

528. Symposium on Gentamicin held at the Royal Society of Medicine, March 22, 1974, <u>Postgrad. Med. J.</u>, 1974, <u>50</u>, 7.

529. B.C. Stratford, S. Dixson, and A.J. Cobcroft, <u>Lancet</u>, 1974, <u>i</u>, 378.

530. M. Barza and M. Lauermann, <u>Clin. Pharmacokin.</u>, 1978, <u>3</u>, 202.

531. J.-C. Pechere and R. Dugal, <u>Clin. Pharmacokin.</u>, 1979, <u>4</u>, 170.

532. R.J. Sawchuck, D.E. Zaske, R.J. Cipolle, W.A. Wargin, and R.G. Strate, <u>Clin. Pharmacol. Ther.</u>, 1977, <u>21</u>, 362.

533. J.H. Hull and F.A. Sarubbi, Jr., <u>Ann. Intern. Med.</u>, 1976, <u>85</u>, 183.

534. R.J. Sawchuk and D.E. Zaske, <u>J. Pharmacokin. Biopharm.</u>, 1976, <u>4</u>, 183.

535. S.M. Bell, <u>Med. J. Austral.</u>, 1976, <u>2</u>, 481.

536. G.H. McCracken, <u>Amer. J. Dis. Children</u>, 1972, <u>124</u>, 884.

537. D.L. Giusti, <u>Drug Intelligence</u>, 1973, <u>7</u>, 540.

538. D.E. Zaske, R.J. Cipolle, J.C. Rotschafer, L.D. Solem, N.R. Mosier, and R.G. Strate, <u>Antimicrob. Ag. Chemother.</u>, 1982, <u>21</u>, 407.

539. J.J. Schentag, M.E. Plaut, and F.B. Cerra, <u>Antimicrob. Ag. Chemother.</u>, 1981, <u>19</u>, 859.

540. S. Pancorbo, C. Compty, and J. Heissler, <u>Biopharm. Drug Dispos.</u>, 1982, <u>3</u>, 83.

541. G.W. Counts, A.D. Blair, K.F. Wagner, and M. Turck, <u>Clin. Pharmacol. Ther.</u>, 1982, <u>31</u>, 662.

542. R.S. Finley, C.L. Fortner, C.A. deJongh, J.C. Wade, K.A. Newman, E. Caplan, J. Britten, P.H. Wiernik, and S.C. Schimpff, <u>Antimicrob. Ag. Chemother.</u>, 1982, <u>22</u>, 193.

543. J.J. Schentag, F.B. Cerra, and M.E. Plaut, <u>Antimicrob. Ag. Chemother.</u>, 1982, <u>21</u>, 721.

544. J.J. Schentag, T.J. Cumbo, W.J. Jusko, and M.E. Plaut, <u>J. Amer. Med. Assoc.</u>, 1978, <u>240</u>, 2067.

545. R.E. Cronin, <u>Clin. Nephrol.</u>, 1979, <u>11</u>, 251.

546. W.A. Colburn, J.J. Schentag, W.J. Jusko, and M. Gibaldi, <u>J. Pharmacokin. Biopharm.</u>, 1978, <u>6</u>, 179.

547. A. Whelton, G.G. Carter, T.J. Craig, H.H. Bryant, D.V. Herbst, and W.G. Walker, J. Antimicrob. Chemother., 1978, 4 (Suppl. A), 13.

548. J.J. Schentag, G. Lasezkay, M.E. Plaut, W.J. Jusko, and T.J. Cumbo, J. Antimicrob. Chemother., 1978, 4 (Suppl. A), 23.

549. G. Kahlmeter, T. Hallberg, and C. Kamme, J. Antimicrob. Chemother., 1978, 4 (Suppl. A), 37.

550. K. Goitein, J. Michel, and T. Sacks, Chemotherapy, 1975, 21, 181.

551. J.J. Rahal, P.J. Hymans, M.S. Simberkoff, and E. Rubinstein, New Engl. J. Med., 1974, 290, 1394.

552. R.W. Angel, New Engl. J. Med., 1974, 291, 533.

553. J.E. Pennington and H.Y. Reynolds, J. Infect. Dis., 1975, 131, 158.

554. J.E. Pennington, D.C. Dale, H.Y. Reynolds, and J.D. MacLowry, J. Infect. Dis., 1975, 132, 270.

555. T.H. Dee and F. Kozin, Antimicrob. Ag. Chemother., 1977, 12, 548.

556. A.J. Kozak, D.N. Gerding, L.R. Peterson, and W.H. Hall, Antimicrob. Ag. Chemother., 1977, 12, 606.

557. C.H. Hsu, T.W. Kurtz, and J.M. Weller, Antimicrob. Ag. Chemother., 1977, 12, 192.

558. B.M. Tune and M. Fernholt, Amer. J. Physiol., 1973, 225, 1114.

559. P.J.S. Chiu, A. Brown, G. Miller, and J.F. Long, Antimicrob. Ag. Chemother., 1976, 10, 277.

560. G.D. Richey and C.J. Schleupner, Antimicrob. Ag. Chemother., 1981, 19, 312.

561. M.E. Bravo, A. Arancibia, S. Jarpa, P.M. Carpentier, and A.N. Jahn, Eur. J. Clin. Pharmacol., 1982, 21, 499.

562. J. Lecompte, L. Dumont, J. Hill, P. Du Souich, and J. Lelorier, J. Pharmacol. Exp. Ther., 1981, 218, 231.

563. I. Sketris, T. Lesar, D.E. Zaske, and R.J. Cipolle, J. Clin. Pharmacol., 1981, 21, 288.

564. S. Korsager, Int. J. Clin. Pharmacol. Ther. Toxicol., 1980, 18, 549.

565. D.R. Myers, J. DeFehr, W.M. Bennet, G.A. Porter, and G.D. Olsen, Clin. Pharmacol. Ther., 1978, 23, 356.

566. J. Kapitulnik, F. Eyal, and A.J. Simcha, Lancet, 1972, ii, 1195.

567. T. Smithivas, P.J. Hymans, and J.J. Rahal, J. Infect. Dis., 1971, 124, Suppl., S106.

568. H. Yoshioka, T. Monma, and S. Matsuda, J. Pediatr., 1972, 80, 121.

569. R.L. Nation, G.W. Peng, W.L. Chiou, and J. Malow, Eur. J. Clin. Pharmacol., 1978, 13, 459.

570. A. Mosegaard, P.G. Welling, and P.O. Madsen, Antimicrob. Ag. Chemother., 1975, 7, 328.

571. M. Adelman, E. Evans, and J.J. Schentag, Antimicrob. Ag. Chemother., 1982, 22, 800.

572. C.A. Friedman, B.R. Parks, and J.E. Rawson, Pediat. Pharmacol., 1982, 2, 189.

573. J.J. Schentag and W.J. Jusko, Clin. Pharmacol. Ther., 1977, 22, 364.

574. J.J. Schentag, W.J. Jusko, J.W. Vance, T.J. Cumbo, E. Abrutyn, M. DeLattre, and L.M. Gerbracht, J. Pharmacokin. Biopharm., 1977, 5, 559.

575. K. Dvořáček, O. Schmidt, and Z. Modr, Progr. Chemotherapy, 1974, 1, 605.

576. G.E. Schumacher, Amer. J. Hosp. Pharm., 1975, 32, 299.

577. R. Wise, D.S. Reeves, H.R. Ingham, and J.A.N. Emslie, Brit. Med. J., 1972, iv, 732.

578. R.A. Chan, E.J. Benner, and P.D. Hoeprich, Ann. Int. Med., 1972, 76, 773.

579. T.W. Wilson, W.A. Mahon, T. Inaba, G.E. Johnson, and D. Kadar, Clin. Pharmacol. Ther., 1973, 14, 815.

580. G.E. Schumacher, J. Clin. Pharmacol., 1975, 15, 656.

581. G.E. Mawer, R. Ahmad, S.M. Dobbs, and J.A. Tooth, Postgrad. Med. J., 1974, 50, 31.

582. D. Kaye, M.E. Levison, and E.D. Lavovitz, J. Infect. Dis., 1974, 130, 150.

583. J.G. Wagner, J.I. Northam, C.D. Alway, and O.S. Carpenter, Nature, 1965, 207, 1301.

584. L.D. Bechtol and H.R. Black, Amer. J. Med. Sci., 1975, 15, 656.

585. E.L. Goodman, J. Van Gelder, R. Holmes, A.R. Hull, and J.P. Sanford, Antimicrob. Ag. Chemother., 1975, 8, 434.

586. J.G. Dahlgren, E.T. Anderson, and W.L. Hewitt, Antimicrob. Ag. Chemother., 1975, 8, 58.

587. G. Prout, J. Antimicrob. Chemother., 1977, 3, 371.

588. J. Stressman, J. Michel, and T. Sacks, Chemotherapy, 1977, 23, 142.

589. T.G. Christopher, D. Korn, A.D. Blair, A.W. Forrey, M.A. O'Neill, and R.E. Cutler, Kidney Internat., 1974, 6, 38.

590. M. Danish, R. Schultz, and W.J. Jusko, Antimicrob. Ag. Chemother., 1974, 6, 841.

591. G. Jaffe, B.R. Meyers, and S.Z. Hirschman, Antimicrob. Ag. Chemother., 1974, 5, 611.

592. R.F. Malacoff, F.O. Finkelstein, and V.T. Andriole, Antimicrob. Ag. Chemother., 1975, 8, 574.

593. B.A. Halpren, S.G. Axline, N.S. Coplon, and D.M. Brown, J. Infect. Dis., 1976, 133, 627.

594. T.G. Christopher, A.D. Blair, A.W. Forrey, and R.E. Cutler, J. Pharmacokin. Biopharm., 1976, 4, 427.

595. L. Letourneau-Saheb, L. Lapierre, R. Daigneault, M. Prud'Homme, G. St.-Louis, G. Sirois, Int. J. Clin. Pharmacol., 1977, 15, 116.

596. W.J. Jusko, T. Baliah, K.H. Kim, L.M. Gerbracht, and S.J. Yafie, Kidney Internat., 1976, 9, 430.

597. S. Pancorbo and C. Comty, Antimicrob. Ag. Chemother., 1981, 19, 605.

598. P. Somani, R.S. Shapiro, H. Stockard, and J.T. Higgins, Clin. Pharmacol. Ther., 1982, 32, 113.

599. P.H. Whiting, H.E. Barber, and J. Petersen, Brit. J. Clin. Pharmacol., 1981, 12, 795.

600. D.H. Lawson, W.J. Tilstone, J.M.B. Gray, and P.K. Srivastava, J. Clin. Pharmacol., 1982, 22, 254.

601. L.S. Young, G. Decker, and W.L. Hewitt, Chemotherapy, 1974, 20, 212.

602. M. Davies, J.R. Morgan, and C. Anand, Antimicrob. Ag. Chemother., 1975, 7, 431.

603. L.K. Pickering and P. Gearhart, Antimicrob. Ag. Chemother., 1979, 15, 592.

604. L.J. Riff and G.G. Jackson, Arch. Int. Med., 1972, 130, 887.

605. F.R. Ervin, W.E. Bullock, Jr., and C.E. Nuttall, Antimicrob. Ag. Chemother., 1976, 9, 1004.

606. J. Murillo, H.C. Standiford, S.C. Schimpff, and B.A. Tatem, J. Amer. Med. Assoc., 1979, 241, 2401.

607. C. Mariel, P. Veyssier, J.-C. Pechere, and E. De Cerner, Brit. Med. J., 1972, ii, 406.

608. A.-M. Gyselynck, A. Forrey, and R. Cutler, J. Infect. Dis., 1971, 134, Suppl., S70.

609. W.E. Evans, S. Feldman, M. Ossi, R.H. Taylor, S. Chaudhary, E.T. Melton, and L.F. Barker, J. Pediatr., 1979, 94, 139.

610. H. Sardemann, H. Colding, J. Hendel, J.P. Kampmann, E.F. Hvidberg, and R. Vejlsgaard, Clin. Pharmacol. Ther., 1976, 20, 59.

611. E. Farago, J. Kiss, A. Gömöry, J. Aranyosi, I. Juhász, and L. Mihóczy, Int. J. Clin. Pharmacol. Biopharm., 1979, 17, 421.

612. W.L. Dull, M.R. Alexander, and J.E. Kasik, Antimicrob. Ag. Chemother., 1979, 16, 767.

613. C. Carbon, A. Contrepois, and S. Lamotte-Barrillon, Antimicrob. Ag. Chemother., 1978, 13, 368.

614. D.J. Breidis and H.G. Robson, Antimicrob. Ag. Chemother., 1978, 13, 1042.

615. M.L. Kornguth and C.M. Kunin, <u>Antimicrob. Ag. Chemother.</u>, 1977, <u>11</u>, 974.

616. P. Federspil, W. Schatzle, and E. Tiesler, <u>J. Infect. Dis.</u>, 1976, <u>134</u>, (Suppl.), S200.

617. T.G. Cleary, L.K. Pickering, W.G. Kramer, S. Culbert, L.S. Frankel, and S. Kohl, <u>Antimicrob. Ag. Chemother.</u>, 1979, <u>16</u>, 829.

618. W.G. Kramer, T. Cleary, L.S. Frankel, S. Kohl, and L.K. Pickering, <u>Clin. Pharmacol. Ther.</u>, 1979, <u>26</u>, 635.

619. B. Vogelstein, A. Kowarski, and P.S. Lietman, <u>J. Pediatr.</u>, 1977, <u>91</u>, 333.

620. J.M. Lanao, A. Dominguez-Gil, A.A. Dominguez-Gil, S. Málaga, M. Crespo, and F. Nuño, <u>Eur. J. Clin. Pharmacol.</u>, 1982, <u>23</u>, 155.

621. T.G. Cleary, L.K. Pickering, W.G. Kramer, S. Culbert, L.S. Frankel, and S. Kohl, <u>Antimicrob. Ag. Chemother.</u>, 1979, <u>16</u>, 829.

622. F. Daschner, E. Reiss, and J. Engert, <u>Antimicrob. Ag. Chemother.</u>, 1977, <u>11</u>, 1081.

623. R.A. Yates, M. Mitchard, and R. Wise, <u>J. Antimicrob. Chemother.</u>, 1978, <u>4</u>, 335.

624. J.M. Walker, R. Wise, and M. Mitchard, <u>J. Antimicrob. Chemother.</u>, 1979, <u>5</u>, 95.

625. J.M. Lano, A. Dominguez-Gil, J.M. Tabernero, and L. Corbacho, <u>Eur. J. Clin. Pharmacol.</u>, 1981, <u>19</u>, 367.

626. M.A. French, F.B. Cerra, M.E. Plaut, and J.J. Schentag, <u>Antimicrob. Ag. Chemother.</u>, 1981, <u>19</u>, 147.

627. H. Yasuhara, S. Kobayashi, K. Sakamoto, and K. Kamijo, <u>J. Clin. Pharmacol.</u>, 1982, <u>22</u>, 403.

628. L.A. Bauer, R.A. Blouin, W.O. Griffen, Jr., K.E. Record, and R.M. Bell, <u>Amer. J. Hosp. Pharm.</u>, 1980, <u>37</u>, 519.

629. J.M. Lanao, A. Dominguez-Gil, J.M. Tabernero, and H.D. Molina, <u>Int. J. Clin. Pharmacol. Ther. Toxicol.</u>, 1982, <u>20</u>, 271.

630. J.T. Clarke, R.D. Libke, C. Regamey, and W.M.M. Kirby, <u>Clin. Pharmacol. Ther.</u>, 1974, <u>15</u>, 610.

631. J. Levy and J. Klastersky, <u>J. Clin. Pharmacol.</u>, 1975, <u>15</u>, 705.

632. J. Pijck, T. Hallynck, H. Soep, L. Baert, R. Daniels, and J. Boelaert, <u>J. Infect. Dis.</u>, 1976, <u>134</u>, (Suppl.), S331.

633. J. Plantier, A.W. Forrey, M.A. O'Neill, A.D. Blair, T.G. Christopher, and R.E. Cutler, <u>J. Infect. Dis.</u>, 1976, <u>134</u>, (Suppl.), S323.

634. M.C. McHenry, J.G. Wagner, P.M. Hall, D.G. Vidt, and T.L. Gavan, <u>J. Infect. Dis.</u>, 1976, <u>134</u>, (Suppl.), S343.

635. J.M. Lanao, A. Dominguez-Gil, J.M. Tabernero, and S. De Castro, <u>Int. J. Clin. Pharmacol. Biopharm.</u>, 1979, <u>17</u>, 171.

636. J.M. Lanao, A. Dominguez-Gil, J.M. Tabernero, and J.A. Sanchez Tomero, <u>Int. J. Clin. Pharmacol. Biopharm.</u>, 1979, <u>17</u>, 357.

637. L. Regeur, H. Colding, H. Jensen, and J.P. Kampmann, Antimicrob. Ag. Chemother., 1977, 11, 214.

638. D.C. Blair, D.U. Duggan, and E.T. Schroeder, Antimicrob. Ag. Chemother., 1982, 22, 376.

639. J.A. Jahre, K.P. Fu, and H.C. Neu, Clin. Pharmacol. Ther., 1978, 23, 591.

640. J.-C. Pechere, R. Dugal, and M.-M. Pechere, Clin. Pharmacol. Ther., 1978, 23, 677.

641. M. Chung, R. Costello, and S. Symchowicz, Antimicrob. Ag. Chemother., 1980, 17, 184.

642. D.J. Edwards, A. Mangione, T.J. Cumbo, and J.J. Schentag, Antimicrob. Ag. Chemother., 1981, 20, 714.

643. T. Bergan and H. Michalsen, Infection, 1982, 10, 153.

644. H. Michalsen and T. Bergen, Antimicrob. Ag. Chemother., 1981, 19, 1029.

645. P. Martinetto, A. Valtz, E. Pessione, S. Olivero, C. Sciascia, and A. Foco, Drugs Exptl. Clin. Res., 1981, 7, 521.

646. P.G. Welling, A. Baumueller, C.C. Lau, and P.O. Madsen, Antimicrob. Ag. Chemother., 1977, 12, 328.

647. J.-C. Pechere, R. Dugal, and M.-M. Pechere, Clin. Pharmacokin., 1978, 3, 395.

648. F.C. Luft, D.R. Brannon, L.L. Stropes, R.J. Costello, R.S. Sloan, and D.R. Maxwell, Antimicrob. Ag. Chemother., 1978, 14, 403.

649. R.N. Brogden, R.M. Pinder, P.R. Sawyer, T.M. Speight, and G.S. Avery, Drugs, 1976, 12, 166.

650. B.R. Meyers and S.Z. Hirschman, J. Clin. Pharmacol., 1972, 12, 321.

651. C. Regamey, R.C. Gordon, and W.M.M. Kirby, Clin. Pharmacol. Ther., 1973, 14, 396.

652. V.K. Simon, E.U. Mösinger, and V. Malerczy, Antimicrob. Ag. Chemother., 1973, 3, 445.

653. G.P. Bodey and T. Pan, Curr. Ther. Res., 1980, 28, 394.

654. D.B. Haughey, D.M. Janicke, M. Adelman, and J.J. Schentag, Antimicrob. Ag. Chemother., 1980, 17, 649.

655. L.A. Bauer and R.A. Blouin, Antimicrob. Ag. Chemother., 1981, 20, 587.

656. H.B. Kelly, R. Menendez, L. Fan, and S. Murphy, J. Pediatr., 1982, 100, 318.

657. F.P. Furgiuele, J.P. Smith, and J.G. Baron, Amer. J. Ophthalmol., 1978, 85, 121.

658. M.M. Uwaydah and B.M. Faris, Arch. Ophthalmol., 1976, 94, 1173.

659. R.E. Brummett, D. Himes, B. Saine, and J. Vernon, Arch. Otolaryngol., 1972, 96, 505.

660. G. Kahlmeter, S. Jonsson, and C. Kamme, J. Antimicrob. Chemother., 1978, 4 (suppl. A), 5.

661. J.J. Schentag, G. Lasezkay, T.J. Cumbo, M.E. Plaut, and W.J. Jusko, Antimicrob. Ag. Chemother., 1978, 13, 649.

662. R.A. Blouin, H.J. Mann, W.O. Griffen, L.A. Bauer, and K.E. Record, Clin. Pharmacol. Ther., 1979, 26, 508.

663. W.R. Lockwood and J.D. Bower, Antimicrob. Ag. Chemother., 1973, 3, 125.

664. K.G. Naber, S.R. Westenfelder, and P.O. Madsen, Antimicrob. Ag. Chemother., 1973, 3, 469.

665. J.M. Kaplan, G.M. McCracken, M.L. Thomas, L.J. Horton, and N. Davis, Amer. J. Dis. Children, 1973, 125, 656.

666. S.R. Westenfelder, P.G. Welling, and P.O. Madsen, Infection, 1974, 2, 76.

667. J.C. Pechere and R. Dugal, J. Infect. Dis., 1976, 134, (Suppl.), S118.

668. J.S. Tobias, P.F.M. Wrigley, S. Korde, and E.J. Shaw, J. Antimicrob. Chemother., 1977, 3, 305.

669. C. Simon, V. Maleryzk, and W. Ahlendorf, Int. J. Clin. Pharmacol., 1978, 16, 145.

670. F. Meunier-Carpentier, M. Staguet, and J. Klastersky, J. Clin. Pharmacol., 1976, 16, 625.

671. J.-C. Pechere, M.-M. Pechere, and R. Dugal, Eur. J. Clin. Pharmacol., 1976, 10, 251.

672. P.G. Welling, A. Mosegaard, and P.O. Madsen, J. Clin. Pharmacol., 1974, 14, 567.

673. M. Chung, J.J. Schrogie, and S. Symchowicz, J. Pharmacokin. Biopharm., 1981, 9, 535.

674. A. Mosegaard, P.G. Welling, F.L.S. Tse, and P. Madsen, Infection, 1975, 3, 143.

675. S. Roth, K. Naber, M. Scheer, G. Gruenwaldt, and H. Lange, J. Clin. Pharmacol., 1976, 10, 357.

676. J.-C. Pechere, M.-M. Pechere, and R. Dugal, Antimicrob. Ag. Chemother., 1976, 9, 761.

677. J.T. Doluisio, L.W. Dittert, and J.C. LaPiana, J. Pharmacokin. Biopharm., 1973, 1, 253.

678. B.M. Orme and R.E. Cutler, Clin. Pharmacol. Ther., 1969, 10, 543.

679. W.A. Ritschel, M. Banarer, E.F. Lau Chang, Int. J. Clin. Pharmacol., 1977, 15, 121.

680. J.K. Healy, P.J. Drum, and A.J. Elliott, Austral. NZ J. Med., 1973, 3, 474.

681. B.R. Knowles, S.B. Lucas, G.E. Mawer, R.M. Stirland, and J.A. Tooth, Brit. J. Pharmacol., 1971, 43, 481P.

682. G.E. Mawer, S.B. Lucas, B.R. Knowles, R.M. Stirland, and J.A. Tooth, *Lancet*, 1972, *i*, 12.

683. G.H. McCracken, Jr. and N. Threlkeld, *J. Pediatr.*, 1976, *89*, 313.

684. G.J. Yakatan, R.B. Smith, R.D. Leff, and J.L. Kay, *Clin. Pharmacol. Ther.*, 1978, *24*, 90.

685. H. Lentzen, E.U. Kölle, and F. Daschner, *Arzneim.-Forsch.*, 1981, *31*, 1967.

686. K.J. Breen, R.E. Bryant, J.D. Levinson, and S. Schenker, *Ann. Int. Med.*, 1972, *76*, 211.

687. J.A. Barrowman, A. D'Mello, and A. Herxheimer, *Eur. J. Clin. Pharmacol.*, 1973, *5*, 199.

688. J.S. Prasad and K. Krishnaswamy, *Chemotherapy*, 1978, *24*, 333.

689. W.A. Craig and P.G. Welling, *Clin. Pharmacokin.*, 1977, *2*, 252.

690. T. Mori, M. Aoki, Y. Aoki, K. Shirai, K. Chiba, and T. Oda, *J. Antibiotics*, 1972, *25*, 634.

691. F. Follath, *J. Antimicrob. Chemother.*, 1979, *5*, 97.

692. T.B. Vree, Y.A. Hekster, J.E. Damsma, M. Tijhuis, and W.T. Friesen, *Eur. J. Clin. Pharmacol.*, 1981, *20*, 283.

693. J.K. Seydel and E. Wempe, *Arzneim.-Forsch.*, 1971, *21*, 187.

694. G.D. Chisholm, P.M. Waterworth, J.S. Calnan, and L.P. Garrod, *Brit. Med. J.*, 1973, *i*, 569.

695. H. Nolte and H. Büttner, *Chemotherapy*, 1973, *18*, 274.

696. S.A. Kaplan, R.E. Weinfeld, C.W. Abruzzo, K. McFaden, M.L. Jack, and L. Weissman, *J. Infect. Dis.*, 1973, *128, Suppl.*, S547.

697. K.C. Gupta, N.K. Desai, T. Paul, and U.K. Sheth, *Int. J. Clin. Pharmacol. Ther. Toxicol.*, 1980, *18*, 536.

698. K. Naber, H. Vergin, and W. Weigand, *Infection*, 1981, *9*, 239.

699. D.S. Reeves, M.J. Bywater, D.W. Bullock, and H.A. Holt, *J. Antimicrob. Chemother.*, 1980, *6*, 647.

700. J.N. Bruun, N. Østby, J.E. Bredesen, P. Kierulf, and P.K.M. Lunde, *Antimicrob. Ag. Chemother.*, 1981, *19*, 82.

701. H. Nolte and H. Büttner, *Chemotherapy*, 1974, *20*, 321.

702. C.M. Wilfert and L.T. Gutman, *Canad. Med. Assoc. J.*, 1975, *112*, 73S.

703. F.B. Eatman, A.C. Maggio, R. Pocelinko, H.G. Boxenbaum, K.A. Geitner, W. Glover, T. Macasieb, A. Holazo, R.E. Weinfeld, and S.A. Kaplan, *J. Pharmacokin. Biopharm.*, 1977, *5*, 615.

704. R. Schulz, *Arch. Pharmacol.*, 1972, *272*, 369.

705. P. Sharpstone, J. Pickard, and R. Williams, 'Proceedings of the 7th Congress on Chemotherapy', Prague, 1971. University Press, 1972, Vol. 1, p. 1269.

706. J. Rieder, D.E. Schwartz, and O. Zangaglia, Chemotherapy, 1974, 20, 65.

707. P.E.J. Pohjanpelto, T.J. Sarmela, and T. Raines, Brit. J. Ophthalmol., 1974, 58, 606.

708. O. Ladefoged, Acta Pharmacol. Toxicol., 1977, 41, 507.

709. T. Bergan and E.K. Brodwall, Acta Med. Scand., 1972, 192, 483.

710. T. Bergan and E.K. Brodwall, Chemotherapy, 1972, 17, 320.

711. R. Baethke, G. Golde, and G. Gahl, Eur. J. Clin. Pharmacol., 1972, 4, 233.

712. W.R. Adam, M. Henning, and J.K. Dawborn, Austral. NZ J. Med., 1973, 3, 383.

713. P.G. Welling, W.A. Craig, G.L. Amidon, and C.M. Kunin, J. Infect. Dis., 1973, 128, (Suppl.), S556.

714. W.A. Craig and C.M. Kunin, Ann. Int. Med., 1973, 78, 491.

715. E. Singlas, J.N. Colin, J. Rottembourg, J.P. Meessen, A. de Martin, M. Legrain, and P. Simon, Eur. J. Clin. Pharmacol., 1982, 21, 409.

716. P.R.W. Tasker, G.A. MacGregor, H.E. deWardener, R.D. Thomas, and N.F. Jones, Lancet, 1975, i, 1216.

717. B. Horn and P. Cottier, Schweiz. Med. Woch., 1974, 104, 1809.

718. S. Kalowski, R.S. Nanra, T.H. Mathew, and P. Kincaid-Smith, Lancet, 1973, i, 394.

719. J. Rieder and D.E. Schwartz, Arzneim.-Forsch., 1975, 25, 656.

720. P. Männistö, J. Tuomisto, N.-E. Saris, and T. Lehtinen, Chemotherapy, 1973, 19, 289.

721. H. Vergin and E. Fritschi, J. Antimicrob. Chemother., 1979, 5, 103.

722. D.S. Reeves, J.M. Broughall, M.J. Bywater, and H.A. Holt, J. Antimicrob. Chemother., 1979, 5, 119.

723. H.J. Peters, G.B. Bishop-Freudling, M. Gregorian, W. Weigand, and H. Vergin, Int. J. Clin. Pharm. Res., 1982, 2, 259.

724. H. Vergin, F.W. Reutter, R. Sieber, and H. Ferber, Arzneim.-Forsch., 1980, 30, 313.

725. F.W. Reutter, H. Vergin, R. Sieber, and H. Ferber, J. Antimicrob. Chemother., 1979, 5, 149.

726. G.W.A. Slywka, A.P. Melikian, A.B. Straughn, P.L. Whyatt, and M.C. Meyer, J. Pharm. Sci., 1976, 65, 1494.

727. D.C. Bloedow and W.L. Hayton, J. Pharm. Sci., 1976, 65, 328.

728. D.C. Bloedow and W.L. Hayton, J. Pharm. Sci., 1976, 65, 334.

729. S.S. Chrai and J.R. Robinson, J. Pharm. Sci., 1976, 65, 437.

730. R.A. Shastri, Brit. J. Clin. Pharmacol., 1980, 10, 499.

731. S. Øie, J.G. Gambertoglio, and L. Fleckenstein, J. Pharmacokin. Biopharm., 1982, 10, 157.

732. T.J. Mikkelson, S.S. Chrai, and J.R. Robinson, J. Pharm. Sci., 1973, 62, 1648.

733. S.A. Kaplan, R.E. Weinfeld, C.W. Abruzzo, and M. Lewis, J. Pharm. Sci., 1972, 61, 773.

734. G.L. Mattock and I.J. McGilveray, J. Pharm. Sci., 1972, 61, 746.

735. M. Nakano, M. Itoh, K. Juni, H. Sekikawa, and T. Arita, Int. J. Pharmaceut., 1980, 4, 291.

736. E.J. Triggs, R.I. Nation, A. Long, and J.J. Ashley, Eur. J. Clin. Pharmacol., 1975, 8, 55.

737. B. Lumholtz, K. Siersbaek-Nielson, L. Skovsted, T. Kampmann, and J.M. Hansen, Clin. Pharmacol. Ther., 1975, 17, 731.

738. D.J. Chapron and M.R. Blum, J. Clin. Pharmacol., 1976, 16, 338.

739. D.J. Chapron, P.A. Kramer, and S.A. Mercik, Clin. Pharmacol. Ther., 1980, 27, 104.

740. G.R. Gordon, A.G. Shafizadeh, and J.H. Peters, Xenobiotica, 1973, 3, 133.

741. K.A. McMahon and W.J. O'Reilly, J. Pharm. Sci., 1972, 61, 518.

742. H. Schröder, Ph.D. Thesis, University of Uppsala, 1973.

743. A.K.A. Khan, S.C. Truelove, and J.K. Aronson, Brit. J. Clin. Pharmacol., 1982, 13, 523.

744. T.R. Bates, H.P. Blumenthal, and H.J. Pieniaszek, Jr., Clin. Pharmacol. Ther., 1977, 22, 917.

745. K.M. Das and R. Dubin, Clin. Pharmacokin., 1976, 1, 406.

746. M.C.B. Van Oudtshoorn and F.J. Potgieter, J. Pharm. Pharmacol., 1972, 24, 357.

747. T. Talseth and K.H. Landmark, Eur. J. Clin. Pharmacol., 1977, 11, 33.

748. E. Fischer, Amer. Heart J., 1973, 86, 280.

749. W.R. Adam, D.J. Brown, P. Hales, and J.K. Dawborn, Med. J. Austral., 1973, 1, 936.

750. E. Fischer, Lancet, 1972, ii, 210.

751. W.A. Craig, P.G. Welling, J.P. Wagnild, and C.M. Kunin, Proceedings of the 8th International Congress of Chemotherapy, Athens, September 8 - 15, 1973, 256.

752. D. Nadeau and C. Marchand, Drug Metab. Dispos., 1975, 3, 565.

753. C. Marchand and D. Nadeau, Brit. J. Pharmacol., 1973, 47, 69.

754. Y.A. Hekster, T.B. Vree, J.E. Damsma, and W.T. Friesen, J. Antimicrob. Chemother., 1981, 8, 133.

755. A. Traeger and G. Stein, Int. J. Clin. Pharmacol., 1977, 15, 315.

756. A. Devriendt, F.H. Jansen, and I. Weemaes, Eur. J. Clin. Pharmacol., 1970, 3, 36.

757. M.A. Moustafa, A.R. Ebian, S.A. Khalil, and M.M. Motawi, J. Pharm. Pharmacol., 1971, 23, 868.

758. S.A. Khalil, M.A. Moustafa, A.R. Ebian, and M.M. Motawi, J. Pharm. Sci., 1972, 61, 1615.

759. N. Khalafallah, S.A. Khalil, and M.A. Moustafa, J. Pharm. Sci., 1974, 63, 861.

760. R.J. Withey, G.R. Van Petten, and H.F. Lettau, J. Clin. Pharmacol., 1972, 12, 190.

761. H.S. Kaumeier, Arzneim.-Forsch., 1980, 30, 1794.

762. A. Melander, E. Wahlin, K. Danielson, and C. Rerup, Acta Med. Scand., 1976, 200, 497.

763. W.G. Crouthamel, L. Diamond, L.W. Dittert, and J.T. Doluisio, J. Pharm. Sci., 1975, 64, 664.

764. M.J. Mattila, J. Jussila, and S. Takki, Arzneim.-Forsch., 1973, 23, 583.

765. E. Gladtke, Arzneim.-Forsch., 1973, 23, 191.

766. E.E. Ohnhaus and P. Spring, J. Pharmacokin. Biopharm., 1975, 3, 171.

767. P. Brühl, G. Gundlach, P. Bastian, and W. Schellenberg, Int. J. Clin. Pharmacol., 1973, 8, 69.

768. P.G. Welling, H. Huang, P.F. Hewitt, and L.L. Lyons, J. Pharm. Sci., 1978, 67, 764.

769. R. Mäntylä, A. Ailio, H. Allomen, and J. Kanto, Ann. Clin. Res., 1978, 10, 258.

770. J. Rutland, N. Berend, and G.E. Marlin, Brit. J. Clin. Pharmacol., 1979, 8, 343.

771. L.D. Bechtol, C.T. Bessent, and M.B. Perkal, Curr. Ther. Res., 1979, 25, 618.

772. P.G. Welling, R.L. Elliott, M.E. Pitterle, H.P. Corrick-West, and L.L. Lyons, J. Pharm. Sci., 1979, 68, 150.

773. C.H. Nightingale, J. Amer. Pharm. Assoc., 1976, NS16, 203.

774. P. Nicholas, New York State J. Med., 1977, 77, 2088.

775. P.J. McDonald, L.E. Mather, and M.J. Story, J. Clin. Pharmacol., 1977, 17, 601.

776. A.R. Disanto and D.J. Chodos, Antimicrob. Ag. Chemother., 1981, 20, 190.

777. B.G. Boggiano and M. Gleeson, J. Pharm. Sci., 1976, 65, 497.

778. D.R. Holland and J.F. Quay, J. Pharm. Sci., 1976, 65, 417.

779. A. Philipson, L.D. Sabath, and D. Charles, Clin. Pharmacol. Ther., 1976, 19, 68.

780. W.A. Colburn, A.R. DiSanto, and M. Gibaldi, J. Clin. Pharmacol., 1977, 17, 592.

781. L.E. Mather, K.L. Austin, C.R. Philpot, and P.J. McDonald, Brit. J. Clin. Pharmacol., 1981, 12, 131.

782. P.G. Welling and F.L.S. Tse, J. Antimicrob. Chemother., 1982, 9, 7.

783. P.D. Kroboth, A. Brown, J.A. Lyon, F.J. Kroboth, and R.P. Juhl, Antimicrob. Ag. Chemother., 1982, 21, 135.

784. G.J. Yakatan, W.J. Poynor, R.G. Harris, A. Martin, R.G. Leonard, A.H. Briggs, and J.T. Doluisio, J. Pharmacokin. Biopharm., 1979, 7, 355.

785. R.G. Wiegand and A.H.C. Chun, J. Pharm. Sci., 1972, 61, 425.

786. S.M. Bell, Med. J. Austral., 1971, 2, 1280.

787. J. Nolan and W.H. Lyle, Trans. Ophthal. Soc. U.K., 1976, 96, 338.

788. A.R. DiSanto, K.Y. Tserng, D.J. Chodos, K.A. Desante, K.S. Albert, and J.G. Wagner, J. Clin. Pharmacol., 1980, 20, 437.

789. P. Patamasucon, S. Kaojarern, H. Kusmiesz, and J.D. Nelson, Antimicrob. Ag. Chemother., 1981, 19, 736.

790. G.J. Yakatan, W.J. Poynor, S.A. Breeding, C.E. Lankford, S.V. Dighe, A.N. Martin, and J.T. Doluisio, J. Clin. Pharmacol., 1980, 20, 625.

791. T.C. Coyne, S. Shum, A.H.C. Chun, L. Jeansonne, and H.C. Shirkey, J. Clin. Pharmacol., 1978, 18, 194.

792. G.H. McCracken, C.M. Ginsburg, J.C. Clahsen, and M.L. Thomas, Pediatrics, 1978, 62, 738.

793. A.-S. Malmborg, Curr. Ther. Res., 1980, 27, 733.

794. S.P. Patel and C.I. Jarowski, J. Pharm. Sci., 1975, 64, 869.

795. J. Barré, R. Zini, and J.P. Tillement, Infection, 1982, 10, S113.

796. G.A. Dette, Infection, 1982, 10, S92.

797. M. Del Tacca, M. Ducci, G. Soldani, G. Fedi, C. Bernardini, and A. Bertelli, Drugs Exptl. Clin. Res., 1981, 7, 555.

798. Y. Brun, F. Forey, J.P. Gamondes, A. Tebib, J. Brune, and J. Fleurette, J. Antimicrob. Chemother., 1981, 8, 459.

799. T. Bergan, K.B. Hellum, A. Schreiner, A. Digranes, and K. Josefsson, Curr. Ther. Res., 1982, 32, 597.

800. T. Bergan and H. Gjφnnaess, Curr. Ther. Res., 1981, 30, 597.

801. T. Bergan, A. Engeset, W. Olszewski, K. Josefsson, and N. Larsen, J. Antimicrob. Chemother., 1982, 10, 319.

802. L. Sundberg, T. Edén, and S. Ernstson, Infection, 1982, 10, S102.

803. L. Sundberg, T. Edén, and S. Ernstson, Infection, 1982, 10, S105.

804. H. Blenk, K. Simm, B. Blenk, and G. Jahneke, Infection, 1982, 10, S108.

805. P.G. Welling and W.A. Craig, J. Pharm. Sci., 1978, 67, 1057.

806. K.L. Austin, L.E. Mather, C.R. Philpot, and P.J. McDonald, Brit. J. Clin. Pharmacol., 1980, 10, 273.

807. K. Josefsson, T. Bergan, and L. Magni, Brit. J. Clin. Pharmacol., 1982, 13, 685.

808. K. Josefsson, M. Steinbakk, T. Bergan, T. Midtvedt, and L. Magni, Chemotherapy, 1982, 28, 176.

809. L. Manzo, C. Gregotti, P. Richelmi, A. Di Nucci, and F. Bertè, Chemotherapy, 1980, 26, 164.

810. A. Iliopoulou, K. Downey, D. M. Chaput de Saintonge, and P. Turner, Eur. J. Clin. Pharmacol., 1982, 23, 435.

811. P. Chelvan, J.M.T. Hamilton-Miller, and W. Brumfitt, Brit. J. Clin. Pharmacol., 1979, 8, 233.

812. R.M. DeHaan, C.M. Metzler, D. Schellenberg, W.D. VandenBosch, and E.L. Masson, Int. J. Clin. Pharmacol., 1972, 6, 105.

813. C.B. Walker, J.M. Gordon, H.A. Cornwall, J.C. Murphy, and S.S. Socransky, Antimicrob. Ag. Chemother., 1981, 19, 867.

814. K.S. Albert, K.A. DeSante, R.D. Welch, and A.R. DiSanto, J. Pharm. Sci., 1978, 67, 1579.

815. A.A. Forist, R.M. DeHaan, and C.M. Metzler, J. Pharmacokin. Biopharm., 1973, 1, 89.

816. R.M. DeHaan, W.D. VandenBosch, and C.M. Metzler, J. Clin. Pharmacol., 1972, 12, 205.

817. R.F. McGehee, C.B. Smith, C. Wilcox, and M. Finland, Amer. J. Med. Sci., 1968, 256, 279.

818. R.M. DeHaan, C.M. Metzler, D. Schellenberg, and W.D. VanderBosch, J. Clin. Pharmacol., 1973, 13, 190.

819. C.M. Metzler, R. DeHaan, D. Schellenberg, and W.D. VanderBosch, J. Pharm. Sci., 1973, 62, 591.

820. F.F. Sun and R.S.P. Hsi, J. Pharm. Sci., 1973, 62, 1265.

821. J.D. Panzer, D.C. Brown, W.L. Epstein, R.L. Lipson, H.W. Mahaffey, and W.H. Atkinson, J. Clin. Pharmacol., 1972, 12, 259.

822. G.L. Simon, D.M. Richmond, F.P. Tally, M. Barza, and S.L. Gorbach, J. Antimicrob. Chemother., 1981, 8, 59.

823. G. Ziv and F.G. Sulman, Brit. Vet. J., 1973, 129, 83.

824. B. Stéen and A. Rane, Brit. J. Clin. Pharmacol., 1982, 13, 661.

825. J.E.L. Sales, M. Sutcliffe, and F. O'Grady, Chemotherapy, 1973, 19, 11.

826. A. Philipson, L.D. Sabath, and D. Charles, New Engl. J. Med.,
      1973, 288, 1219.

827. P. Nicholas, B.R. Meyers, R.N. Levy, and S.Z. Hirschman,
      Antimicrob. Ag. Chemother., 1975, 8, 220.

828. R.M. DeHaan and D. Schellenberg, J. Clin. Pharmacol., 1972, 12,
      74.

829. J.B. Eastwood and P.E. Gower, Postgrad. Med. J., 1974, 50, 710.

830. A.M. Joshi and R.M. Stein, J. Clin. Pharmacol., 1974, 14, 140.

831. A.P. Roberts, J.B. Eastwood, P.E. Gower, C.M. Fenton, and J.R.
      Curtis, Eur. J. Clin. Pharmacol., 1978, 14, 435.

832. B.A. Peddle, E. Dann, and R.R. Bailey, Austral. NZ J. Med.,
      1975, 5, 198.

833. R.H.K. Eng, S. Gorski, A. Person, C. Mangura, and H. Chmel, J.
      Antimicrob. Chemother., 1981, 8, 277.

834. D.R. Hinthorn, L.H. Baker, D.A. Romig, K. Hassanein, and C. Liu,
      Antimicrob. Ag. Chemother., 1976, 9, 498.

835. J.C. Rotschafer, K. Crossley, D.E. Zaske, K. Mead, R.J. Sawchuk,
      and L.D. Solem, Antimicrob. Ag. Chemother., 1982, 22, 391.

836. R.A. Blouin, L.A. Bauer, D.D. Miller, K.E. Record, and W.O.
      Griffen, Jr., Antimicrob. Ag. Chemother., 1982, 21, 575.

837. D.J. Krogstad, R.C. Moellering, Jr., and D.J. Greenblatt, J.
      Clin. Pharmacol., 1980, 20, 197.

838. D.P. Krontz and L.J. Strausbaugh, Antimicrob. Ag. Chemother.,
      1980, 18, 882.

839. M.S. Engineer, D.-H.W. Ho, and G.P. Bodey, Sr., Antimicrob. Ag.
      Chemother., 1981, 20, 718.

840. H.E. Nielsen, H.E. Hansen, B. Korsager, and P.E. Skov, Acta
      Med. Scand., 1975, 197, 261.

841. R.H. Glew, R.A. Pavuk, A. Shuster, and H.J. Alfred, Int. J.
      Clin. Pharmacol. Ther. Toxicol., 1982, 20, 559.

842. R.B. Smith, W.L. Lummis, R.E. Monovich, and K.A. DeSante, J.
      Clin. Pharmacol., 1981, 21, 411.

843. E. Novak, T.G. Vitti, J.D. Panzer, C. Schlagel, and M.S.
      Hearron, Clin. Pharmacol. Ther., 1971, 12, 793.

844. S.A. Kaplan, J. Pharm. Sci., 1970, 59, 309.

845. H.L. Newmark and J. Berger, J. Pharm. Sci., 1970, 59, 1246.

846. H.L. Newmark, J. Berger, and J.T. Carstensen, J. Pharm. Sci.,
      1970, 59, 1249.

847. B. Boon, M. Gilbert, and F. Lamy, Thérapie, 1973, 28, 367.

848. M.B. Roberfroid and P.A. Dumont, J. Antibiotics, 1972, 25, 30.

849. A.D.J. Watson, Res. Vet. Sci., 1974, 16, 147.

850. H.A. Koeleman and M.C.B. Van Oudtshoorn, S. African Med. J., 1973, 47, 94.

851. R.E. Kauffman, M.C. Thirumoorthi, J.A. Buckley, M.K. Aravind, and A.S. Dajani, J. Pediatr., 1981, 99, 963.

852. M.C. Nahata and D.A. Powell, Clin. Pharmacol. Ther., 1981, 30, 368.

853. J.E. Burton and L.S. Schanker, Proc. Soc. Exp. Biol. Med., 1974, 145, 752.

854. J.R. Koup, A.H. Lau, B. Brodsky, and R.L. Slaughter, Antimicrob. Ag. Chemother., 1979, 15, 651.

855. G.J. Burckart, F.F. Barrett, A.B. Straughn, and S.R. Ternullo, J. Clin. Pharmacol., 1982, 22, 49.

856. A.P.S. Narang, D.V. Datta, N. Nath, and V.S. Mathur, Eur. J. Clin. Pharmacol., 1981, 20, 479.

857. W.W. Weber and D.W. Hein, Clin. Pharmacokin., 1979, 4, 401.

858. V. Prát, J. Grafnetterová, O. Schück, and E. Kotanová, Int. J. Clin. Pharmacol., 1976, 13, 71.

859. O. Schück, V. Prát, J. Grafnetterová, I. David, E. Kotanová, and V. Reitschlägerová, Int. J. Clin. Pharmacol., 1974, 10, 33.

860. L.E. Davis, C.A. Neff, J.D. Baggot, and T.E. Powers, Amer. J. Vet. Res., 1972, 33, 2259.

861. J. Traeger, J. Moskovchenko, J.C. Momer, and P. Zach, Postgrad. Med. J., 1974, 50, 39.

862. V. Monafo, A. Gazzaniga, F. Azzollini, and E. Lodola, Postgrad. Med. J., 1974, 50, 41.

863. H.F. Von Oldershausen, I. Hartmann, R. Ilg, H.P. Menz, H.J. Bezler, and G.C. Burck, Postgrad. Med. J., 1974, 50, 44.

864. D.D. Bella, M. Veronese, G. Marca, and R. Franceschinis, Arzneim.-Forsch., 1974, 24, 1.

865. B. Hoener and S.E. Patterson, Clin. Pharmacol. Ther., 1981, 29, 808.

866. T.R. Bates, J.A. Sequeira, and A.V. Tembo, Clin. Pharmacol. Ther., 1974, 16, 63.

867. H.A. Rosenberg and T.R. Bates, Clin. Pharmacol. Ther., 1976, 20, 227.

868. J.M. Jaffe, J. Pharm. Sci., 1975, 64, 1729.

869. A.R. DiSanto, D.J. Chodos, J.P. Philips, K.A. DeSante, R.G. Stoll, Int. J. Clin. Pharmacol., 1976, 13, 220.

870. C.A. Hirst and R.C. Kaye, J. Pharm. Pharmacol., 1971, 23, Suppl., 246S.

871. I.J. McGilveray, G.L. Mattok, and R.D. Hossie, Rev. Canad. Biol., 1973, 32, Suppl., 99.

872. G.L. Mattok, R.D. Hossie, and I.J. McGilveray, Canad. J. Pharm. Sci., 1972, 7, 84.

873. M.C. Meyer, G.W.A. Slywka, R.E. Dann, and P.L. Whyatt, J. Pharm. Sci., 1974, 63, 1693.

874. E.L. Parrott and L.E. Matheson, Jr., J. Pharm. Sci., 1977, 66, 955.

875. R.G. Stoll, T.R. Bates, and J. Swarbrick, J. Pharm. Sci., 1973, 62, 65.

876. J.D. Conklin, R.J. Sobers, and D.L. Wagner, Brit. J. Pharmacol., 1973, 48, 273.

877. H. Maier-Lenz, L. Ringwelski, and A. Windorfer, Arzneim.-Forsch., 1979, 29, 1898.

878. J.W. Sullivan, A.J. Bueschen, and J.U. Schlegel, J. Urology, 1975, 114, 343.

879. W. Zilly, D.D. Breimer, and E. Richter, Clin. Pharmacokin., 1977, 2, 61.

880. S. Virtanen and E. Tala, Clin. Pharmacol. Ther., 1974, 16, 817.

881. P. Mannisto, Clin. Pharmacol. Ther., 1976, 21, 370.

882. D.I. Siegler, M. Bryant, D.M. Burley, K.M. Citron, and S. Standen, Lancet, 1974, ii, 197.

883. H. Iwainsky, K. Winsel, E. Werner, and H. Eule, Scand. J. Resp. Dis., 1974, 55, 229.

884. G.H. McCracken, Jr., C.M. Ginsburg, T.C. Zweighaft, and J. Clahsen, Pediatrics, 1980, 66, 17.

885. G.L. Archer, B.C. Armstrong, and B.J. Kline, Antimicrob. Ag. Chemother., 1982, 21, 800.

886. G. Ziv and F.G. Sulman, Antimicrob. Ag. Chemother., 1974, 5, 139.

887. G. Boman and A.-S. Malmborg, Eur. J. Clin. Pharmacol., 1974, 7, 51.

888. S. Kenwright and A.J. Levi, Lancet, 1973, ii, 1405.

889. R.J. Fallon, G.W. Allan, A.W. Lees, J. Smith, and W.F. Tyrrell, Lancet, 1975, ii, 792.

890. G. Binda, E. Domenichini, A. Gottardi, B. Orlandi, E. Ortelli, B. Pacini, and G. Fowst, Arzneim.-Forsch., 1971, 21, 1938.

891. M. T. Kenny and B. Strates, Drug Metab. Rev., 1981, 12, 159.

892. G. Curci, N. Bergamini, F. Delli Veneri, A. Ninni, and V. Nitti, Chemotherapy, 1972, 17, 373.

893. E. Pozzi and P. Menghini, Int. J. Clin. Pharmacol. Ther. Toxicol., 1974, 10, 44.

894. G. Acocella, V. Pagani, M. Marchetti, G.C. Baroni, and F.B. Nicolis, Chemotherapy, 1971, 16, 356.

895. V. Nitti, F.D. Veneri, A. Ninni, and G. Meola, Chemotherapy, 1972, 17, 121.